Immunological Methods

Immunological Methods

v. 1

EDITED BY

IVAN LEFKOVITS

Basel Institute for Immunology
Basel, Switzerland

BENVENUTO PERNIS

Health Sciences Center
Columbia University
New York, New York

ACADEMIC PRESS New York San Francisco London 1979

A Subsidiary of Harcourt Brace Jovanovich, Publishers

ACADEMIC PRESS, INC.
111 Fifth Avenue, New York, New York 10003

United Kingdom Edition published by
ACADEMIC PRESS, INC. (LONDON) LTD.
24/28 Oval Road, London NW1   7DX

Library of Congress Cataloging in Publication Data
Main entry under title:

Immunological methods.

    Includes bibliographies and index.
    1. Immunology--Laboratory manuals.   2. Immunology,
Experimental.   I. Lefkovits, Ivan.   II. Pernis,
Benvenuto.
QR183.I43   599'.02'9028   78–3342
ISBN 0–12–442750–2

PRINTED IN THE UNITED STATES OF AMERICA

80 81 82 83 84 9 8 7 6 5 4 3 2

Contents

7 Isotachophoresis of Immunoglobulins

Andreas Ziegler and Georges Köhler

8 The Chemical Modification of Proteins, Haptens, and Solid Supports

Hansruedi Kiefer

9 Reagents for Immunofluorescence and Their Use for Studying Lymphoid Cell Products

Luciana Forni

10 Radiolabeling and Immunoprecipitation of Cell-Surface Macromolecules

J. Richard L. Pink and Andreas Ziegler

15 The MLR Test in the Mouse

Tommaso Meo

16 A Sensitive Method for the Separation of Rosette-Forming Cells

Bruce E. Elliott

17 The Use of Protein A Rosettes to Detect Cell-Surface Antigens

Judith Johnson

18 Hapten–Gelatin Gels Used as Adsorbents for Separation of Hapten-Specific B Lymphocytes

Werner Haas

19 Assay for Plaque-Forming Cells

Ivan Lefkovits and Humberto Cosenza

20 Plaquing and Recovery of Individual Antibody-Producing Cells

Marc Shulman

21 Assay for Specific Alloantigen-Binding T Cells Activated in the Mixed Lymphocyte Reaction

Bruce E. Elliott, Zoltán Nagy, and Markus Nabholz

22 Assay for Antigen-Specific T-Cell Proliferation in Mice

Şefik Ş. Alkan

List of Contributors

Numbers in parentheses indicate the pages on which the authors' contributions begin. Affiliations listed are current. All but the two contributors, whose names are preceded by an asterisk, were at the Basel Institute for Immunology, 487, Grenzacherstrasse, Postfach CH-4005, Basel 5, Switzerland, at the time the chapters were written.

Şefik Ş. Alkan (309), Basel Institute for Immunology

Domenico Bernoco (217), University of California at Los Angeles, Medical School, Los Angeles, California 90024

*Daniel Ch. Brandt (43), University of Geneva, Geneva, Switzerland

Dietmar G. Braun (107, 123, 345), Basel Institute for Immunology

Humberto Cosenza (277), Basel Institute for Immunology

Bruce E. Elliott (241, 291), Division of Cancer Research, Department of Pathology, Queen's University, Kingston, Ontario K7L 3N6, Canada

C. Garrison Fathman (207), Department of Immunology, Mayo Medical School, Rochester, Minnesota 55901

Luciana Forni (151), Basel Institute for Immunology

Ruedi Frech (403), Basel Institute for Immunology

Werner Haas (181, 269), Basel Institute for Immunology

Kerstin Hild (107), Basel Institute for Immunology

Norman N. Iscove (379), Basel Institute for Immunology

Jean-Claude Jaton (43), Department of Pathology, University of Geneva, Geneva, Switzerland

Judith Johnson (197, 261), Basel Institute for Immunology

Hansruedi Kiefer (137), Basel Institute for Immunology

Georges Köhler (131, 391, 397), Basel Institute for Immunology

Ivan Lefkovits (277, 355), Basel Institute for Immunology

Alma L. Luzzati (335), Basel Institute for Immunology

Tommaso Meo (227), Basel Institute for Immunology

B. A. Moss (69), CSIRO Animal Genetics, Delhi Road, North Ryde, New South Wales, Australia

Markus Nabholz (291), ISREC, Lausanne, Switzerland

Zoltán Nagy (291), Academy of Sciences, Budapest, Hungary

Alberto Piazza (419), Istituto di Genetica Medica dell'Università di Torino, Via Santena 19, 10126 Torino, Italy

J. Richard L. Pink (169), Department of Pathology, University of Geneva, Geneva, Switzerland

Helmut M. Pohlit (181, 403), Basel Institute for Immunology

Wolfgang Schalch (123), Basel Institute for Immunology

Max H. Schreier (327, 371, 379), Basel Institute for Immunology

Marc Shulman (287), Basel Institute for Immunology

S. Fazekas de St.Groth (1), CSIRO Animal Genetics, Delhi Road, North Ryde, New South Wales, Australia

John W. Stocker (217), Basel Institute for Immunology

Béla Takács (81), Hoffmann–La Roche, Inc., Grenzacherstrasse 124, Basel, Switzerland

Michael J. Taussig (317), Agricultural Research Council, Institute of Animal Physiology, Barbraham, Cambridge, United Kingdom

Reet Tees (387), Basel Institute for Immunology

*Pierre Vassalli (43), University of Geneva, Geneva, Switzerland

Harald von Boehmer (181), Basel Institute for Immunology

Bernd J. Weimann (371), Basel Institute for Immunology

Jürg Widmer (403), Basel Institute for Immunology

Andreas Ziegler (107, 131, 169), MRC Laboratory of Molecular Biology, Hills Road, Cambridge CB2 2QH, United Kingdom

Preface

Far more than with most disciplines, the fortunes of modern immunology have been closely tied to the evolution of methodology suited to its array of paramount issues. Beginning about the time of the mid-1950's revolution in the biologic sciences, this discipline has been especially fortunate in having amongst its practitioners many who were innovative and ingeneous in devising procedures for coping with basic issues that emerged in the study of transplantation, autoimmunity, tolerance, immune reconstitution, and cancer. In addition to the continued expansion of the analytic attributes of biophysical and biochemical technology, those involved in cell transfer and tissue culture approaches proved especially adept at devising means for handling immunocompetent and accessory cells.

The resultant massive technology now accounts for a great deal of the sustained vigor, dynamism, and continued expansion of the frontiers of this discipline. There is no lack of books devoted to immunological methods, but most concern themselves with established procedures that have become traditional to this discipline. The conception of the present volume arose from the unique situation that pertains at the Basel Institute for Immunology inasmuch as it has become a kind of international crossroads for the immunological community. More often than not, colleagues who spent a period at the Institute on short as well as long term visits have contributed to the more permanent staff unusual, valuable technology ranging from better, more practical ways of conducting standard procedures to utterly basic novel means of managing key operations. From this rich store of experience at the Basel Institute for Immunology, we have selected an array of procedures we judge to be especially useful and important for modern immunology laboratories.

This book, then, is a compendium of basic research techniques in current use in one of the largest immunology research institutes, with particular emphasis given to new methodology. The procedures have been described by individuals judged to be highly expert in their specialties. In many instances the methods developed or adapted to unique uses by the contributors have not previously been described in detail.

The thirty-four chapters cover techniques for detection, isolation, and purification of antibodies (including dansylation, two-dimensional chromatography, isoelectric focusing, polyacrylamide gel electrophoresis, and isotachophoresis); measurement of equilibrium constants (equilibrium dialysis, filtration, and sedimentation); isotope and fluorescent labeling and detection of cell-surface components; isotope laboratory maintenance; chemical modification of proteins, haptens, and solid supports, and haptenation of viable biological carriers; production of antisera against allotypes and histocompatibility antigens and production of antibody with clonal dominance; histocompatibility and MLR testing; cell separation by haptenated gels and by velocity sedimentation of rosette-forming cells; detection of antibody-secreting and alloantigen-binding cells; immune responses *in vitro* and their analysis by limiting dilution; production of T-cell factors; hybridoma production by cell fusion; maintenance of cell lines and cloning in semisolid media; and the mathematical analysis of immunological data.

The authors have been encouraged to present their contributions in ways each felt to be most appropriate and in a manner that reflects their actual laboratory working habits—in essence, their personalities. Nonetheless, we had extensive discussions with many of the authors in seeking to harmonize the varied segments of this volume.

We believe that this book will prove useful to investigators and to technicians involved in basic and applied immunological research. The utilization of immunological methods as research tools by scientists in other disciplines is now of a very high order and continues to increase exponentially. The details of immunological methods, notably much information that tends to be passed on only by "word of mouth," could prove to be a valuable resource to this diverse group of "non-immunologists." This volume should also be helpful in the teaching of immunological methodology.

We are deeply indebted to the many colleagues who, in various ways, helped us realize the unusual quality of this laboratory guide: to Dr. Maurice Landy, who played an important role in the conception and development of this work and who suggested and subsequently considered and discussed with us its format and main features; to the authors for their efforts to present in a lucid and maximally informative way the spectrum of immunological methods required to fulfill the unique aims of this project, and for their patience in undertaking revisions as requested; to Steven Fazekas de St.Groth, for his deep interest in the development of the book and for the time he devoted in making valuable revisions and suggestions; to Charles Steinberg whose assistance was so freely given; to David Steward, Katie Perret, and Margaret Maraggiulo for the extensive typing and retyping of drafts; and, finally, to the staff of Academic Press for their invaluable assistance in smoothly effecting the transition from typescript to printed volume.

This volume reflects still another facet of the benefits that accrue from the generous support provided by the Hoffmann–La Roche organization in promoting and nurturing basic research in immunology at the Basel Institute. That broad comprehensive research program that has evolved over the years is inextricably intertwined with the laboratory methods detailed in this book.

Ivan Lefkovits
Benvenuto Pernis

Abbreviations List

AFC	antibody-forming cell
ALS	anti-lymphocyte serum
B	bursa equivalent derived or bone marrow derived
BBS	borate-buffered saline
BDB	bis-diazobenzidine
Bicine	N,N-bis(2-hydroxyethyl)-glycine
Bis	N,N-methylenebisacrylamide
BPB	bromphenol blue
BSA	bovine serum albumin
BSS	balanced salt solution
BrdU	5′-bromodeoxyuridine
B6	C57BL/6
C	complement
Cap	ϵ-aminocaproic acid
Ci	curie
CFA	complete Freund's adjuvant
CML	cell-mediated lympholysis
DATD	N,N'-diallyltartaryldiamide
DCC	dicyclohexylcarbodiimide
DEAE	diethylaminoethyl
DMEM	Dulbecco's modified Eagle's medium
DMF	dimethylformamide
DNBS	2,4-dinitrobenzene sulfonate
DNP	dinitrophenyl
EA	erythrocyte–antibody complex
EAC	erythrocyte–antibody–complement complex
EBSS	Eisen's balanced salt solution or Earle's balanced salt solution
EDIA	ethylene diacrylate

EDTA   ethylenediaminetetraacetic acid
FCS   fetal calf serum
FITC   fluorescein isothiocyanate
FSRBC   formalinized sheep red blood cells
g   acceleration due to gravity
GPC   guinea pig complement
HAT   hypoxanthine–aminopterin–thymidine
HAU   hemagglutinating units
Hepes   *N*-2-hydroxyethylpiperazine-*N'*-2-ethanesulfonic acid
HGPRT   hypoxanthine–guanine phosphoribosyltransferase
HRBC   horse red blood cells
HS   horse serum
HT   hypoxanthine–thymidine
IEF   isoelectric focusing
Ig   immunoglobulin
ITP   isotachophoresis
KLH   keyhole limpet hemocyanine
LPS   lipopolysaccharide
MEM   minimal essential medium
MHC   major histocompatibility complex
MLC   mixed lymphocyte culture
MLR   mixed lymphocyte reaction
MW   molecular weight
NHS   *N*-hydroxysuccinimide
NIP   4-hydroxy-3-iodo-5-nitrophenyl
NMS   normal mouse serum
NRS   normal rabbit serum
ONS   *N*-hydroxysuccinimidyl ester radical
PBL   peripheral blood lymphocytes
PBS   phosphate-buffered saline
PFC   plaque-forming cell
PFU   plaque-forming unit
PMSF   phenylmethylsulfonyl fluoride
POPOP   1,4-bis[2-(5-phenyloxazolyl)]benzene
PPO   2,5-diphenyloxazole
PRC   primed responder cell

R	roentgen
RBC	red blood cell
RFC	rosette-forming cell
SDS	sodium dodecyl sulfate
SI	stimulation index
SpA	protein A from *Staphylococcus aureus*
SRC	sheep red cells
T	thymus derived
TCA	trichloroacetic acid
TEA	triethylamine
TEMED	N,N,N',N'-tetramethylethylenediamine
THF	tetrahydrofuran
TK	thymidine kinase
TLC	thin-layer chromatography
TLD	thermoluminescence detector
TNP	trinitrophenyl
TNPS	trinitrophenyl sulfonate
TPCK	tosyl-L-phenylalanine chloromethyl ketone
Tris	tris(hydroxymethyl)aminomethane
TRITC	tetramethylrhodamine isothiocyanate
Trizma	trade name for Tris produced by Sigma Chemical Co.

The Quality of Antibodies and Cellular Receptors

S. Fazekas de St.Groth

I. INTRODUCTION

Conventional titrations define an end point which depends on both the quantity and quality of reactants. The reaction can be made of practically zero order by working in great excess of one component, and the quantity of the other may then be estimated independently. Quality cannot be assayed in such systems because either it appears confounded with quantity or its effects are eliminated altogether. This holds equally for binary reactions (such as precipitin tests in solution or in gels, active or passive agglutination, complement fixation, etc.) and for ternary systems where an

IMMUNOLOGICAL METHODS

acceptor and an indicator compete for the third component (such as inhibition of any binary reaction, neutralization of toxins or pathogens, etc.).

The simplest overall measure of the forces holding epitope and paratope together, that is, of quality in the immunological sense, is the *equilibrium constant*. When not only the extent but also the nature of these forces is to be investigated, thermodynamic parameters (such as changes in enthalpy, entropy, heat capacity, etc.) must be determined. All this, however, amounts to no more than measuring equilibrium constants under different environmental conditions (commonly at different temperatures, less frequently by varying pressure or volume experimentally). This chapter deals, therefore, with the theory and practice of estimating equilibrium constants in immune systems.

II. SIMPLE EQUILIBRIA

A. Theory

1. Monovalent Reactants

Consider the reaction between epitopes at concentration $[E]$ and paratopes at concentration $[P]$. Both reagents are in thermal motion and have a calculable chance of colliding with each other. Epitope–paratope complexes, x, will be formed at a rate proportional to the concentration of *free* reagents ($[E - x]$ and $[P - x]$ and to the rate of effective collisions, k_1. Formally, the concentration of complexes will increase with time as

$$\frac{d[x]}{dt} = k_1[E - x][P - x] \tag{1}$$

The formed complexes dissociate at a rate of k_2, and hence their concentration decreases with time as

$$-\frac{d[x]}{dt} = k_2[x] \tag{2}$$

The overall rate is obtained by combining Eqs. (1) and (2):

$$\frac{d[x]}{dt} = k_1[E - x][P - x] - k_2[x] \tag{3}$$

Equilibrium is defined as the state where $d[x]/dt = 0$, that is, where association and dissociation exactly balance each other (Note 1). Thus, at equilibrium we have

$$k_1[E - x][P - x] - k_2[x] = 0 \tag{4}$$

NOTE 1. The approach to equilibrium is obtained by integrating Eq. (3). Thus, the concentration of epitope–paratope complexes at time t is

$$[x_t] = \frac{x_1(x_0 - x_2) - x_2(x_0 - x_1) \exp\{(x_1 - x_2)k_1(t - t_0)\}}{(x_0 - x_2) - (x_0 - x_1) \exp\{(x_1 - x_2)k_1(t - t_0)\}}$$

or, conversely, the time required to reach a particular concentration of complexes, x_t, is

$$t = \frac{1}{k_1(x_1 - x_2)} \ln \frac{(x_t - x_1)(x_0 - x_2)}{(x_t - x_2)(x_0 - x_1)}$$

where x_0 is the concentration of complexes at zero time and x_1, x_2 are the roots of Eq. (5), $x_1, x_2 = \frac{1}{2}\{E + P + K + [(E + P + K)^2 - 4EP]^{1/2}\}$. The equilibrium concentration, x, reached at t_∞, is obviously x_2, the smaller root of Eq. (5).

The equilibrium constant, K, is simply the ratio of k_2 and k_1, as seen by rearranging Eq. (4):

$$\frac{k_2}{k_1} = \frac{[E - x][P - x]}{[x]} = K = \frac{[\text{free epitopes}][\text{free paratopes}]}{[\text{complexes}]} \tag{5}$$

The equilibrium constant has the dimensions of concentration and is conventionally expressed in terms of molarity (moles per liter). With biological material, such as cells, it is more meaningful to use cgs units, that is, to speak of topes per cubic centimeter (cf. Jerne *et al.*, 1974). Since there are 6.023×10^{23} molecules per mole, and thus 6.023×10^{20} in 1 cm^3 of a molar solution, the two notations are readily interconvertible: $K_{cgs} = 6.023 \times 10^{20} K_{mol}$.

(Some immunochemists define K as

$$\frac{k_1}{k_2} = \frac{[x]}{[E - x][P - x]}$$

a formally unobjectionable alternative which, however, imparts to K the quaint dimension of liters per mole. This may stun those accustomed to thinking in concentrations and has to be inverted in any case for conventional thermodynamic calculations.)

2. Multivalent Reactants

Equation (5) holds for monovalent reagents, such as small haptens and F_{ab} fragments. Considering the valency of whole antibody molecules, that is, a number n of paratopes/antibody (making $P = nA$), the equilibrium equation becomes

$$\frac{[E - x][nA - x]}{[x]} = K \tag{5a}$$

For large multivalent antigens (such as cells, bacteria, viruses) of concentration $[C]$, each carrying n epitopes, the corresponding equation is

$$\frac{[nC - x][P - x]}{[x]} = K \tag{5b}$$

(The valency of antibodies can usually be ignored in this situation. To check the correctness of this practice, the behavior of whole Ig molecules may be compared with F_{ab} fragments derived from them.)

3. Microscopic Equilibria

Equation (5b) does not take into account the fact that epitopes are found on a large particle and thus occur in parcels of n. It can be shown, however, that in the absence of interaction between epitopes their behavior is the same, irrespective of whether they occur singly or as part of the surface of large carriers (Note 2).

NOTE 2. Consider the microscopic equilibrium between the $(i - 1)$th and the ith epitope on, say, a red cell:

$$k_i = \frac{x_i[P - x]}{x_{i-1}} \tag{6}$$

Here x_i denotes the sum of all $\binom{n}{i}$ classes in which i out of n sites can be occupied. Note that

$$x_i = \frac{x_{i-1}K_i}{[P - x]} = \frac{\left(C - \sum_1^n x_i\right)\prod_1^i K_i}{[P - x]^i} \tag{7}$$

If all sites are identical and equivalent, a single equilibrium constant, K, characterizes all associations and $K_i = K[n - (i - 1)]/i$, since there are $n - (i - 1)$ ways of adding an antibody molecule to make x_i out of x_{i-1} and i ways in which a molecule can dissociate from x_i to make x_{i-1}. Equation (7) may be rewritten accordingly as

$$x_i = \binom{n}{i}\left(C - \sum_1^n x_i\right)\left(\frac{K}{P - x}\right)^i \tag{7a}$$

The average number of antibody molecules bound to a cell is

$$\frac{\text{Number of sites occupied}}{\text{Number of cells}} = \frac{x}{C} = \frac{x_1 + 2x_2 + \cdots + nx_n}{\left(C - \sum_1^n x_i\right) + x_1 + x_2 + \cdots + x_n} \tag{8}$$

Substituting the function (7a) and simplifying by the zero term, we have

$$\frac{x}{C} = \frac{\sum_1^n i \binom{n}{i} [K/(P - x)]^i}{1 + \sum_1^n \binom{n}{i} [K/(P - x)]^i} \tag{9}$$

The denominator here is the binomial expansion of $[1 + K/(P - x)]^n$ and the numerator is its derivative with respect to $K/(P - x)$. Thus,

$$\frac{x}{C} = \frac{n[1 + K/(P - x)]^{n-1}}{[1 + K/(P - x)]^n} = \frac{n}{1 + K/(P - x)} \tag{10}$$

which is directly rearranged to give

$$\frac{[nC - x][P - x]}{[x]} = K$$

a result identical with Eq. (5b).

B. Practical Restrictions

Equation (5) can be solved numerically for any set of observations. The quadratic form (cf. Note 1), however, is not convenient for plotting and especially not for statistical estimation of parameters. The parabola will have to be transformed into a straight line as soon as it is decided what we wish to estimate.

1. Separation of Terms

For practical measurement, at least one of the three components making up the equilibrium mixture (free epitopes, free paratopes, or epitope–paratope complexes) must be separated from the other two. If there are reasonable differences in size, the separation presents no problems. Thus, haptens will diffuse through membranes which retain antibody, yielding a compartment representing $[E - x]$. With particulate antigens, $[P - x]$, the antibody remaining free can be separated either in the form of a supernatant after centrifuging or as a filtrate after passing the equilibrium mixture through a sieve retaining the antigen and, hence, a fortiori, antigen–antibody complexes. When the two reactants are of comparable size, for example, in idiotope–antiidiotope reactions, simple mechanical separation will not work, but there are alternative techniques (labeling one or the other reactant and using a precipitating agent directed against one of them; following the formation of complexes by some physical, usually optical, change in the system; or attaching one of the reactants to a solid or particulate carrier and thus reducing the problem to mechanical separation).

In either case, the separated compartment, that is, $[E - x]$ or $[P - x]$, will have to be estimated and compared to the input concentration $[E]$ or $[P]$. It is customary therefore to express x as a fraction of the input. In most cases this practice becomes mandatory since only titers (unknown multiples of absolute concentrations) can be determined, with $[E]$ or $[P]$ themselves as parameters to be estimated.

2. Linear Transforms

Since the equilibrium equation is symmetric in E and P, the formal treatment is the same for both. Here we shall take as an example a cell with n epitopes on it, that is, an input concentration of $[nC]$ epitopes reacting with $[P]$ paratopes. In this system, the separated compartment will be free antibody, and we define therefore $x \equiv \alpha P$ (i.e., a fraction $0 < \alpha < 1$ of antibody is bound in epitope–paratope complexes) and rewrite Eq. (5b) as

$$\frac{[nC - \alpha P][P - \alpha P]}{[\alpha P]} = K = [nC - \alpha P]\frac{1 - \alpha}{\alpha} \tag{11}$$

Equation (11) has six possible linear transforms, obtained by multiplying both sides by a factor and rearranging to the general form $y = a + bx$ (Note 3).

Note 3

Multiplier	Linear form			
	y	$=$ a	$+$	$b \cdot x$

$$\frac{\alpha}{(1 - \alpha)K} \qquad \frac{\alpha}{1 - \alpha} = \frac{nC}{K} - \frac{P}{K}\alpha \tag{11a}$$

$$\frac{1}{(1 - \alpha)K} \qquad \frac{1}{1 - \alpha} = -\frac{P}{K} + \frac{nC}{K}\frac{1}{\alpha} \tag{11b}$$

$$\frac{K}{nC} \qquad \frac{1}{\alpha} = \frac{P}{nC} + \frac{K}{nC}\frac{1}{(1 - \alpha)} \tag{11c}$$

$$\frac{1}{nC} \qquad \frac{1 - \alpha}{\alpha} = \frac{K}{nC} + \frac{P}{nC}(1 - \alpha) \tag{11d}$$

$$\frac{1}{P} \qquad 1 - \alpha = -\frac{K}{P} + \frac{nC}{P}\frac{1 - \alpha}{\alpha} \tag{11e}$$

$$\frac{\alpha}{(1 - \alpha)P} \qquad \alpha = \frac{nC}{P} - \frac{K}{P}\frac{\alpha}{1 - \alpha} \tag{11f}$$

In equilibrium dialysis tests [where Eq. (5a) is used], the concentration of free hapten is called c ($c = [E - x]$, in our notation), and the ratio of bound to total antibody r ($r = x/A$, in our notation). The equilibrium constant is defined as k_1/k_2. The unknown parameters are usually estimated by one of two linear transforms. The first,

$$\frac{r}{c} = Kn - Kr$$

or

$$\frac{\alpha}{A(1 - \alpha)} = \frac{n}{K} = \frac{E}{AK} \cdot \alpha$$

in our notation, is clearly Eq. (11a), scaled by the factor $1/A$. The second equation,

$$\frac{1}{r} = \frac{1}{ncK} + \frac{1}{n}$$

becomes

$$\frac{A}{\alpha E} = \frac{K}{[nE(1 - \alpha)]} + \frac{1}{n}$$

in our notation and is seen to be equivalent to Eq. (11c), scaled by A/E. These linear forms are occasionally referred to by special names (Lineweaver–Burk plot, Scatchard plot, etc.). Perpetuation of proprietary names for trivial transforms is a tiresome conceit.

3. The Informative Range

Each of these equations can be used to estimate the parameters from the y intercept a and the slope b. (In case of emergency, the x intercept $c = -a/b$ may also be used.) We wish then to choose the plots which provide the greatest precision, that is, estimate intercepts with minimal extrapolation and have a slope close to unity. Each equation will be examined therefore from this aspect once the *optimal range of concentrations for the reactants* has been set. We have here two considerations to guide us. First, the system should be far from saturation, to avoid interactions between sites. In the example, this means that most epitopes should remain free. This sets $[nC] \geq 10[\alpha P]$. Second, the separated reactant should be a small fraction of the input, to make the difference highly significant. This sets $\alpha \geq 0.9$. These two conditions define the relations between the parameters over the most informative range of equilibrium tests. Thus, $P \sim K$ and $nC \sim 10K$.

Figure 1 illustrates the course of the six linear transforms on varying the concentration of antigen over a tenfold range. For the plots, nC was taken as constant and its dilution factor d ($1 \leq d \leq 10$) was incorporated into the appropriate variables.

4. Problems of Estimation

Equations (11a) and (11f) have, statistically speaking, the most to recommend them. Both have slopes that can be estimated with precision, while the y intercept of Eq. (11a) and the x intercept of Eq. (11f) are

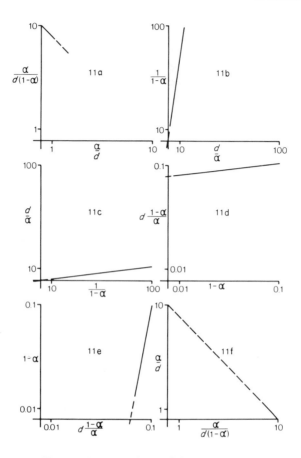

Fig. 1. Linear transforms of the mass equation.

reached by minimal extrapolation and differ greatly from zero. The information extracted from either of these is the same, as they happen to be inverse functions of each other. Their common shortcoming is that P cannot be estimated independently and will always carry the error of K, too.

The next pair, Eqs. (11d) and (11e), gives satisfactory estimates of K (contained in their y and x intercepts, respectively) but are poor estimators of P, even though the slope is independent of K.

The last pair, (11b) and (11c), have both their x and y intercepts close to the origin and will therefore give reliable estimates of P only if the experimental points are not scattered widely about the theoretical line. Of the two, Eq. (11c) is preferable because it estimates the parameters P and K independently.

C. Complications

1. Heterogeneity

Since even the simplest antigen may interact with and stimulate a large variety of cells, the observed immune response is the sum of a number, usually an unknown number, of clonal responses. Equation (5) does not take this into account, and thus the *observed equilibrium constant*, K_0, is in fact the central measure of an unknown distribution of particular equilibrium constants, K_i ($1 \leq i \leq n$), where the number n itself is unknown.

As is usual in such situations, a normal distribution was assumed for the free energies of association (Pauling *et al.*, 1944), that is, log-normal for K (Note 4).

NOTE 4. While this assumption is certainly wrong in its limits, it also seems intuitively inappropriate as there are more ways of obtaining poor than perfect fits. Indeed, each of the few reports analyzing subpopulations of antisera (Fazekas de St.Groth, 1967; Werblin and Siskind, 1972; Werblin *et al.*, 1973; Kim *et al.*, 1974) demonstrated distributions heavily skewed toward antibodies of low affinity. The true form of the distribution, however, is still not known and, what is worse, it is known to change with time even in the same individual, as the response "matures." Under the circumstances, then, the normal assumption is retained as the most convenient compromise; it is found also to work in practice, provided the tests do not cover extreme ranges.

The measure of heterogeneity, σ, was defined as the square root of the estimated variance. Since the value of σ is obtained by cumbersome empirical fitting, the usual treatment fits a distribution which is *similar* to the normal, but more manageable. Of the many distributions which approximate the normal, the choice of immunochemists (Nisonoff and Pressman, 1958) fell on one of the distributions proposed by Sips (1948) (Note 5).

NOTE 5. The Sips function,

$$\frac{r}{n} = \frac{(K_0 c)^a}{1 + (K_0 c)^a}$$

stated here in immunochemical terms, amounts to a late rediscovery of the logistic distribution, whose metametric transformation is $P = e^Y/(1 + e^Y)$. In the Sips formulation, P defines the chance of a single paratope being occupied, while Y (the *logit of P*) is equated to $a \ln K_0 c$.

This is by far not the best approximation (it deviates seriously from the normal around $\pm\sigma$ and becomes increasingly inappropriate with the distance from the mean beyond $\pm 2\sigma$) and is also unsuited to routine statistical estimation of precision. But it has the redeeming virtue of being stated in the same terms as have been historically used in the treatment of equilibrium data (cf. Note 3). Thus,

$$\log \frac{r}{n-r} = a \log K_0 + a \log c \tag{12}$$

The *heterogeneity index*, a, can be read off the slope of the straight line and K_0 worked out from the y intercept or, better, obtained directly from the x intercept. The value of a lies between 0 and 1, homogeneity being indicated by $a = 1$.

The equilibrium equation underlying Eq. (12) would read, in our notation,

$$\frac{[E - x]^a [P - x]}{[x]} = K_0^a$$

and the linear transform suitable for estimating a

$$\log \left(\frac{nA}{\alpha E} - 1 \right) = a \left(\log \frac{K_0}{E} \right) + a \left(\log \frac{1}{1 - \alpha} \right) \tag{12a}$$

Equations (12) and (12a) use all the information for the estimation of a and K_0 and can be solved only if all other parameters ([E], [P], and [x]) are known.

2. Incestuous Combinations

The simple treatment of equilibria assumes independence of epitopes and paratopes. In fact, immunoglobulin molecules found in sera are multivalent and so are most natural antigenic molecules and particles. It should be considered, therefore, that some of the n-valent antibody molecules already attached by one of their paratopes may form a second, third, ... nth epitope–paratope bond with the same antigenic particle. That such complexes exist has been well known since the 1960s (Lafferty, 1963; Lafferty and Oertelis, 1963; Almeida et al., 1963; Greenbury et al., 1965; Klinman and Karush, 1967; Feinstein and Munn, 1969), but their rate of formation and the proportion present in a particular equilibrium mixture are not known. The problem is difficult as not only the number and flexibility of paratope-bearing limbs on the globulin molecule but also the topography of epitopes on the antigen will influence the outcome. Experimental tests on one system (Klinman et al., 1967; Hornick and Karush, 1969, 1972; Gopalakrishnan and Karush, 1974) showed that incestuous bonds occurred with high probability and thus the observed K_0 for IgG was close to the square of K_0 measured for single attachments. In another system, van Regenmortel and Hardie (1976) found that, depending on the concentration of the reactants, the frequency of incestuous combinations could be varied to involve from practically none to practically all IgG molecules.

The danger of this phenomenon lies in its insidious effect on estimates of heterogeneity which, by their very nature, are estimates at different concentrations of reactants. The way out is simple: F_{ab} fragments of a particular antibody population have the same affinity and heterogeneity as the parent population, but cannot form incestuous complexes. Thus, the difference in K_0 and a of an antiserum and the F_{ab} preparation obtained from it is the measure of incestuous combinations.

3. Interaction between Sites

The most common interaction between antibodies landing on neighboring sites is electrical. If such interactions are present, an additional term for electrostatic free energy change arises and the observed K will not remain constant but appear as a function of the density of epitope–paratope complexes (Note 6).

NOTE 6. If all the epitopes on an antigenic particle are equivalent and there is no interaction between them, the equilibrium constant characterizing the binding of the ith paratope is $K_i = (n - i + 1)K/i$ [cf. Eqs. (6) and (7a)]. The corresponding change in standard free energy is

$$-\Delta F° = RT \ln K_i = RT \ln [K(n - i + 1)/i]$$

As may be derived from the Debye–Hückel theory, electrostatic interaction will change the free energy by

$$\Delta F°_{electr} = - \frac{N\epsilon^2 z^2}{2D} \left(\frac{1}{r} + \frac{\kappa}{1 + \rho\kappa} \right) (2i - 1)$$

where N is Avogadro's number, ϵ the electronic charge, z the charge on the antibody molecule, D the dielectric constant, ρ the radius of nearest approach of opposed ions, and $1/\kappa$ the thickness of the ionic atmosphere as defined in the Debye–Hückel theory. Thus,

$$K_i = \frac{n - i + 1}{i} K e^{-(2i-1)w}$$

if we write w for the constant term

$$\frac{N\epsilon^2 z^2}{2RTD} \left(\frac{1}{r} + \frac{\kappa}{1 + \rho\kappa} \right)$$

Katchalsky and Spitnik (1947), as well as Scatchard (1949), have proposed a very simple approximation which, when written in a form analogous to Eq. (5b), reads

$$\frac{[nC - x][P - x]}{[x]} = K e^{2wx/C} \tag{13}$$

It can be shown to carry a maximal error of less than $\pm 1.2\%$ when $n = 3$, less than $\pm 0.3\%$ when $n = 4$, and one that is entirely negligible with the number of epitopes on large carriers such as cells.

Interactions become manifest only near saturation (i.e., when x/nC approaches unity). The effect is an apparent gradual increase in K and hence a curve concave toward the ordinate when plotting one of the transforms where K appears as a multiplier of the independent variable, such as Eq. (11f). Since the slope at low values of x/nC still gives a valid estimate of K_0, its exponential term [(cf. Eq. (13)] is best evaluated by plotting $2\alpha P/C$ (twice the ratio of complexes to cells) against $\ln\{[(1 - \alpha)/\alpha]$ $(nC - \alpha P)\}$ (the logarithm of the concentration of free epitopes multiplied by the ratio of free to bound paratopes). The slope gives directly the value of w and the line is constrained to cut the ordinate at $\ln K$, as derived from the plot of Eq. (11f). The functional relationship is

$$\ln\left(\frac{1 - \alpha}{\alpha} [nC - \alpha P]\right) = \ln K + w \frac{2\alpha P}{C} \tag{14}$$

For interactions of unknown mechanism and undefined magnitude (such as steric inhibition or allosteric changes in the neighborhood of an occupied epitope), an "apparent equilibrium constant" may be found according to Wyman (1948) by plotting $\ln[(nC/\alpha P) - 1]$ against $\ln[P(1 - \alpha)]$. The x intercept (where $nC = 2\alpha P$, i.e., the point of 50% saturation) represents this value. A slope greater than unity at the intercept reveals positive interactions between sites; slopes less than unity suggest negative interactions, although the existence of some positive interactions is not excluded here. The magnitude of the interaction at particular levels of saturation may be gauged by comparing the "apparent equilibrium constant" with K_0 obtained from plots of Eqs. (11a)–(11f) far from saturation.

D. Practice

1. Equilibrium Dialysis

a. Principle. Equilibrium dialysis relies on the retention of antibodies by semipermeable membranes that freely pass the antigen. Dialyzable antigens (i.e., molecules of molecular weight less than 3000, preferably less than 1000) are, generally, not immunogenic. They are haptens, capable of combining with antibodies but incapable of inducing the production of antibodies. The method of equilibrium dialysis thus implies the nonidentity of immunogen and test antigen. It is well to keep this fact in mind as it restricts equilibrium dialysis to the study of heterologous reactions, nonidentiy of immunogen and test antigen being the formal definition of a cross reaction.

Apart from this restriction, the method yields unequivocal answers: Free hapten appears on one side of the membrane and, knowing the input concentrations of hapten and antibody, the average equilibrium constant may be calculated from a set of such data by substituting into any of Eqs. (11a)–(11f). This holds for the ideal case where (1) equilibrium is attained,

(2) the equilibrium is not distorted by osmotic effects, and (3) the membrane or, generally, the equipment does not interact with any of the reactants. None of these conditions is automatically fulfilled in practical systems; the ways of recognizing and correcting potential systematic errors will be given below.

b. Equipment. Some of the classical equilibrium measurements have been performed in dialysis bags tied at both ends and dangled in a solution of hapten. Nowadays the technique is both more economical in materials and less accident prone.

Diffusion chambers of 1.5-ml capacity are commercially available[1] or can be homemade by cutting off the top third of 5-ml antibiotic vials and grinding their cut surfaces flat. Before putting them into service, the chambers are cleaned in hot nitric acid or KOH–ethanol, thoroughly rinsed in distilled water, and siliconed to cut down adsorption. Washing under the tap followed by a distilled-water rinse is usually sufficient between runs. The chambers are dried and stored in a dust-free container, such as a large Petri dish. A pair of diffusion chambers may be clamped together (Quickfit JC-19 clamps) or mounted in an appropriate brass frame (Drummond Scientific Co., Broomall, Pennsylvania).

Dialyzing membranes (20/32–32/32, Visking Corp., Chicago, Illinois) are cut to convenient size, say 10×10 cm², and soaked in distilled water. After an hour, the water is brought to boiling and allowed to cool over the next hour. Then the membranes are rinsed in cold distilled water, three changes of 30 min each, and finally stored in 0.01 M NaN_3 (0.06% in H_2O), ready for use.

Since concentration gradients during dialysis are to be minimized, the assembled cells must be agitated. A simple device for this purpose is a vertical disk rotating at 5–10 rpm, as used in tissue culture laboratories. It will accommodate 20–60 assembled dialysis units and can be mounted on a bench top. For critical thermodynamic work, more accurate temperature control is required than can be achieved in incubators or constant-temperature rooms. Commercially available agitators have either insufficient capacity or improper action, but a simple and effective rotating device has been designed by Karush and Karush (1971), holding 36 dialysis units and fitting readily available refrigerated constant-temperature baths.

c. Performance of Test. The dialysis cells are assembled the night before the test. First the ground-glass flanges are given a *thin* coating of silicone

---

[1] Bellco Glass Co., Vineland, New Jersey. Micro equipment, operating with 50- to 100-μl volumes, may be obtained from Gateway Serum Co., Cahokia, Illinois.

grease (e.g., Merck, Darmstadt, Art. 7921) and placed, face up, on the bench. Then a sheet of dialyzing membrane is blotted between two sheets of lint-free absorbent paper (e.g., Photowipes, Sorg Paper Co., Middletown, Ohio) and disks of a size exactly fitting the dialysis cell are punched out with a sharp cork borer. (A sheet of 10×10 cm^2 is meant to give 16 disks of 22.5-mm diameter.) A membrane free of visible imperfections is placed on top of each half-cell, smoothed out, covered with the other half-cell, and the assembly clamped together. As a check for invisible imperfections and imperfect sealing at the edges, the top halves are filled with 1 ml of water and connected to a source of compressed air or nitrogen through a rubber stopper fitting the mouth of the cells. The pressure is set at 0.1 atm (1.5 psi) and any significant leak through the membrane or between the membrane and the top compartment should show up within 5 min. After that the pressure is released, the dialyzing unit inverted, and the pro-cedure repeated to test the seal between the membrane and the bottom compartment. If the experiment is to be performed in a water bath, the joining perimeter of the two half-cells is painted with molten paraffin wax (melting point, 62°–65°C; heated to ca. 100°C) to prevent lateral seepage during dialysis. The assembled cells, lying on their sides, are stored overnight at room temperature. The small residue of water, usually less than 0.1 ml, evaporates during this period and the cells are ready for use.

Before setting up an equilibrium test the dialysis units are labeled. Then the various hapten solutions are measured in with volumetric pipettes and the top half-cell is sealed. The commercial cells have screw caps and these we found unsatisfactory on two accounts. First, tightening the caps occasionally twists the cell and thereby distorts or tears the membrane; even if great care is taken to avoid such damage, the sealing itself puts the cell under positive pressure. Second, the caps collect water between the threads and, unless they are sealed with wax (i.e., by an extra operation), this water will dilute the samples to be assayed after completion of the run. We use, therefore, the rubber stoppers employed in sealing antibiotic vials. The stopper is first pierced through its center by a 15-mm (⅝th-in.) 22-gauge needle (to allow equalization of pressure during insertion) and then pressed into the cell to give a flush fit. After all solutions have been delivered, the needles are withdrawn and the units inverted. Measuring in the antibody solutions and sealing their compartments are done similarly. The dialysis units are then mounted on the rotating device and diffusion is allowed to proceed for a predetermined time.

After the equilibration period the neck of the cells is blotted, a needle inserted into the stopper of the hapten compartment, and the stopper removed. The sample is withdrawn with a Pasteur pipette by slightly tilting the cell and touching its side (*not* the membrane!) with the tip of the pipette. By this technique usually not more than 0.05 ml of fluid is left in the cell. While the exact contents are difficult to assess, the error will be only of the order of $\pm 2\%$ by using a correction of $+0.05$ ml for the capillary layer of fluid left behind. Even though in most tests only the concentration of hapten is to be determined, the antibody compartment is drained in a similar fashion and the yield of fluid recorded.

d. Experimental Design and Controls. Since one of the reactants, the hapten, is usually monovalent, the precautions aimed at avoiding interaction between sites (cf. Section II,C,3) may be relaxed for equilibrium dialysis. There are, however, other considerations that limit the scope of informative tests. First, the concentration of epitope–paratope complexes is obtained as a difference, by subtracting free from total hapten. This calls for special care in determining the input concentrations, since their imprecision will enter as systematic error into the estimate of complexes. It also demands that the difference between free and bound hapten be made as large as possible, their error variances being additive. In practice, this amounts to setting the antibody concentration above the equilibrium constant, to ensure better than 50% binding (Note 7).

NOTE 7. Since animal sera are about 10^{-4} M in immunoglobulin and hyperimmune globulin contains only a few percent of specific antibody, measurement of equilibrium constants above 10^{-6} M (or 6.10^{14} in cgs units) becomes an expensive hobby. It can also become a dangerous hobby, partly because at such high concentrations nonspecific binding starts to interfere—some of the best-liked haptens are known to bind also outside the paratope—and partly because the Donnan effect may become significant—globulins being polyions, the concentration of charged groups retained by the membrane may not be negligible compared to the freely diffusible species.

Nonspecific binding may be assessed by setting up control cells with nonantibody globulin at a concentration equal to that of the test cell. A positive result is more of a danger signal than an exact measure of nonspecific binding: Particular preparations, especially monoclonal antibodies, may deviate from the average control globulins considerably and in either direction.

The *Donnan effect* is usually swamped by the ions present in physiological buffers (~ 0.16 M). It may bias the results when working with highly concentrated antibody preparations, that is, when measuring affinities above $10^{-4.5}$ M. The bias is not obvious from the course of the binding curves: It has the same effect as increased heterogeneity among the poorer antibodies. Unequal volumes recovered from the two half-cells is a warning sign; a diagnostic sign is finding significant differences in the concentration of free hapten when replicate tests are set up in buffers of, say, 0.10 and 0.20 M. The remedy is the inclusion of a macromolecular polyion in the hapten compartment. It is understood that the remedy should not be worse than the disease: The balancing macromolecule must not interact with the hapten.

There is also a second reason for aiming at equilibria of high bound-to-free hapten ratios. Dialyzing membranes will themselves bind a fraction of the ligand and this fraction, a correction factor in the evaluation of results, should be kept as low as possible. And that not only because the error of measuring hapten lost by adsorption adds to the error of estimating hapten specifically bound by antibody, but mainly because dialyzing membranes are inhomogeneous and even accurately determined correction curves cannot fully account for the vagaries of manufacture. Since the quantity of hapten bound to the membrane depends, by and large, on the concentration of free hapten, shifting the equilibrium in favor of binding will keep this error within bounds, too.

When starting work on a system of unknown parameters, *sighting experiments* must first be performed. To begin with, the *equilibration period* has to be set. This is done by filling replicate half-cells with hapten solution ranging in concentration from 10^{-4} M to the detection limit of the assay, say, 10^{-7} M. The other half-cells are filled with buffer. A pair of dialysis units is taken down at intervals (after 12, 24, 36, and 48 hr is the usual timing) and the concentration of hapten on either side of the membrane is determined. In most systems the asymptote will be reached within 24 hr, but at least an extra 12 hr should be allowed for equilibration in the main experiments as the total transport through the membrane will be greater when the bulk of hapten is bound by antibody.

The same preliminary test gives information also on the *quantity of hapten retained by the membranes*. This quantity is estimated as the difference between observed and expected hapten concentrations, that is, between the average concentration found in the two half-cells and half of the input concentration. The preliminary experiment is no substitute for a proper correction curve, but it is sufficient for setting the concentrations of antibody and hapten. Thus, if at a hapten input of, say, 10^{-8} mole (1.0 ml of a 10^{-5} M solution) 0.10×10^{-8} mole is found to be bound by the membrane, an antibody concentration binding more than 0.5×10^{-8} mole will give results of sufficient precision.

The *concentration of antibody* to be used is determined in a second experiment. The highest dose of antibody one can afford, say, 10^{-8} mole per unit, and one-tenth of this quantity are set up against hapten concentrations of 10^{-5}, 10^{-6}, and 10^{-7} M. After an equilibration period defined by the first experiment, the free hapten concentrations are determined and the fraction bound to antibody is calculated, taking into account the nonspecific binding by the membrane (roughly known from the first experiment). The choice for the main tests is that dose of antibody which binds half the hapten at an input concentration tenfold above the level of detection. This will ensure both valid results and an economy of reagents (Note 8).

NOTE 8. *Example:* From a range-finding experiment, we calculate the following percentages of hapten bound.

Antibody input (mole)	Hapten input		
	$10^{-5} M$	$10^{-6} M$	$10^{-7} M$
10^{-8}	73	90	91
10^{-9}	9	38	49

At the higher input, antibody binds more than half of the hapten over the whole range. This level would be satisfactory, therefore, even at hapten concentrations somewhat above $10^{-5} M$, but its use extravagant. The lower dose gives 50% binding at $10^{-7} M$ hapten and would be satisfactory only over hapten concentrations below that, where measurements of free hapten are not practicable. The choice of antibody input is 3 to 5×10^{-9} mole (1.0 ml of a 3 to $5 \times 10^{-6} M$ solution), equilibrated against hapten in the range of 8×10^{-6} to $2 \times 10^{-6} M$.

The preliminary test which governs the choice of antibody input defines also the corresponding *span of hapten concentrations.* Assuming antibody populations of the usual heterogeneity, the informative range of equilibria extends from the concentration at which half of the hapten is bound to a concentration about fourfold below that.

The *main test* is performed in 20 dialysis units, assembled the day before. The antibody dilution (Note 9) and the series of hapten dilutions (Note 10)

NOTE 9. For the main test, 12 ml of antibody dilution is needed, at a concentration defined by the range-finding experiment. The equilibrium controls require 1 ml, at twice the experimental concentration.

As diluent we use a solution of 0.138 M NaCl, 0.02 M phosphate buffer at pH 7.25, and 0.01 M NaN$_3$ in quartz-distilled water, passed through a sintered glass filter. The azide is included to prevent microbial growth during the experiment. The buffer solution is self-sterilizing and keeps indefinitely at room temperature.

NOTE 10. Two series of hapten dilutions are required: one for the main test (five tubes containing 3.20 ml of buffer each) and one for the controls (six tubes containing 2.00 ml of buffer). First, 20 ml of hapten stock is made up, at a concentration expected to give 50% binding with the chosen antibody input. The starting stock is serially diluted in five tubes, carrying 10.0 ml into 3.20 ml. The series of $4^{1/5}$-fold dilutions covers a fourfold range for the main test. The concentrations, in terms of the starting dilution (i.e., the hapten stock), are 1.00, 0.76, 0.57, 0.43, 0.33, and 0.25. These are *expected* concentrations and are by no means an excuse for not determining the *actual* concentrations with the greatest care.

For the control set, 3.0 ml is carried into 2.0 ml of buffer, providing a series of six $10^{1/5}$-fold steps over a tenfold range. The expected concentrations, in terms of the hapten stock, are 0.60, 0.38, 0.23, 0.15, 0.09, and 0.06.

The equilibrium controls require 1 ml of hapten stock diluted with an equal volume of buffer.

are made up first. Then the top compartment of 12 units is filled, in duplicate, with 1.0 ml of the six experimental hapten dilutions. The half-cells are sealed, the units inverted, and 1.0 ml of the antibody dilution is measured into each. After inserting the stoppers into the antibody compartments, the dialyzing units are mounted on the rotating device.

The six units which will serve to establish the control curve receive 1.0 ml of the control hapten series in one compartment and 1.0 ml of buffer in the other.

The remaining two units, the equilibrium controls, receive 0.50 ml of half-strength hapten stock plus 0.50 ml of double-strength antibody stock in one compartment and 1.0 ml of buffer in the other.

When testing several haptens against the same serum, or testing the same combination of hapten and antibody at different temperatures, a complete set of controls is needed for each hapten and at each temperature. When several antibody preparations are tested against the same hapten, only one series of controls is required, but in this case the number of units used for control purposes may be increased, either by setting up duplicates or, better, by covering the same range in smaller steps. The two equilibrium control units are obligatory, whatever the design of the experiment.

e. Evaluation. The data available for evaluation are the input concentration of antibody, $[A]$; the six input concentrations of hapten, $[H]_1$ to $[H]_6$; and the six input concentrations of the control series, $[C]_1$ to $[C]_6$—all of these are determined at the beginning of the experiment. At its completion, we obtain also six duplicates of free hapten concentration, $[h]_1$ to $[h]_6$; six pairs of control hapten concentrations, $[c_t]_1$ to $[c_t]_6$ from the top compartments and $[c_b]_1$ to $[c_b]_6$ from the bottom compartments; and a duplicate free hapten concentration from the two equilibrium control units, $[q]$.

The first move is to compare $[q]$ with $[h]_6$. If these are not equal within the error of the assay for hapten, equilibrium has not been reached and the test is invalid. (For a comparison of means, see Chapter 34).

The next move is to compare the pairs of hapten concentrations of the control series ($[c_t]_i$ versus $[c_b]_i$): At equilibrium they are expected to be indistinguishable, within the error of measurement. If they are, a *correction curve* is established by entering the average free hapten concentrations, $\frac{1}{2}[c_t + c_b]_i$, on the abscissa and entering the corresponding concentration corrections, $[C]_i - [c_t + c_b]_i$ on the ordinate. A smooth curve may be fitted to the experimental points by eye; a less subjective procedure is fitting a logarithmic function of the form $y = a + b \ln x$, where x is the free hapten concentration and y the concentration correction. Use of the theoretical curve also serves to relieve the anguish of graphical interpolation (for fitting and testing regression curves, see Chapter 34.)

Before constructing the *binding curve*, the concentration corrections corresponding to particular free hapten values, $[h]_i$, are subtracted from the respective $[H]_i$ values, giving the operative epitope input $[E]_i$. For the conventional treatment, the molar ratio of bound hapten and antibody, r, must be worked out $[r_i = ([E]_i - 2[h]_i)/A]$. When fitting one of Eqs. (11a)–(11f), the values of $\alpha_i = 1 - (2[h]_i/[E]_i)$ are required. In the latter case, the input values refer to the total volume of the test; that is, $[E]_i/2$ and $[A]/2$ are to be used in the calculations (Note 11).

NOTE 11. The experimental readings are best entered on an appropriately ruled data sheet. If the calculations are to be performed on a computer, the raw data are sufficient; otherwise, the computed values can be worked out on the same sheet. An example, estimating the quantity and quality of monoclonal anti-TNP γ_1-globulin produced by a hybrid cell line, is given in Fig. 2.

The experimental data are fitted here to Eq. (11a), that is, $x = \alpha E = [E] - [h]$ and $y = \alpha/(1 - \alpha) = x/[h]$. The binding curve shows no significant departure from linearity, which, if mere inspection would fail to convince, can also be seen from the high r^2 value: 99.16% of the variation is accounted for by the regression (for tests of linearity, see Chapter 34). The clonal antibody thus scores as homogeneous, and its quantity and quality are estimated by this test with an accuracy rather better than ±3%.

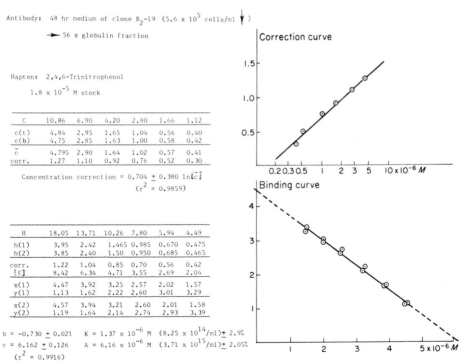

Fig. 2. Working sheet of an equilibrium dialysis test.

If the fitted data fall on a straight line, the parameters of interest, K and either $[A]$ or n, are unambiguously defined. If the regression turns out to be nonlinear, the same data are used for estimating the index of heterogeneity (cf. Section II,C,1) after the value of n or $[A]$, as the case may be, has been obtained by extrapolating the binding curve. Even K_0 may be derived from this curve: It is the concentration of free reagent at the point where $\alpha = (1 - \alpha) = 0.5$ or, alternatively, where $r = 0.5n$.

f. Scope and Limitations. Both the points for and against equilibrium dialysis follow from the way free antigen is separated from the other components of the system. The pore limit of dialyzing membranes is small and hence only small molecules can be used as ligands. This has the advantage that the usual complications besetting equilibrium tests of multivalent antigens (cf. Section II,C) do not arise here and observations can be interpreted in a straightforward manner. However, the lack of complications is a mixed blessing: It underlines the artificiality of a system where immunogen and test antigen are not the same, where the ligand fills only a small fraction of the paratopic cavity, and where the firmness of binding remains several orders of magnitude below that found with most large antigenic molecules.

Equilibrium dialysis has also its own complications, due largely to the cellulose membranes used. Diffusion, especially through membranes, is a slow process and the long period of equilibration precludes any kinetic studies in this system. What is worse, there is always some nonspecific binding of the ligand, and this forces the tests into the region of high antibody concentrations, with its electroosmotic and economic sequelae.

2. Equilibrium Filtration

a. Principle. Equilibrium filtration relies on the retention of particulate antigens by filter membranes that freely pass antibodies. Since macroglobulins are partly retained by pores of less than 20-nm diameter and commercial filters, contrary to the manufacturers' claims, vary by at least 15% about their nominal values, the smallest average pore size safe to use in the separation of antibodies and particulate antigens is 25 nm. This sets the lower limit of the antigenic particle at 30-nm diameter or about 10^7 molecular weight, corresponding to the size of small viruses. As a rule, such antigens are made up of repeating subunits and mostly of more than one kind of subunit. Since even one subunit may display several different epitopes, all complications listed in Section II,C should be considered and either eliminated or accounted for.

Antigen and antibody are brought together in a test tube, and equilibration is thus more rapid than in equilibrium dialysis. The separation of free antibody takes only about a minute, allowing also kinetic measurements in this system.

The criteria of validity (Note 12) (reversible combination of antigen and antibody, attainment of equilibrium, and absence of interaction between the equipment and any of the reactants) are the same as in any equilibrium test. Data from a valid assay allow unambiguous definition of the average equilibrium constant and one other parameter, such as the number of antibody molecules or antigenic particles or the valency of either.

NOTE 12. If it is not intuitively clear that filtration (i.e., reducing the volume of the compartment containing free and occupied epitopes) does not alter the equilibrium, it can be formally proven by writing out Eq. (5) explicitly, that is, without using square brackets to indicate concentrations. Thus, if the initial volume of the equilibrium mixture was v and this is reduced by filtration to w $(0 < w < v)$, we have

$$\frac{E-x}{v} \cdot \frac{P-x}{v} \bigg/ \frac{x}{v} = K \; \therefore \; (E-x)(P-x) - vxK = 0$$

before filtration and the same after filtration:

$$\frac{E-x}{w} \cdot \frac{P-x}{v} \bigg/ \frac{x}{w} = K \; \therefore \; (E-x)(P-x) - vxK = 0$$

b. Equipment. Any kind of filter assembly is suitable, such as Swinney adapters[2] fitted to Yale-lock syringes and taking 13- or 25-mm-diameter filter membranes. Special equipment designed for the purpose (Fazekas de St.Groth and Webster, 1961)[3] allows simultaneous handling of sets of 24 filters, has a dead volume of less than 0.05 ml per unit, and is free from the usual troubles of Swinney adapters, such as air locks above the membrane and leaks between syringe and filter.

Membranes of 25-, 50-, or 100-nm average pore size are commercially available.[4] The Sartorius filters, made of fully substituted cellulose acetate, bind considerably less globulin than do the Millipore membranes. Such nonspecific binding can be reduced to negligible levels either by floating the membranes on a solution of 0.1% serum globulin or by passing about 1 ml of the same solution through them.

[2] Millipore Co., Bedford, Massachusetts, Cat. Nos. XX30 012 00, SX00 013 00, and SX00 025 00. Sartorius Membranfilter GmbH., Goettingen, West Germany, Cat. Nos. 162 22, 162 14, and 165 17.

[3] Obtainable from W. Junghans Feinmechanik, Basel, Switzerland.

[4] Millipore Cat. Nos. VC WP013 00, VM WP013 00, VS013 00, VC WP 025 00, VM WP 025 00, and VS 025 00. Sartorius Cat. Nos. SM 113 09, SM 113 10, and, on special order, SM 111 09 and SM 111 10, made of cellulose triacetate.

Gasket sets, containing a flat and an O-section Teflon ring and a nickel or stainless steel crib plate, are available.[5] These can be reused many times, provided the filters are not excessively tightened. Use of a small torque wrench (e.g., Dual Signal Tension Wrench, Warren and Brown Pty. Ltd., Sydney, Australia), set at 100 cm/kg (18 in./lb), will ensure both proper sealing and long gasket life.

c. Performance of Test. The filter units are assembled by placing the flat washer, crib plate, filter membrane, and ring gasket (in that order) in the lower part of the filter housing and screwing on the upper part.

Mixtures of antigen and antibody are set up in a series of small test tubes (13 × 75 mm). A convenient final volume is 1.20 ml, allowing recovery of about 1.1 ml of filtrate. The dilutions of antigen are made up first, by delivering 1–24 standard drops[6] of a stock antigen suspension and complementing to 24 drops with buffer. Then an equal volume (0.60 ml) of the antibody solution is measured in, best in the form of twelve 50-μl drops, and the tubes are well shaken.

After the period of equilibration, the mixtures are poured into the filter device, the air line is fitted, and the pressure, preset at 0.6 atm (10 psi), turned on. Filtration of 1.2 ml through 25-, 50-, or 100-nm pore membranes takes about 110, 50, or 20 sec, respectively.

d. Experimental Design and Controls. As equilibrium filtration is expected to estimate equilibrium constants and count the number of epitopes or paratopes in a system of both multivalent and heterogeneous reactants, the tests must be done over a range where distorting complications are negligible, that is, where most epitopes remain free. Even when interactions between neighboring sites are to be studied, the baseline is set by measurements done far from saturation or, formally, where $[E] > 10[x]$.

The precision of the assay, on the other hand, demands that most of the antibody be bound, that is, $[x] > 0.9[P]$. Both prerequisites are met by an experimental arrangement where $[E] > 10K$ and $K \sim [P]$. In practice, this means setting the antibody input at about 100 times the sensitivity of the method of detection so that, assuming 90 to 99% binding, the filtrates will give titers between 10 and 1.

This represents the ideal case, where *nonspecific binding* is negligible. To test for this, several dilutions of antibody (ranging in titer from 1 to 50) are filtered and the titers before and after filtration are compared. If some of the antibody is found to be retained by the membrane, the experiment is

[5] Millipore Cat. No. XX 30 012 03.

[6] Cooke Laboratory Products, Alexandria, Virginia, Cat. Nos. M5, M17 and M35, M36 for droppers delivering 25 and 50 μl, respectively.

repeated with pretreated filters: The membranes are floated (*not* immersed!) on a solution of 0.2% gelatin in buffer for 10 min at room temperature and blotted between two sheets of absorbent paper before mounting in the filter device. Such treatment usually reduces nonspecific binding to acceptable levels, but it will approximately double the time required for filtration. If this treatment is not quite satisfactory, the membranes are floated on a 0.1% solution of nonantibody globulin homologous to the test preparation. The latter procedure is more expensive and further reduces the rate of filtration, but will practically eliminate nonspecific binding. After either gelatin or globulin pretreatment, the membranes may be stored dry (between two sheets of filter paper) and used whenever convenient.

The *equilibration period* is relatively short in this system: We incubate the antigen–antibody mixtures for 1 hr at room temperature or above and for 2–4 hr at lower temperatures. For an objective assessment of the time required, a single mixture of antigen and antibody (aiming at about 99% binding) is made up and aliquots are filtered at intervals, say, after 15, 30, 60, 120, and 240 min. The period of preincubation chosen for the main experiment is at least twice that needed for reaching the asymptote. Choice of longer equilibration periods will, of course, not influence the results.

The *concentration of antibody* to be used is governed by three independent criteria. First, the concentration of antibody must be at least ten times lower than the concentration of epitopes in the test, to ensure conditions far from epitope saturation even at $>90\%$ binding of antibody. Second, the lowest free antibody concentration must still lie within the sensitivity of the assay. Third, the assay used for detection must measure the quantity of antibodies only and not a compound of quantity and quality. Compliance with the third criterion is an absolute requisite of valid tests since with heterogeneous antibody populations the filtrate will *always* have a lower average affinity than the input population. The most sensitive assay techniques, such as neutralization of bacteriophages through a coupled antigen or conventional radioimmunoassays, do not meet this requirement and will give systematically biased results, overestimating affinities and underestimating the concentration of topes. Plainly, the third criterion is irrelevant to equilibria of monoclonal antibodies, where among equally precise assays the most sensitive is also the best.

Given an appropriate assay, then, the antibody input is set at about 100-fold above its limit of detection. If this happens to be too high in terms of epitope concentration, the antigen input will have to be raised to maintain the ratio of 10:1 between the two reactants.

Since the equilibrium constant is not known beforehand, the *range of antigen concentrations* must be determined in a preliminary test. To this end, antigen dilutions are set out in threefold steps, from about 10^{11} to 10^{14}

epitopes/ml, and 0.6 ml of each is mixed with an equal volume of an antibody dilution giving a titer of 100. After an appropriate period of equilibration, the mixtures are filtered and the points of 90 and 99% binding are noted. The corresponding antigen concentrations will cover the range to be used in the main test (Note 13). Such a range-finding experiment is mandatory for each antibody preparation to be tested. False economy at this level will have to be paid for by uninformative equilibrium tests, yielding either unmeasurable free antibody concentrations if the guessed range was set too low or nonlinear binding curves if it was set too high.

NOTE 13. With antibodies of low affinity, the informative range of antigen doses may include some that will block the filter. For instance, 10^{10} influenza virus particles, representing 2×10^{13} epitopes, will cover at close packing an area of 0.64 cm², that is, the whole available surface of a 13-mm-diameter filter membrane. The blocking effect may be overcome, at least partly, by adding 100 mg of Kieselguhr to the equilibrium mixtures, thus creating a primitive prefilter. The right way out is to change to a method that is not affected by the mass of antigen present, such as equilibrium sedimentation.

The antigen stock to be used in the *main test* is that dilution which gave about 96–98% binding in the range-finding experiment. Ten dilution steps, covering a sixfold range, are conveniently made up from 4 ml of stock by distributing 24, 21, 18, 15, 12, 10, 8, 6, 5, and 4 25-μl drops in 10 tubes and complementing each to 24 drops with buffer. Two control tubes receive buffer only. Then 0.60 ml of the antibody stock (8 ml of titer 100 is required) is added to each tube, the contents well mixed and incubated at the chosen temperature for a period of equilibration found adequate in the preliminary tests. A few minutes before the end of this period, each tube is emptied into a filter unit and eventually filtered under 0.6 atm pressure. The filtrates are sufficient for duplicate titrations, starting with undiluted samples. The remainder of the antibody stock is also titrated, providing a control for nonspecific binding by the membrane: The titers of the two filtered antibody samples and of the unfiltered stock are expected to be the same.

e. Evaluation. The data available for evaluation are all in the form of titers, that is, some unknown multiple of absolute concentrations. One task of an equilibrium test, therefore, is to find the factor by which a titer can be transformed into the number of antibody molecules. The other task is estimating the equilibrium constant. Since from a linear regression only two parameters can be estimated, this implies that the third parameter, the concentration of epitopes, is known. Indeed, it better be known accurately, as its error will be incorporated into and increase the error of all estimates. Evaluation of the experimental data proceeds in three steps. First, the titers of the filtrates, that is, of free antibody, are expressed as fractions of the input. Since titers are usually given as logarithms, this involves subtracting the average titer of the control tubes from each of the experimental titers, to give $\log(1 - \alpha)$ and, looking up the antilogarithms, to obtain $(1 - \alpha)$. The corresponding dilution factors of the antigen inputs and the α values are also entered.

The second step is choosing one of Eqs. (11a)–(11f) and preparing the variables to be plotted.[7]

The third step is fitting the theoretical curve to the data and, provided the regression has passed the tests of validity, deriving estimates of the equilibrium constant and the concentration of antibody molecules, as well as of their errors (Note 14).

NOTE 14. For fitting regression lines, see Chapter 34. All computations needed can be conveniently performed on a small electronic pocket calculator. The programmable kinds also have sufficient capacity to perform the transformations of steps 1 and 2 and then use the supplied machine program for fitting a linear regression.

A Fortran program, written specifically for virus–antibody equilibria but readily adapted to other equilibrium filtration data, is available on request. Operating on an input of raw experimental data, it performs the maximum likelihood fitting of all six of Eqs. (11a)–(11f), applies tests of validity, works out the best combined (weighted) estimates of the parameters of interest, tests the significance of the regression and of deviations from linearity in an analysis of variance, and also does thermodynamic calculations on sets of data obtained at different temperatures.

f. Scope and Limitations. Equilibrium filtration has some major advantages. First, it can be applied to homologous systems; that is, it uses the same antigen as was used for immunization. Second, it works with unpurified reagents. Third, it is economical: 10 μl of a hyperimmune serum and, in the case of viruses, one-tenth of the output of an egg or a tissue culture bottle are sufficient for a test. Fourth, it is easy to perform: 20 complete tests, involving 240 filtrations, can be set up and evaluated in half a day. Fifth, it is rapid, allowing kinetic measurements on dilute systems.

The disadvantages are equally numerous. First, the acceptable size of antigenic particles is limited, downward by the smallest pore size still passing antibodies and upward by the need to provide the required epitope density without blocking the filter. Second, it is unsuited to measuring low affinities, again because larger masses of antigen will block the filter. Third, it is beset by all the complications following from the multivalence of large antigenic particles. Fourth, it is based on comparing antibody titers and hence cannot match the precision of chemical measurements. Fifth, it requires special assays that do not confound quantity and quality.

[7] Numerical tables for the solution of equilibrium equations, listing the values of α and $(1 - \alpha)$ between 0.001 and 0.999, in steps of 0.001, and of the derived variables $1/\alpha$, $1/(1 - \alpha)$, $\alpha/(1 - \alpha)$, $(1 - \alpha)/\alpha$, and $\alpha(1 - \alpha)$, are available (Fazekas de St.Groth, 1961). That paper also contains a worked example of evaluating an equilibrium filtration test.

3. Equilibrium Sedimentation

a. Principle. Equilibrium sedimentation relies on pelleting antigenic particles in gravitational fields where antibody remains in the supernatant. Since the largest immunoglobulin has a sedimentation constant of 19 S, the lower limit of antigenic size corresponds to that of ribosomes or small viruses when working in an ultracentrifuge or to bacterial or mitochondrial size when the separation is done in an ordinary centrifuge. There is no upper limit on antigenic size. Such large particles are, as a rule, antigenically both multivalent and heterogeneous; they are unlikely to enter uncomplicated equilibria except far from epitopic saturation.

The reactants are mixed directly and, after a period of equilibration, antigen and antigen–antibody complexes are spun down. Since the time taken for centrifuging is comparable to the equilibration period, the system is not suited to kinetic measurements.

Of all equilibrium techniques, sedimentation is least subject to nonspecific binding by the equipment used to separate the free reactant. If equilibrium is reached, the test will give an unbiased estimate (Note 15) of the average equilibrium constant and one other parameter of the system.

NOTE 15. An equilibrium, established in volume v, is unchanged by creating two compartments, one of volume $v - w$ containing the fraction $(v - w)/v$ of a free reactant, and the other of volume w containing the remainder together with the other two reactants:

$$\frac{E - x}{v} \cdot \frac{P - x}{v} \bigg/ \frac{x}{v} = K = \frac{E - x}{w} \cdot \frac{(w/v)(P - x)}{w} \bigg/ \frac{x}{w}$$

b. Equipment. While any centrifuge tube is suitable for equilibrium tests, parsimony prompts the use of small-volume equipment, such as polyethylene tubes of 0.5- or 1.5-ml capacity (Eppendorf tubes, obtainable from any laboratory supply house) and minifuges (e.g., Microfuge, Beckman Instrument Co., Fullerton, California; Minifuge, Heraeus AG, Osterode, West Germany), although nowadays most laboratory centrifuges have fittings to take large numbers of small tubes. In the ultracentrifuge range, the choice is between standard equipment (unfit for handling small volumes or many samples) or ad hoc apparatus (requiring precision-engineering facilities). To the latter class belong the Perspex or nylon inserts fitting 38.5-ml centrifuge tubes, each with six drilled cups 6 mm in diameter and 30 mm deep (Fazekas de St.Groth and Webster, 1963). These can be used as a cluster of centrifuge tubes, so that 72 or 60 equilibrium mixtures of 0.60 ml are spun simultaneously in a Beckman Spinco 30 or 60 rotor, respectively.

The only other piece of special equipment is a Pasteur pipette whose tip (the last 2–3 mm) is bent in a flame, indispensable for collecting supernatants from small tubes without disturbing the pellet.

c. Performance of Test. Antigen–antibody mixtures of 1.20 ml are made up in 13 × 75-mm tubes, exactly as for equilibrium filtration (cf. Section II,D,2,c). This is preferable to making them up directly in centrifuge tubes, as adequate mixing in small tubes filled to the brim is hardly possible. In addition, with large particulate antigens such as cells, the mixtures must be agitated to prevent settling and thus the slowing down of the approach to equilibrium. After the period of equilibration, each mixture is transferred to a 1.5-ml tube for low-speed centrifugation or split between two 0.60-ml tubes for high-speed centrifugation. At the end of the run, the supernatants are carefully pipetted off, leaving about 0.1 ml over the pellet.

d. Experimental Design and Controls. The considerations governing experimental design are the same as in equilibrium filtration (cf. Section II,D,2,d): For a test free of complications, the concentration of epitopes must be kept well above the equilibrium constant, and the concentration of antibody as low as the assay of detection will permit. As antibodies of higher affinity are preferentially bound, the supernatants will be qualitatively different from the input. Unbiased estimates of the average equilibrium constant and of the concentrations of epitopes or paratopes can be expected only when the method of titration is quantitative, that is, equally sensitive to antibodies of high or low affinity.

Nonspecific binding is no problem in equilibrium sedimentation, but the *separation of free antibody* is. With submicroscopic particles, sedimenting only somewhat faster than antibodies, preliminary experiments are required to demonstrate that the two special criteria of a valid test are satisfied, namely, that the supernatant contains no antigen and that it contains all of the free antibody. Knowing the sedimentation constant of the antigen will reduce the time spent on preliminary centrifugal runs, but this is no excuse for not checking the predictions experimentally. Once the minimal time and centrifugal force needed for sedimenting >99% of the antigen are established, the same conditions are applied to several dilutions of antibody. If the top and bottom thirds of the supernatants have the same titers, the second criterion is also satisfied.

The period needed for equilibration as well as the concentrations of antigen and antibody to be used are worked out in the same way as for equilibrium filtration tests, except that there is no limitation on the mass of antigen that can be used in a test. The protocol for the main experiment is also the same (cf. Section II,D,2,d), with the only difference that equilibrium mixtures containing antigenic particles of the size of cells must be shaken during the incubation period.

e. Evaluation. The experimental data are handled exactly as those obtained in equilibrium filtration tests. Rather than repeating what has been said in Section II,D,2,e, a practical example will be given in which the technique is used for estimating the epitope density on cells and for comparing the affinities of antibody for free and bound haptens.

Trinitrophenylsulfonate (TNPS)-coupled red cells are equilibrated against the monoclonal antibody preparation, whose concentration and affinity were determined by equilibrium dialysis (see Fig. 2). The input is a 1:100 dilution of the same preparation, that is, 3.71×10^{13} antibody molecules/ml, mixed with an equal volume of TNPS-coupled erythrocytes, starting at 2.4×10^9 cells /ml (Fig. 3).

The first column, the dilution factor d, is conveniently expressed as the number of drops of stock cell suspension in the equilibrium mixtures, while the second column gives the duplicate hemagglutinin titers of the supernatants in $\log_2$ units. These are the experimental data.

The first stage of evaluation consists of computing the fractions of antibody bound (α) and free ($1 - \alpha$). To this end, the four control titers are averaged and their mean is subtracted from each of the experimental titers: Column 3 shows the mean differences, $\log_2(1 - \alpha)$. The values of $(1 - \alpha)$ and α are obtained by transforming the entries of column 3 into common logarithms (i.e., multiplying by $\log 2 = 0.3010 \ldots$), looking up their antilogarithms (column 4), and subtracting this figure from 1 (column 5).

In the second stage, the variables for one or the other of Eqs. (11a)–(11f) are derived. The computer program by which the entries of Fig. 3 were prepared fits each of Eqs. (11a)–(11f). Here we choose Eq. (11c), to demonstrate that with reasonably precise data even this, the least promising of the six transforms, is adequate. In Eq. (11c) the number of epitopes is nC, n standing for the number of epitopes/cell and C for the number of cells. But we varied the number of cells by the factors d, so that the number of epitopes will be dnC. Since the dilution factors should appear only in the variables, we multiply both sides of Eq. (11c) by d, making the two variables $1/(1 - \alpha)$ and d/α. These are worked out and entered in columns 6 and 7, respectively.

Finally, the binding curve is plotted and its slope (b) and intercept (a) are estimated. (A plot of columns 6 and 7 is shown in Fig. 3.) The three lowest points do not seem to fall on a straight line, but statistical evaluation of the data (see Chapter 34) tells that only the last two deviate significantly from linearity, that is, that complications of various kinds have become manifest from about 40% binding upward. The slope and intercept are estimated therefore from the first eight entries only; the best-fitting regression line, as drawn in Fig. 3, is also based on these eight pairs of data. The slope of this line $b = K/nC = 2.669$ and its intercept $a = P/nC = 1.903$. The paratope concentration $P = \frac{1}{2}$ (antibody input)(valency) $= 3.71 \times 10^{13}$ and $C = \frac{1}{2}$ (cell stock)/(dilution factor) $= 5 \times 10^7$. (Halving the input concentrations accounts for making up the equilibrium mixtures from equal parts of the two reactants.) By substituting these values, we estimate the epitope density as 3.9×10^5 TNP molecules per red cell and the average equilibrium constant as 5.2×10^{13} (or $1.16 \times 10^7 \ M^{-1}$), that is, almost a 16 times higher affinity than found by equilibrium dialysis against the free hapten, trinitrophenol. The equilibrium constant is still only an average value because, even though the antibody preparation was homogeneous, the same cannot be assumed about the epitopes.

f. Scope and Limitations. Equilibrium sedimentation is virtually free from nonspecific effects and in that respect superior to other equilibrium

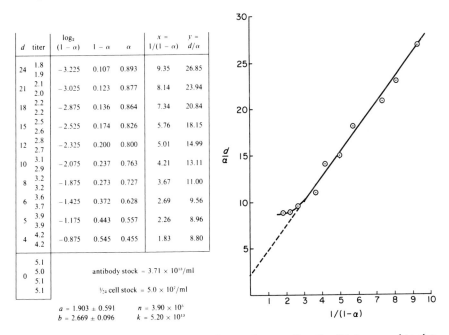

d	titer	$\log_2$ $(1 - \alpha)$	$1 - \alpha$	α	$x = 1/(1 - \alpha)$	$y = d/\alpha$
24	1.8 1.9	-3.225	0.107	0.893	9.35	26.85
21	2.1 2.0	-3.025	0.123	0.877	8.14	23.94
18	2.2 2.2	-2.875	0.136	0.864	7.34	20.84
15	2.5 2.6	-2.525	0.174	0.826	5.76	18.15
12	2.8 2.7	-2.325	0.200	0.800	5.01	14.99
10	3.1 2.9	-2.075	0.237	0.763	4.21	13.11
8	3.2 3.2	-1.875	0.273	0.727	3.67	11.00
6	3.6 3.7	-1.425	0.372	0.628	2.69	9.56
5	3.9 3.9	-1.175	0.443	0.557	2.26	8.96
4	4.2 4.2	-0.875	0.545	0.455	1.83	8.80
0	5.1 5.0 5.1 5.1					

antibody stock $= 3.71 \times 10^{13}$/ml

$\frac{1}{24}$ cell stock $= 5.0 \times 10^7$/ml

$a = 1.903 \pm 0.591 \qquad n = 3.90 \times 10^5$
$b = 2.669 \pm 0.096 \qquad k = 5.20 \times 10^{13}$

Fig. 3. Working sheet of an equilibrium sedimentation test. Equation (11c) was used to plot the graph.

techniques in use. While, in principle, it could be applied to all problems solved by dialysis or filtration, separations in high gravitational fields imply equipment not suited to handling many small samples.

Equilibrium sedimentation comes into its own in the size range of antigenic particles that can be spun down in low- and medium-speed centrifuges. It is therefore uniquely suited to the immunological study of cell surface components, whether they are, for example, antibodylike recognition structures, antigenic markers, or receptors for lectins, etc. The technique itself is both simple and economical in reagents and, in the range of gravitational fields of 10,000 g or less, requires no special equipment.

Kinetic measurements, however, do not fall within the scope of equilibrium sedimentation, nor will it be successful in dealing with low affinities, as the required high epitope concentrations are usually unattainable when the antigenic determinant represents only a vanishingly small part of the total mass of the particle. Large particles raise also the specter of all complications that go with multivalent, heterogeneous surfaces.

III. COMPETITIVE EQUILIBRIA

A. Theory

1. Competitive Inhibition

Consider a reaction scheme in which two different epitopes, at concentrations $[E]$ and $[I]$, can reversibly combine with the same paratope, $[P]$.

$$
\begin{array}{c}
E \rightleftharpoons x \\
+ \\
P \\
+ \\
I \rightleftharpoons y
\end{array}
$$

The two kinds of complex, x and y, will be formed at rates defined by Eq. (3), with the only difference that the two reactions share a common pool of free paratopes, $[P - (x + y)]$. Thus

$$
\left.
\begin{aligned}
\frac{dx}{dt} &= k_1[E - x][P - (x + y)] - k_2[x] \\
\frac{dy}{dt} &= l_1[I - y][P - (x + y)] - l_2[y]
\end{aligned}
\right\}
\tag{15}
$$

At equilibrium, where $dx/dt = dy/dt = 0$, we have, by analogy to Eq. (5),

$$\left.\begin{aligned} \frac{[E-x][P-(x+y)]}{[x]} &= \frac{k_2}{k_1} = K \\[2mm] \frac{[I-y][P-(x+y)]}{[y]} &= \frac{l_2}{l_1} = L \end{aligned}\right\} \tag{16}$$

Note that, at low paratopic occupancy (where $(x + y) \ll P$, i.e., $[P - (x + y)] \sim [P]$), the two equations become effectively independent (Note 16) and competition will not be observed. Standard competition tests

NOTE 16. Note also that, by dividing the first equation by the second, we have

$$K/L = [(E - x)/x]\,[(I - y)/y]$$

that is, the *ratio* of the two equilibrium constants can always be worked out from the two binding ratios, irrespective of the concentration of free epitopes.

therefore imply an excess of one component, ensuring that the shared reactant is largely bound—in our system, that $[P - (x + y)] \ll [P]$. This means that one of the complexes, say $[y]$, must nearly equal $[P]$, and that can be achieved only if both $[I] > [P]$ and $[I] > L$. We may therefore simplify the second equation by writing $[I]$ for the practically constant inhibitor concentrations. But under these conditions, the concentration of free paratopes will be numerically lower than K, the equilibrium constant of the competitor, and hence a second simplification follows, namely, that $[E - x] \sim [E]$, as $[E] \gg [x]$. With these simplifications, Eq. (16) is restated as

$$\left.\begin{aligned} \frac{[E][P-(x+y)]}{[x]} &= K \\[2mm] \frac{[I][P-(x+y)]}{[y]} &= L \end{aligned}\right\} \tag{16a}$$

Expressing y from the first equation and substituting into the second, we have

$$[x] = \frac{L[E][P]}{K([I] + L) + L[E]} \tag{17}$$

Since in practical tests the concentration of inhibitor will be the independent variable, Eq. (17) may be arranged to give

$$\frac{1}{[x]} = \frac{[E] + K}{[E][P]} + \frac{K[I]}{L[E][P]} \tag{17a}$$

This is the equation of a straight line from whose slope and intercept the two equilibrium constants can be estimated. Note that in the absence of competition, where $[I] = 0$, Eq. (17a) reduces to the common reciprocal form of the mass equation

$$\frac{1}{[x_0]} = \frac{[E] + K}{[E][P]}$$

2. Noncompetitive Inhibition

If an antigen–antibody reaction is affected by an inhibitor combining with the antibody molecule outside the paratope (such as in some idiotope–antiidiotope systems), there will be four reactions running simultaneously

$$
\begin{array}{c}
E \rightleftharpoons x + I \\
+ \\
P \qquad \qquad \searrow z \\
+ \\
I \rightleftharpoons y + E
\end{array}
$$

with the ternary product either inactive or inaccessible by one route. The corresponding mass equations can be simplified in the same way as in the case of competitive inhibition, by recognizing that $[E - (x + z)] \sim [E]$ and $[I - (y + z)] \sim [I]$. Accordingly,

$$
\left.
\begin{aligned}
\frac{[E][P - (x + y + z)]}{[x]} &= K \\[2mm]
\frac{[I][P - (x + y + z)]}{[y]} &= L \\[2mm]
\frac{[E][y]}{[z]} &= K \\[2mm]
\frac{[I][x]}{[z]} &= L
\end{aligned}
\right\}
\tag{18}
$$

The assignment of identical equilibrium constants to the secondary reactions is gratuitous and implies independence of sites. Altering these would make no difference to the general form of the results.

By the same treatment as used for competitive inhibition, we derive

$$[x] = \frac{L[E][P]}{(L + [I])(K + [E])} \tag{19}$$

and

$$\frac{1}{[x]} = \frac{[E] + K}{[E][P]} + \left(1 + \frac{K}{[E]}\right)\frac{[I]}{L[P]} \tag{19a}$$

yielding a linear equation for the estimation of the two equilibrium constants.

As a check, note that by setting $[I] = 0$, that is, in the absence of competition, the second term vanishes and Eq. (19a) reduces to the reciprocal form of the mass equation.

3. Steric Inhibition

An inhibitor may interfere with the formation of antigen–antibody complexes by occupying the paratope (competitive inhibition), by rendering it unoccupiable through some allosteric change (noncompetitive inhibition), or by doing neither but simply being in the way. Such steric inhibition was first observed in the neutralization of enzymes by antibodies, and a mathematical model developed in the same paper (Fazekas de St.Groth, 1963). It is likely to operate whenever independent reactions are insufficiently separated in space, for instance, when antibodies of several specificities are simultaneously reacting with a mosaic of epitopes, say, on a cell.

Consider, therefore, a cell surface made up of n *domains*, each centered on an epitope and containing also s sites at which an inhibitor may bind. The inhibitor, I (considered to be in excess), combines at random with its binding sites, so that at equilibrium we have

$$\frac{[snC - y][I]}{[y]} = L \tag{20}$$

The average occupancy is $y/snC = [I]/([I] + L)$, and the efficiency of the inhibitor in blocking epitopes is taken to be proportional to the occupancy through a factor p $(0 < p < 1)$ (Note 17). Thus, at a particular occupancy, the fraction $p[I]/([I] + L)$ of domains will be inaccessible and $\{1 - p[I]/([I] + L)\}$ free.

NOTE 17. The steric factor p may be thought of as each inhibitor unit blocking a sector of approach to the epitope. Such a problem in geometric probability has been proposed and solved by Stevens (1939) as follows.

On a circle of unit circumference, mark out n arcs of length x $(x < 1)$, at random. The probability that the arcs cover the whole circumference is

$$P = 1 - \binom{n}{1}(1 - x)^{n-1} - \binom{n}{2}(1 - 2x)^{n-1} - \cdots - \binom{n}{j}(1 - jx)^{n-1}$$

where $jx < 1 \le (j + 1)x$.

The asymptotic value of the probability that the circumference is not covered is $1 - P = n(1 - x)^{n-1}$, and is in fact a good approximation over a fairly wide range of x and n.

The equilibrium between an excess of paratopes and epitopes is

$$\frac{[nC - x - nCpI/(I + L)][P]}{[x]} = K \tag{21}$$

where the concentration of free epitopes is made up of the total domains, diminished by the number actually occupied by paratopes (x) and those that are unoccupiable $[nCpI/(I + L)]$. Accordingly, the concentration of paratopes bound in the presence of inhibitor is

$$[x] = \frac{[nC][P]}{K + [P]} \left(1 - \frac{p[I]}{[I] + L}\right) \tag{22}$$

In the absence of inhibitor, Eq. (22) reduces to $x = [nC] [P]/(K + [P])$, the standard mass equation, in excess of paratopes. The reciprocal form,

$$\frac{1}{[x]} = \frac{K + [P]}{[nC][P]} \left(1 + \frac{p[I]}{(1 - p)[I] + L}\right) \tag{22a}$$

is less useful in this case, partly because it is not linear and partly because it contains the extra parameter, p. However, it will be noted that, by increasing the inhibitor concentration, the term in parentheses asymptotes to $1/(1 - p)$, whereas at low inhibitor concentrations it will approximately equal $1 + (p[I]/L)$, thus allowing estimation of all parameters.

4. Discrimination between Mechanisms

Since each of Eqs. (17), (19), and (22), defining the three types of competition, contains a common term, it is best to eliminate this term first and then discriminate between the rest. We define therefore R, the ratio of epitope–paratope complexes in the absence and presence of inhibitor, as

$$R_{\text{comp}} = \frac{x_0}{x_{\text{comp}}} = 1 + \frac{K[I]}{L(K + E])}$$

$$R_{\text{noncomp}} = \frac{x_0}{x_{\text{noncomp}}} = 1 + \frac{[I]}{L} \tag{23}$$

$$R_{\text{steric}} = \frac{x_0}{x_{\text{steric}}} = 1 + \frac{p[I]}{(1 - p)[I] + L}$$

All three plots have the same intercept, and the first two are linear when $[I]$ is the independent variable. Steric inhibition can be identified by this criterion, as long as the value of p is not too high. In that case, it will not be readily distinguished from noncompetitive inhibition.

By varying $[E]$, competitive inhibition stands apart from the other two as only R_{comp} is a function of the epitope input. This holds over the whole range where competition is observable, since there $[E]$ cannot become negligible in terms of K. Noncompetitive and steric inhibition can still be distinguished, even if $p \sim 1$, by comparing the slopes of the R plots: It is $1/L$ for the former and p/L for the latter. But this implies independent and precise estimation of the equilibrium constants, which is certainly not the simplest way out.

We define, therefore, a second set of discriminants, D, as the difference between paratopic occupancies in the presence and absence of inhibitor. Thus,

$$D_{comp} = \frac{[P]}{x_{comp}} - \frac{[P]}{x_0} = \frac{K[I]}{L[E]}$$

$$D_{noncomp} = \frac{[P]}{x_{noncomp}} - \frac{[P]}{x_0} = \left(1 + \frac{K}{[E]}\right)\frac{[I]}{L} \tag{24}$$

$$D_{steric} = \frac{[P]}{x_{steric}} - \frac{[P]}{x_0} = \left(\frac{p[I]}{(1-p)[I] + L}\right)\frac{K + [P]}{[E]}$$

The D plots for competitive inhibition pass through the origin, whether $[I]$ or $[E]$ is the independent variable. For noncompetitive inhibition, the same holds when $[I]$ is varied, but on varying $[E]$ the intercept $[I]/L$ significantly differs from zero since $[I] > L$, if competition is to be observed. The D plot for steric inhibition is nonlinear on varying $[I]$, is linear and passing through the origin on varying $[E]$, and is also a function of $[P]$, which the other two are not.

B. Practice

1. Compartmental Assays

a. Principle. By separating one of the free reactants from a ternary equilibrium, the nature of competition and its parameters may be assessed. Such tests can be based on each of the three equilibrium techniques treated in Section II,D. The only additional problem likely to arise is that the compartment (dialysate, filtrate, or supernatant), which in simple equilibria contained only one of the free reactants, may here contain two. This problem is most acute in equilibrium dialysis, where the concentration of one hapten has to be determined in an excess of the other. Yet, some closely similar haptens can be distinguished spectrophotometrically or, if that fails, the minority competitor may be labeled, measuring then the overall concentration of free epitopes optically and the minority as radioactivity. With the other two techniques, the problem arises only when two antibodies are set up in competition for the same antigen. In such cases, at least one of the antibodies must be specifically purified and labeled, unless the two can be distinguished by some special property (such as sensitivity to S—S-breaking reagents, fixation of complement, allotype, etc.).

Assuming these problems can be overcome, ternary equilibria will allow the estimation of two parameters (e.g., the two equilibrium constants, the number of epitopes or paratopes, or some measure of heterogeneity). This is sufficient since preliminary and control tests, establishing the behavior of the system in the absence of competition, leave only the second equilibrium constant (denoted by L in the theoretical part) to be determined. The remaining information is best used for assessing heterogeneity, as a check that the two competitors share the whole of the target.

b. Design and Controls. While the concentration of epitope–paratope complexes is the dependent variable in all equilibrium tests, the separated compartment contains free epitopes by equilibrium dialysis and free paratopes by the other two techniques. This difference is reflected in the design of competitive tests.

In equilibrium dialysis, the concentrations of the minority competitor and antibody must be so adjusted that, in the absence of competition, the concentration of free hapten is about at the limit of detection. In this way, reduction of binding will still give free hapten concentrations that are significantly below the input, while nonspecific binding by the membrane remains a small fraction only of specific binding. In equilibrium filtration and sedimentation, on the other hand, the aim is to bind, in the absence of competition, as little antibody as is compatible with a valid test. In this way, the fraction taken up by the inhibitor will still leave detectable amounts of antibody in the separated compartment. In practice, this means increasing the antibody input about tenfold, remembering that simple equilibrium tests of this kind were designed to work at minimal concentrations of antibody.

As competition experiments are, presumably, not even considered without having determined first the equilibrium parameters of at least one of the competitors, only the effective range of inhibitor concentrations will have to be set by a *preliminary test*. In equilibrium dialysis, this means starting with a hapten input that will be about 95% bound and leaves a just measurable concentration in the free hapten compartment. Inhibitor inputs of 10-, 100-, and 1000-fold higher will usually cover the range over which the fraction of free test hapten rises from 5 to 50%. This is the span to be used in the main experiment. For equilibrium filtration and sedimentation, the baseline is an antibody input of titer 1000 and a test antigen input that will reduce this titer 20- to 50-fold, that is, will bind 95–98% of the antibody in the absence of competition. The range of inhibiting antigen lies between the concentrations at which the titer further drops by 5- to 20-fold.

In the *main test*, the concentration of both competitors must be varied, to allow discrimination between mechanisms. Since the intercepts of the binding curves are either known from preliminary experiments or are theoretically defined, it is sufficient to replicate only the controls (equilibrium mixtures not containing inhibitor). The range of effective inhibitor concentrations, as established in the sighting test, is covered in four dilution steps. Thus, a subset, with the inputs of $[E]$ and $[P]$ constant, takes six experimental units. The second variable, $[E]$ (the competitor whose unbound fraction is to be measured), is varied over a threefold range, in the ratio $1:2:3$. The main test requires therefore 18 units. To this are to be added six adsorption controls in equilibrium dialysis or a pair of antibody controls for each serum dilution in filtration or sedimentation tests.

The competitors are measured into the same compartment in equilibrium dialysis, and antibody is placed in the other. By the other two techniques, the two competitors are measured in first, followed by the target. In all other particulars, competition tests are conducted in the same way as tests of simple equilibria.

c. Evaluation. First the equilibrium constant K is estimated, either from the data of preliminary experiments or from the controls, in the same manner as in tests of simple equilibria (cf. Section II,D:1e, 2e, and 3e). With this knowledge, the intercept of the binding curves can be predicted and, in a valid assay, the estimated intercept is expected to be the same, within statistical error.

In the linear regression fitted to the data, the concentration of the inhibitor, $[I]$, will be the independent variable and some function of the concentration of epitope–paratope complexes the dependent variable. If $1/[x]$ is chosen, the binding curves will follow Eq. (17a), (19a), or (22a). It is usually more convenient to use the directly measured concentration of free epitopes or paratopes as the dependent variable. The corresponding equations are

$$\frac{1}{1-\alpha} = \left(1 + \frac{[E]}{K}\right) + \frac{[I]}{L} \tag{17b}$$

$$\frac{1}{1-\alpha} = \left(1 + \frac{[E]}{K}\right) + \left(1 + \frac{[E]}{K}\right)\frac{[I]}{L} \tag{19b}$$

$$\frac{1}{1-\alpha} = \left(1 + \frac{[P]}{K}\right) + \left(1 + \frac{[P]}{K}\right)\frac{p[I]}{(1-p)[I] + L} \tag{22b}$$

where $(1 - \alpha)$ is the fraction of free reactant, as defined in Section II,B,2.

If the binding curve is flattening and eventually parallels the abscissa, the inhibition is steric and the value of p can be worked out from the asymptote as

$$p = 1 - x \frac{[P] + K}{[E][P]} \quad \text{or} \quad p = 1 - (1 - \alpha) \frac{[P] + K}{K}$$

respectively. The value of p may then be used to estimate L from the initial slope, but this is better done by plotting the R discriminant and finding L from its initial slope, which is p/L whether the ratio x_0/x or $(1 - \alpha_0)/(1 - \alpha)$ is plotted.

If the binding curve is linear or, in any case, does not asymptote, the D discriminant is plotted, with $[E]$ as the independent variable. With competitive inhibition, the regression will pass through the origin, whereas noncompetitive inhibition will give the positive intercept of I/L, from which L can be estimated directly. The best estimate of L in noncompetitive inhibition is derived from the original binding curve, where $1/(1 - \alpha)$ was plotted against $[I]$: The slope here is $1/L$.

2. Plaque Assays

a. Principle. A hemolytic plaque assay (Jerne and Nordin, 1963) detects single antibody-producing cells by plating them in a medium of hapten-carrying erythrocytes and complement. A plaque is the disk of lysed red cells, centered on the lymphocyte from which the antibody emanates. Theory and practice of the technique have been reviewed (Jerne *et al.*, 1974; see also Chapter 19). The following points are relevant to the assessment of quality in this system.

1. The assay is quantal; that is, it deals in numbers, not concentrations.
2. The number of plaques is relatively small: They must be kept within countable limits and overlaps are to be avoided.
3. The distribution of plaque size is truncated: Below a certain rate and level of production an antibody-producing cell will not be detected.
4. The size of plaques depends on both the quantity and quality of antibodies released: Given the same number of molecules, high-affinity antibody will produce a smaller plaque than low-affinity antibody.
5. The size of plaques also depends on the epitope density of the indicator system: Given a number of antibody molecules, the plaques will be smaller the higher the epitope density of the cells.
6. The system is open: At the center of the plaque antibody is generated and beyond its edge, well within the diffusion limit, the concentration is too low to cause appreciable lysis.

The first and last points rule out any direct measurement of quality, even if points 3, 4, and 5 would not act as sufficient deterrent. What remains is the use of the discriminants R or D [see Eqs. (23) and (24)], that is, assessing affinity as well as the nature of competition in *plaque reduction tests*. In fact, even the mechanism is restricted to competitive inhibition, since the indicator system does not lend itself to equilibrium measurements and the only parameter left to determine is L, the equilibrium constant of the antibody–inhibitor interaction.

Assuming that both stationary diffusion and equilibrium are reached (Note 18) early in the assay period, the competition for antibody between free and cell-bound epitopes will follow Eq. (15) and, since both competitors are in excess, the fraction of paratopes bound to cells, x, is given by Eq. (17). Jerne *et al.* (1974) have shown, both theoretically and on examples from the literature, that within any one assay the number of plaques is proportional to s, say, px. They have also shown that the radius of a plaque is similarly a direct function of x, and that this function is linear with unit slope over the practical range of plaque sizes.

Note 18. The steady state is attained when $k_1[E] > 1/t$ in Eq. (15). This condition is fulfilled in the standard assay, since $[E] \sim 10^{13}$ (2×10^8 cells/cm^3 and, say, 5×10^4 epitopes/cell), $k_1 \sim 10^{-16}$, and $t = 7200$ sec.

The time required for equilibration is given by integrating Eq. (3), with epitopes in excess, as

$$x(1 - \exp\{-(k_1[E] + k_2)t\}) = \frac{[E] + K}{[E][P]}$$

This reduces to the standard mass equation when the exponential term approaches zero, that is, when $(k_1[E] + k_2) > 3/t$. Since $k_1[E] \sim 10^{-3}$ and $t = 7200$, dissociation rate constants of $k_2 > 10^{-3}$ meet the requirements, and even the most firmly binding antibodies will hardly contradict the assumptions.

b. *Design and Controls.* The various ways of setting up plaque assays are treated in Chapter 19. The special considerations concerning competitive assays bear on validity and precision. A valid test implies a state of stationary diffusion of antibody, as well as equilibrium between epitopes and paratopes. Both can be checked in a single *preliminary experiment*, by setting up the assay with three red cell concentrations, say 10^8, 2×10^8, and 4×10^8/ml. If $k_1[E] < k_2$ and $(k_1[E] + k_2) > 3/t$, the number of plaques will be the same on the three plates and their size will stand in inverse proportion to the concentration of red cells.

The question of precision has been considered in detail by Jerne *et al.* (1974), and they conclude that, apart from the irreducible random sampling error, a competently conducted plaque assay also carries a procedural error which increases the variance by $0.0044P^2$ (P is the number of plaques counted) (Note 19). Uniform precision over plaque reduction assays demands that the replicates be increased when lower counts are expected, that is, at higher inhibitor concentrations.

NOTE 19. The 95% confidence intervals (in parentheses) for particular counts are: 50 (34–66), 100 (76–124), 200 (161–239), 300 (247–353), and 400 (334–466).

The effective concentration of inhibitor is chosen empirically. Since $[I] >$ $[E]$, if competition is to be observed, and since incestuous combinations are possible with cell-bound but not with single epitopes, the lower limit of inhibitor cannot be much below 10^{14} molecules/ml ($\sim 10^{-7}$ M). The preliminary test is set up, therefore, in the range of 10^{-7} to 10^{-3} M, in tenfold steps, and the concentration giving 50% inhibition of plaques is noted.

The main test requires 10 plates. The number of immunocytes per plate is adjusted to give about 400 plaques in the absence of inhibitor. If four such control plates are set up, two with the full dose of cells and two with half the dose, the expected error of counting will be about ±7%. The competition plates, set up in duplicate, receive the full dose of cells in 0.5, 1, or 2 times the concentration of inhibitor found to give 50% plaque reduction in the preliminary test. In every other detail, the test is performed and read as a simple plaque assay (see Chapter 19).

c. *Evaluation.* The smallest recognizable plaque corresponds to the angular resolution of the human eye, about 0.1 mm; hence, the minimal plaque radius r_0 is 0.05 mm. A 50% plaque reduction amounts therefore to lowering the median plaque size, r, to somewhat less than r_0. Since the function $f(x, r)$ is linear and of unit slope over the experimental range (cf. Section III,B,2,a), reducing the number of plaques by half equals also an r_0/r-fold change in the number of paratopes bound to indicator cells. Thus, by Eq. (17),

$$\frac{[x]}{[P]} = \frac{[E]}{(K + [E])}$$

in the absence of inhibitor and

$$\frac{[x]r_0}{[P]r} = \frac{L[E]}{\{K(I_{50} + L) + L[E]\}}$$

in the presence of I_{50}, the concentration of inhibitor reducing the number of plaques by half. Dividing the first equation by the second and rearranging, we have

$$\frac{r}{r_0} = 1 + \frac{I_{50}}{L}\left(\frac{K}{K + [E]}\right) \qquad (25)$$

Jerne *et al.* (1974), by ignoring the term in parentheses, arrived at a very simple formula for the equilibrium constant: $L = r_0 I_{50}/(r - r_0)$. Some of the time saved by this formula may well be spent on repeating the assay with a different cell concentration. If the results are the same (i.e., $[E] \ll K$), the formula is valid; if on changing the epitope concentration the estimate of L changes, the formula is invalid. Still, the extra effort does not go unrewarded: By defining median inhibitory concentrations at several cell densities, we arrive at a linear equation,

$$\frac{r_0}{r - r_0} = \frac{L}{I_{50}} + \frac{L}{I_{50}K}[E] \qquad (26)$$

the intercept of which unambiguously defines L. The slope, in its turn, may be used for the estimation of K, provided the concentration of cell-bound epitopes can be determined. That this is more than a pious wish has been shown in Section II,D,3,e.

REFERENCES

Almeida, J. D., Cinader, B., and Howatson, A. (1963). *J. Exp. Med.* **118**, 327.

Fazekas de St.Groth, S. (1961). *Aust. J. Exp. Biol.* **39**, 563.

Fazekas de St.Groth, S. (1963). *Ann. N.Y. Acad. Sci.* **103**, 674.

Fazekas de St.Groth, S. (1967). *Cold Spring Harbor Symp. Quant. Biol.* **32**, 525.

Fazekas de St.Groth, S., and Webster, R. G. (1961). *Aust. J. Exp. Biol.* **39**, 549.

Fazekas de St.Groth, S., and Webster, R. G. (1963). *J. Immunol.* **90**, 151.

Feinstein, A., and Munn, E. A. (1969). *Nature (London)* **224**, 1307.

Gopalakrishnan, P. V., and Karush, F. (1974). *J. Immunol.* **113**, 769.

Greenbury, C. L., Moore, D. H., and Nunn, L. A. C. (1965). *Immunology* **8**, 420.

Hornick, C. L., and Karush, F. (1969). *Isr. J. Med. Sci.* **5**, 163.

Hornick, C. L., and Karush, F. (1972). *Immunol. Chem.* **9**, 325.

Jerne, N. K., and Nordin, A. A. (1963). *Science* **140**, 405.

Jerne, N. K., Henry, C., Nordin, A. A., Fuji, H., Koros, A. M. C., and Lefkovits, I. (1974). *Transplant. Rev.* **18**, 130.

Karush, F., and Karush, S. S. (1971). *Methods Immunol. Immunochem.* **3**, 383.

Katchalsky, A., and Spitnik, P. (1947). *J. Polym. Sci.* **2**, 432.

Kim, Y. T., Werblin, T. P., and Siskind, G. W. (1974). *J. Immunol.* **112**, 2002.

Klinman, N. R., and Karush, F. (1967). *Immunochemistry* **4**, 387.

Klinman, N. R., Long, C. A., and Karush, F. J. (1967). *J. Immunol.* **99**, 1128.

Lafferty, K. J. (1963). *Virology* **21**, 76.

Lafferty, K. J., and Oertelis, S. (1963). *Virology* **21**, 91.

Nisonoff, A., and Pressman, D. (1958). *J. Immunol.* **80,** 417.

Pauling, L., Pressman, D., and Grossberg, A. L. (1944). *J. Am. Chem. Soc.* **66,** 784.

Scatchard, G. (1949). *Ann. N.Y. Acad. Sci.* **51,** 660.

Sips, R. (1948). *J. Chem. Phys.* **16,** 490.

Stevens, W. L. (1939). *Ann. Eugen. London* **9,** 315.

van Regenmortel, W. H. V., and Hardie, G. (1976). *Immunochemistry* **13,** 503.

Werblin, T. P., and Siskind, G. W. (1972). *Immunochemistry* **9,** 987.

Werblin, T. P., Kim, Y. T., Quagliata, F., and Siskind, G. W. (1973). *Immunology* **24,** 477.

Wyman, J. (1948). *Advan. Protein Chem.* **4,** 407.

2

The Isolation and Characterization of Immunoglobulins, Antibodies, and Their Constituent Polypeptide Chains

Jean-Claude Jaton, Daniel Ch. Brandt, and Pierre Vassalli

IMMUNOLOGICAL METHODS
Copyright © 1979 by Academic Press, Inc.
All rights of reproduction in any form reserved.
ISBN 0-12-442750-2

I. INTRODUCTION

Ig's consist of a highly heterogeneous group of macromolecules with respect to charge, mass, and biological activity. They represent the most basic globulins of the serum and exhibit the least electrophoretic mobility (for a review, see Eisen, 1973). Their separation from the other serum proteins requires the use of conventional physicochemical means such as salt precipitation, ion-exchange chromatography, gel filtration, preparative zonal electrophoresis, or affinity chromatography, the latter method being particularly well suited to the isolation of specific antibodies from sera. All these methods are fairly rapid and simple and provide Ig's in good yield. Ig's of various species possess different electrical charges and masses and consequently may exhibit different electrophoretic behaviors, which implies that a fractionation procedure particularly successful for the isolation of Ig from one animal species may not necessarily be directly applicable to the isolation of Ig's of another species. Adjustment of the procedure is needed in each case. General methods of fractionation suitable for Ig's of most animal species will be briefly outlined in this chapter.

II. FRACTIONATION WITH NEUTRAL SALTS AT HIGH CONCENTRATION

Ammonium and sodium sulfate are most commonly used to achieve a crude separation of Ig's. This method is applicable to Ig's of most species (Kekwick, 1940). Serum Ig's are precipitated at room temperature or in the cold with $(NH_4)_2SO_4$ or Na_2SO_4 solutions buffered at pH 7.3 to a final saturation of 33 or 18%, respectively. The precipitated proteins, removed by centrifugation, are redissolved in PBS and precipitated a second time with 33% $(NH_4)_2SO_4$ or 12–15% Na_2SO_4, respectively. This step can be repeated a third or fourth time when necessary. The pellet is then dissolved in PBS, and the excess salts are removed by gel filtration through a Sephadex G-25 column or by exhaustive dialysis against PBS (the barium chloride test should be negative). This treatment leads, in general, to fairly pure human and rabbit IgG preparations, which may be slightly contaminated by α-globulins. Reasonably pure chicken Ig's can be rapidly prepared in this way. This method may be used to separate Ig's from other mammalian sera, for example, the guinea pig IgG's that are brought to 40% saturation with $(NH_4)_2SO_4$ for optimal precipitation.

III. PURIFICATION OF Ig's

A. Diethylaminoethyl Cellulose Chromatography

Ion exchange chromatography has proved exceedingly useful for the purification of Ig's (Peterson and Sober, 1956). Most studies have utilized diethylaminoethyl (DEAE) cellulose. Proteins become fixed to the anion exchanger through electrostatic bonds and are easily eluted from the adsorbent by raising the ionic strength and/or by changing the pH toward the isoelectric point of the proteins.

1. Human Ig's

Whole serum (10 ml) is first dialyzed against the starting buffer, 0.01 M potassium phosphate at pH 8.0, clarified by centrifugation, and applied on top of a 2.5 × 20-cm DEAE-cellulose column (about 9 gm of Whatman DE-52 adsorbent) equilibrated with the same buffer (Fahey and Horbett, 1959). Potassium phosphate, 0.015 to 0.3 M, is used for sequential elution of the serum proteins. Three major peaks are recorded. The first peak, which is eluted with 0.02 M phosphate buffer, contains more than 80% of the IgG fraction. This fraction is free of other serum proteins. The second peak consists of β- and some α-globulins, whereas the large third peak contains mainly serum albumin. The yield of Ig's recovered from the ion exchanger ranges between 75 and 85%. When only the IgG fraction is desired, 0.02 M phosphate buffer, pH 8.0 may be used and the effluent in the first peak is collected.

The Ig's contained in the ammonium or sodium sulfate cut from 10–20 ml of serum can be further purified on the same column. The human IgM macroglobulins are retained on the DEAE column and require a much higher salt concentration for elution; consequently, the IgM is usually largely contaminated with other protein components, such as α-globulins. (A better and faster method for the isolation of IgM from any species consists of gel filtration on Sephadex G-200 or Bio-Gel P-300 columns, as will be described in Section IV.) The IgA proteins are also retained on the column and are eluted with 0.1 to 0.15 M phosphate buffer. The eluted fractions contain IgA and many other serum components. DEAE-cellulose chromatography per se does not provide pure IgA molecules, except when myeloma IgA sera are used, for which the level of IgA is usually much higher than that of the other Ig's. IgD, which is present in very small amounts in normal serum (30–50 $\mu g/ml$), is usually eluted between IgG and IgA. Its isolation in substantial amount and with a high degree of purity requires the availability of an IgD myeloma serum.

It is important to avoid protein overloading, especially when sera contain large amounts of Ig's (myeloma or Waldenström macroglobulinemic sera), because the proteins may be eluted sooner than expected and, consequently, may be cross-contaminated. Conversely, an excess of adsorbent relative to serum proteins should be avoided in order to reduce nonspecific adsorption of Ig's. As a general rule, a small-scale experiment should be performed before attempting to fractionate a large quantity of protein.

2. Rabbit Ig's

These may be efficiently isolated from an initial 33% $(NH_4)_2SO_4$ precipitation by passage through a DEAE-cellulose column. The crude preparation is dialyzed against 0.0175 M phosphate buffer, pH 6.3 (Levy and Sober, 1960), and eluted with the same buffer. Electrophoretically slow-moving IgG's, free of any other serum proteins, are obtained in high yield. A second fast-moving IgG can be eluted from the column by applying 0.2 M phosphate, pH 8.0. This fraction, however, may be slightly contaminated by α_2-globulin and therefore requires a second run on the same adsorbent.

3. Guinea Pig IgG₁ and IgG₂

The two known subclasses, IgG_2 (slow-moving Ig) and IgG_1 (fast-moving component), may be isolated by ion exchange chromatography on DEAE-cellulose (Oettgen et al., 1965) using a salt gradient for elution (Leslie and Cohen, 1970). Since IgG_1 is present in serum in relatively low concentrations, it is rather difficult to obtain in a pure state, free of IgG_2. Pure IgG_1 and IgG_2 can be obtained by stepwise gradient elution from the DEAE-cellulose column (Whatman DE-52) (Tracey et al., 1976). The 40% $(NH_2)_2SO_4$ cut containing the IgG's from 330 ml of serum is dialyzed against 0.005 M phosphate buffer, pH 8.0, and placed on the column (5.0 × 60 cm), which is eluted stepwise with 0.005 M phosphate buffer, pH 8.0; 0.01 M, pH 6.5; 0.04 M, pH 6.2; 0.06 M, pH 6.1; and 0.3 M, pH 5.3. The IgG_2 fraction elutes with 0.005 M phosphate buffer, pH 8.0, whereas the IgG_1 fraction elutes with 0.06 M phosphate buffer, pH 6.1.

4. Mouse Ig's

These Ig's (IgG_{2a}, IgG_{2b}) may be precipitated with 18% Na_2SO_4 and further purified by DEAE chromatography. Bourgois and Fougereau (1970) used 0.017 M phosphate buffer, pH 7.3, to elute the MOPC 173 mouse myeloma IgG_{2a} from the adsorbent. Nonspecific IgG may be separated first by zonal electrophoresis in 0.054 M barbital buffer, pH 8.6, on Pevikon supporting medium. The IgG peak is then run through a DEAE-cellulose column and pure IgG can be recovered after elution with 0.04 M phosphate buffer, pH 8.0 (Capra *et al.*, 1975). Mouse myeloma IgM proteins are best isolated by gel filtration on Bio-Gel P-300 (or Sephadex G-200) after elution with 0.5 M NaCl–0.02 M phosphate buffer, pH 7.0, or by Pevikon or agarose block electrophoresis (see Section V).

5. Rat Ig's

The purification of three classes and four subclasses of rat Ig's, IgM, IgA, IgE, IgG_1, IgG_{2a}, IgG_{2b}, and IgG_{2c}, respectively, has been described in detail (Bazin *et al.*, 1974). The various steps involve 40–50% $(NH_4)_2SO_4$ precipitation followed by DEAE-cellulose chromatography and gel filtration on Sephadex G-200.

B. Salt-Mediated Hydrophobic Chromatography

An interesting report by Doellgast and Plaut (1976) described the purification of human IgA using salt-mediated hydrophobic chromatography. High concentrations of $(NH_4)_2SO_4$ are used to enhance the interaction of proteins with a hydrophobic ligand covalently bound to Sepharose. Adsorption of IgA from both normal and myeloma sera onto an L-phenylalanine–Sepharose column takes place in the presence of 1 M $(NH_4)_2SO_4$, and desorption occurs as the salt concentration is reduced to 0.8 M $(NH_4)_2SO_4$. In most cases, a second purification step involving gel filtration chromatography is required to remove small amounts of other proteins. This technique is rapid and reproducible and can be used for partial purification of almost any serum protein.

IV. FRACTIONATION BY GEL FILTRATION CHROMATOGRAPHY

This technique involves chromatography on Bio-Gel P-300 or Sephadex G-200, which separates proteins or crude Ig mixtures according to the molecular size of the proteins. The method is largely used for quantitative fractionation of the macroglobulin IgM, which can be isolated free of IgG or IgA proteins by one-step chromatography. The IgM of most animal species is excluded from the gel and recovered in the first elution peak in the presence of a high salt concentration (0.5 M NaCl buffered with 0.02 M phosphate buffer, pH 7.3, or 0.05 M Tris–HCl, pH 8.0). Because of the euglobulin properties of many IgM or Waldenström macroglobulins, dialysis of serum containing these macroglobulins against low ionic strength buffers causes the macroglobulins to precipitate. The washed precipitates are redissolved in buffered 0.5 M NaCl and eluted on a Sephadex G-200 column. The void volume fractions from the gel contain the IgM protein. Mouse and rabbit IgM's isolated in this way are often contaminated by α_2-macroglobulin, which coelutes with IgM. The contaminant is best removed by subjecting the impure IgM preparations to agarose block electrophoresis: IgM migrates toward the cathode, whereas α_2-macroglobulin travels toward the anode (see Section V).

V. ELECTROPHORETIC SEPARATION ON A SOLID SUPPORTING MEDIUM

This is one of the simplest preparative electrophoretic methods and has been used extensively since the late 1960s. Starch and Pevikon, a copolymer of polyvinyl chloride and polyvinyl acetate, were the most commonly used supporting media (Müller-Eberhard and Osterland, 1968). Agarose has now replaced starch and Pevikon because of its ease in handling and the nearly complete absence of the electroendosmotic effect.

Agarose Block Electrophoresis

The major advantages of this method are the high recovery of either isolated Ig's or antibodies from serum and the possibility of successfully separating two or more electrophoretically distinct antibodies of the same class of Ig. In addition, two or more samples can be simultaneously subjected to electrophoresis (Braun and Krause, 1968; Johansson, 1972). One disadvantage of the technique is the limited amount of sample that can be applied on the block, when compared with previously mentioned methods, such as DEAE-cellulose chromatography or gel filtration. Moreover, this method is rather time-consuming, but the reproducibility and the ease of separation from other non-Ig components are among its most outstanding features.

Methodology

a. Material. A schematic representation of the apparatus is shown in Fig. 1. The sample is dialyzed overnight and then its serum components are electrophoretically separated in 0.054 *M* barbital buffer, pH 8.6.

b. Preparation of Agarose. Agarose (Seakem Brand Marine Colloids, Inc., Biomedical Systems, Springfield, New Jersey) at a concentration of 0.5% is heated in a boiling water bath at 100°C until a clear solution is obtained. The agarose is then cooled to 50°C and poured carefully into a 2-liter mold. The solution is allowed to gel at room temperature and is covered with Saran Wrap before storage overnight at 4°C prior to use.

A trough is made by cutting out a 1-cm-wide slice 19 cm from the anodic side (Fig. 1). Since the block is usually split lengthwise into two identical compartments, two troughs are prepared. Up to 14 ml of serum can be applied into each trough.

c. Sample Application. The serum (14 ml) previously dialyzed overnight against 0.054 *M* barbital buffer is heated at 50°C for 5 min and quickly poured into 2 ml of 4% agarose-buffered solution at 50°C so that the final concentration of agarose is 0.5%. The resulting mixture is finally poured into the trough and allowed to set, and 2–5 ml of the 0.5% agarose solution at 50°C is applied on top of the layer to level off the trough. The block is then covered with Saran Wrap and subjected to electrophoresis at 4°C. Two blotters are used on each side of the block to make contact with the barbital

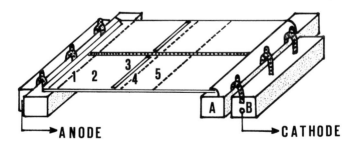

Fig. 1. Schematic representation of the agarose block electrophoresis setup. The mold is made of a Plexiglas plate (50 × 40 × 0.5 cm) surrounded by edges with an outer height of 1.7 cm. It can be split into two or more lengthwise compartments, thus allowing simultaneous electrophoretic separation of various samples. (1) Albumin position; (2) α- and β-globulin position; (3) appplication trough; (4,5) immunoglobulins migrate between these positions. (A) Sodium barbital buffer compartment (0.054 *M*, pH 8.6); (B) sodium phosphate buffer compartment (0.2 *M*, pH 7.5). A and B are connected by glass bridges.

buffer reservoirs (they should cover 5–10 cm of the gel at both ends). A constant voltage of 600 V is applied for 48–72 hr.

d. Recovery of Sample from the Block. After the run, slices of 0.5–1 cm are cut from 15 to 30 cm from the anodic side toward the cathode. They are transferred into centrifuge tubes and kept at $-20°C$ overnight. The tubes are then quickly thawed (freezing and thawing break agarose) and spun at 27,000 *g* for 30 min. The supernatant is collected and the pellets are washed twice with 3 ml of 0.1 *M* Tris–HCl buffer containing 0.5 *M* NaCl and 0.02% NaN_3, pH 8.0. The supernatants are combined and a Lowry protein (Lowry and Hunter, 1945) determination is used to localize peak fractions. These fractions are pooled, concentrated by ultrafiltration, and finally dialyzed extensively against PBS, pH 7.4. The purity of the various peak fractions is assessed by, for example, microzone electrophoresis, isoelectric focusing, or polyacrylamide gel electrophoresis techniques.

A typical agarose-block electrophoretic pattern is shown in Fig. 2 for the isolation of three electrophoretically distinct anti-type III pneumococcal antibodies from the serum of rabbit 4184. This antiserum contains about 15 mg of antibodies/ml of the IgG class. Four major Ig fractions can be isolated. The corresponding isoelectric focusing (IEF) patterns of three of them (Fig. 3) clearly demonstrate the efficiency of the electrophoretic method; it can be seen that fraction 4 contains a predominant antibody component (slowest-moving component) characterized by a pI value

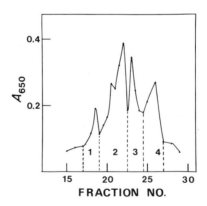

Fig. 2. Elution profile of various antibody components present in the same antiserum after agarose block electrophoresis. Whole anti-type III pneumococcal polysaccharide serum 4184 (14 ml) was applied onto an agarose block and the electrophoresis was done for 48 hr as described in the text. The fraction numbers correspond to a 1-cm slice of gel, which is numbered from the anode (left). The sample was applied in a trough corresponding to fraction 19. Protein eluates were detected by Lowry's method. See the text for details.

between 7.7 and 8.0, whereas fraction 2 (fastest-moving antibody) contains a major component of pI 5.9–6.2. Fraction 3 is contaminated by fraction 2, as is to be expected from the block electrophoretic pattern. Fraction 1 (not shown in Fig. 3) is contaminated by non-Ig components as determined by microzone electrophoresis. The total antibody fractions recovered from the block represent 74.2% of the amount of antibodies present in the serum, as determined by quantitative precipitation analysis with type III pneumococcal polysaccharide.

To obtain completely pure antibody components, a further purification of the contaminated fractions may often be achieved by subjecting each of them to a longer electrophoresis period (72–96 hr).

VI. ISOLATION OF ANTIBODY BY AFFINITY CHROMATOGRAPHY ON SEPHAROSE IMMUNOADSORBENTS

In this method, the antigen is covalently bound to a solid phase, usually Sepharose, type 4B or 6B (Axén et al., 1967; Cuatrecasas and Anfinsen, 1971) and the antigen–Sepharose conjugate is then poured into a chromatography column. The serum containing the corresponding antibodies is run through the column; the specific antibodies will be adsorbed onto the matrix gel and subsequently eluted by either nonspecific means (e.g., acid, high salt concentration) or specific agents (i.e., hapten ligand).

This technique has the advantage of being rapid and specific and provides isolated antibodies in good yield. It affords a means to selectively isolate, from the same serum, several antibody components exhibiting different affinities for an antigen. This method is particularly well suited for the separation of antibodies against protein antigens such as hemocyanin, bovine serum albumin, hapten–protein conjugates, and glycoproteins and of antibodies against polysaccharide antigens as described in Section VI,B.

With high molecular weight polysaccharide antigens, direct coupling to CNBr-activated Sepharose 4B is not possible; thus, a preparation of a suitable polysaccharide–protein conjugate must be prepared, which in turn can be efficiently coupled to the activated Sepharose via the protein moiety, by a standard procedure (Axén et al., 1967).

A. Preparation of the Type III Pneumococcal–Protein Complex

The method of conjugation, based on that described by Goebel and Avery (1931), is applicable to any type of polysaccharide and involves preparing

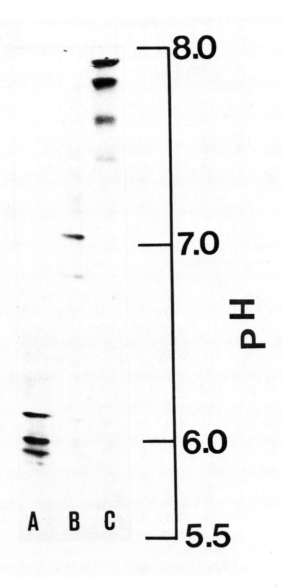

Fig. 3. Isoelectric focusing (IEF) analysis of the antibody fractions recovered from the agarose block after electrophoresis. (A) Fraction 2; (B) fraction 3; (C) fraction 4. The fractions were run in 5% acrylamide gels containing 2% Ampholine (pH range, 5–9) at 450 V for 14 hr and at 600 V for an additional 2 hr. They were stained with bromphenol blue. The experimental details with respect to the analytical IEF technique are described in Chapter 5.

the *p*-nitrobenzylether derivative of the polysaccharide, reducing into the *p*-amino derivative, and then converting this derivative to the diazonium salt, which is in turn coupled by diazotization with any protein containing aromatic residues (Pincus *et al.*, 1970; Jaton *et al.*, 1970). SIII (250 mg) is dissolved in 100 ml of water adjusted to pH 11 with diluted NaOH, and then *p*-nitrobenzyl bromide (1 gm) is added in five portions to the polysaccharide solution at 100°C in a boiling water bath. The pH is maintained between 10 and 11 with 5 *N* NaOH and the reaction mixture is stirred until all nitrobenzyl bromide crystals are dissolved (about 2 hr). The opalescent yellow solution is then extensively dialyzed against distilled water, and the *p*-nitrobenzylether derivative of SIII is reduced into the amino derivative in the presence of an excess of sodium dithionite at 60°C, pH 9. The solution becomes clear after 20–30 min. The *p*-amino derivative is exhaustively dialyzed against distilled water and centrifuged, and the small amount of insoluble material is discarded after centrifugation. The *p*-aminobenzylether derivative of SIII (about 210 mg) is finally lyophilized (yellow powder). It is further suspended in 30 ml of 0.25 *N* HCl and a slight excess of 0.5 *M* sodium nitrite is slowly added in an ice bath with vigorous stirring for 20 min. The diazonium salt solution is then quickly poured into bovine serum albumin (BSA, 500 mg) dissolved in 50 ml of 0.2 *M* borate buffer, pH 9. The solution is vigorously stirred and the pH is kept constant between 9 and 10 with dilute NaOH. The reaction mixture is allowed to stand at 0°C for 4 hr at pH 10. The dark orange solution of SIII–azo-BSA conjugate is finally dialyzed against water and lyophilized after eliminating a small amount of insoluble material by centrifugation. The conjugate contains approximately 30% (w/w) polysaccharide.

B. Coupling of SIII–azo-BSA Conjugate to CNBr-Activated Sepharose 4B

The method of activation of Sepharose 4B has been described elsewhere (Axén *et al.*, 1967; Cuatrecasas and Anfinsen, 1971) (CNBr-activated Sepharose 4B is commercially available from Pharmacia, Uppsala, Sweden). In a typical coupling procedure, freeze-dried CNBr-activated Sepharose 4B (15 gm) is reswollen and washed on a sintered glass filter with 0.001 *M* HCl (about 2 liters). The protein conjugate to be coupled (130 mg) is dissolved in 100 ml of 0.1 *M* NaHCO₃, pH 8.3, containing 0.5 *M* NaCl, and the packed washed gel is added to the protein solution and gently stirred at room temperature for 2 hr or at 4°C overnight. The uncoupled protein is washed with the coupling buffer and filtered through the sintered glass filter; the excess active groups are blocked by reacting with 1 *M* ethanolamine (adjusted to pH 8.5 with HCl) at room temperature for 2 hr.

The excess blocking reagent is washed with the coupling buffer and filtered through the sintered glass filter, followed by alternate washings with 0.1 M acetate buffer, pH 4, containing 1 M NaCl, and 0.1 M borate buffer, pH 8, containing 1 M NaCl. About five alternate washings are required to remove traces of noncovalently adsorbed material, which might interfere with subsequent experiments. The final washing of the immunoadsorbent is carried out with PBS containing 0.02% NaN_3. It should be stored at 4°C without freezing. The amount of conjugate covalently coupled to the Sepharose matrix ranges from 1.5 to 2.5 mg/ml of packed gel as determined by weighing the amount of uncoupled conjugate recovered after coupling.

1. Adsorption of Specific Antibodies onto and Elution from the Immunoadsorbent

The maximal capacity of the immunoadsorbent is determined by saturation experiments with antiserum. When the optimal ratio of antibody to antigen is found, a large-scale experiment is carried out. In a typical experiment, 50 ml of packed immunoadsorbent is poured into a column (1.5 × 30 cm) and the anti-SIII pneumococcal antiserum 3968 (12 ml) containing multiple antibody components is applied to the immunoadsorbent. The column is washed with PBS until the optical density of the effluent reads less than 0.05 at 280 nm. Adsorption is then complete because no antibody can be detected in the effluent. In an attempt to fractionate the various antibody components from the mixture, a gradient of decreasing pH and of increasing ionic strength can be used to elute the

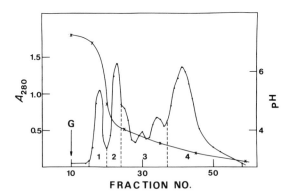

Fig. 4. Elution pattern of various antibody components present in antiserum 3968 from antigen–Sepharose immunoadsorbent. Fractions of 3.5 ml were collected; absorbance of the fractions was measured at 280 nm. ×——×, pH gradient. G, application of the gradient. See the text for details.

antibodies. The mixing chamber contains 250 ml of PBS, whereas the other chamber contains 250 ml of 0.2 N acetic acid–3 M NaCl. The elution pattern is depicted in Fig. 4. Five distinct peaks can be seen. The peak fractions, pooled as indicated in the figure, are dialyzed against PBS, concentrated by ultrafiltration, and analyzed by analytical IEF (Fig. 5). Although they are eluted at quite different pH values (1 pH unit difference), fractions 2 and 4 have very similar, but not identical, IEF patterns since the mixture of both yields an additive banding effect (Fig. 5, gel E). These IEF patterns are very different from that of fraction 3. The overall recovery of antibodies in the fractions is 68% of the total antibody concentration in the serum, as determined by quantitative precipitation analysis. Here, as in the case of the agarose block electrophoresis, none of the fractions is entirely pure. Recycling of selected fractions often yields a homogeneous antibody component whose IEF pattern is indistinguishable from that exhibited by a typical myeloma protein.

2. *Other Means of Elution*[1]

Recovery of antibodies in high yield can be obtained by the use of either stepwise or gradient elution with 0.1 M glycine-HCl buffer, pH 2.5, 3 M ammonium thiocyanate (Dandliker *et al.*, 1967), or 2 M NaI (Avrameas and Ternynck, 1967).

C. Isolation of Specific Anti-Allotypic Antibodies

Affinity chromatography can also be used for the isolation of specific anti-allotypic rabbit antibodies by coupling Ig's or homogeneous antibodies of known allotypic specificities to Sepharose 4B; the subsequent elution may be carried out by using either 4 M guanidine in 0.05 M glycine buffer, pH 3.5 (Aasted *et al.*, 1967), or 0.2 M acetic acid (Jaton *et al.*, 1976).

D. Isolation of Specific Anti-Idiotypic Antibodies

Rabbit anti-idiotypic antibodies can be isolated from whole idiotypic antiserum (9 ml) by affinity chromatography on Sepharose 4B (40 ml) to which the idiotype (20 mg) is covalently coupled. After washing the column with buffered saline, the bound antibody is eluted with 3 M NH₄SCN in buffered saline and passed through a second Sepharose column containing covalently bound pooled rabbit IgG. This step removes nonspecific binding

---

[1] Experiments in progress in our laboratory are aiming at the *specific* elution of anti-polysaccharide antibodies with oligosaccharide ligands of different sizes derived from partial acid hydrolysis of the whole polysaccharide.

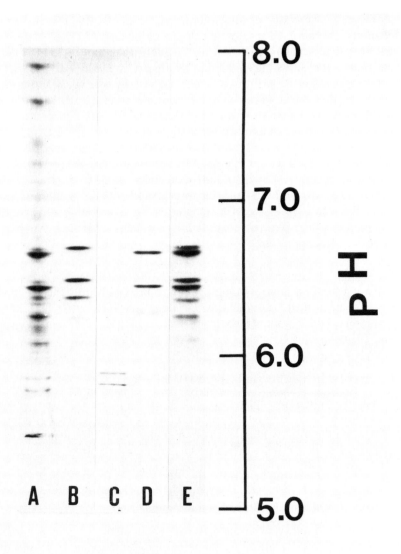

Fig. 5. Isoelectric focusing analysis of the antibody fractions of serum 3968 described in Fig. 4. (A) Serum 3968 prior to fractionation; (B) fraction 2; (C) fraction 3; (D) fraction 4; (E) mixture of equal amounts of fractions 2 and 4.

Ig's present in the eluted fraction. The eluate from the column contains 2.4 mg of the specific anti-idiotypic antibody (Sogn *et al.*, 1976).

E. Isolation of Anti-Hapten Antibodies

Anti-DNP (Ollander and Little, 1975) or anti-phosphorylcholine (Chesebro and Metzger, 1972) antibodies can be successfully isolated by the same method using ad hoc hapten derivatives coupled directly to Sepharose 4B. The elution is carried out in the presence of hapten solutions (Goetzl and Metzger, 1970) and the excess ligand is removed either by dialysis against neutral buffers or, in the case of charged haptens (Little and Eisen, 1966), by chromatography through an ion exchanger.

When the antibodies exhibit a high affinity for a given hapten, a cross-reactive hapten with a lower affinity for the antibodies should be used for coupling to the Sepharose and for the elution of the bound antibodies from the immunoadsorbent. The excess hapten is removed by dialysis and the hapten that remains associated with the antibodies can be eliminated by denaturation in 6 M guanidine-HCl at 4°C. The protein is then renatured by successive dialyses in solutions containing decreasing concentrations of guanidine-HCl and finally in PBS. The percentage recovery of the antibodies during the denaturation–renaturation procedure varies between 73 and 94 in the case of antibodies to digitoxin (Curd *et al.*, 1971).

F. Regeneration of the Immunoadsorbent

To ensure that all antibodies have been eluted, extensive washing with either 0.2 N acetic acid, 0.1 M glycine-HCl, or 3 M thiocyanate is performed, followed by reequilibration of the column in PBS containing 0.2% NaN_3. The material is stored at 4°C.

G. General Considerations on the Purification of Class-Specific Ig's

It should be emphasized that most Ig preparations of a given class are usually not completely free of any other Ig classes with the frequent exception of the IgG class, which is isolated by DEAE-cellulose chromatography, and of the IgM fraction recovered in the first excluded peak from Sephadex G-200 chromatography. It is therefore recommended that the particular Ig fraction should be rerun on the same column under identical conditions or that another fractionation procedure such as agarose block electrophoresis or gel filtration should be used. Affinity chromatography with class-specific antisera can be used to remove contaminating Ig's. Myeloma proteins of the G, A, and M classes and M–Waldenström macroglobulins may be purified in one step by DEAE-cellulose chromatography or zonal electrophoresis as long as they constitute the major Ig component in the serum. The purity of each Ig fraction should be tested by immunoelectrophoresis, double immunodiffusion, or radioimmunoassay with class- or subclass-specific reagents. The pure proteins should be stored at 4°C in the presence of 0.02% NaN₃ or kept frozen at a concentration of 10–30 mg/ml.

H. J Chain

The J chain has been shown to be present in IgM and in polymeric IgA molecules but is not found in monomeric IgA or in subunits of IgM (Morrison and Koshland, 1972). The J chain has been detected in polymeric Ig of many vertebrates, as well as in the shark (see, e.g., Koshland, 1975). This chain, which is similar in size to the L chain, is linked by disulfide bonds to the Fc portion of the α or μ chain and is thought to act as a "joining" protein; that is, it plays a role in the polymerization of Ig's through disulfide bridging. The J chain can be separated from the L chain by virtue of its anodic electrophoretic mobility, which is greater than that of the L chain. Partial separation of the J from the L chain can be achieved because of the lower water solubility of the former. Gel filtration and ion exchange chromatography provide a means of purification on a large scale. Contaminating H chains (α, μ) or L chains can be efficiently removed by affinity chromatography with the appropriate anti-α, anti-μ, or anti-L chain antisera, respectively (Wilde and Koshland, 1973).

VII. IMMUNOADSORBENTS WITH INSOLUBILIZED GLUTARALDEHYDE-TREATED PROTEINS

Using glutaraldehyde as a cross-linking agent, protein antigens or antibodies can be polymerized and made insoluble when the pH of the reaction mixture approaches the isoionic point of the proteins (pH range, 4.5–7.5). The insoluble cross-linked proteins are stable in urea or sodium dodecyl sulfate and can be used as immunoadsorbents for the purification of the corresponding antigens or antibodies, using either a batchwise procedure or a column. This method is rapid and reproducible and can be used for all proteins with free α- or ϵ-amino groups (Avrameas and Ternynck, 1969).

A. Insolubilization of Bovine Serum Albumin (BSA)

BSA (400 mg) is dissolved in 10 ml of 0.2 M sodium acetate buffer, pH 5.0, and 2.5% aqueous glutaraldehyde solution (2 ml) is added dropwise to the antigen solution while stirring. The gel is allowed to stand for 3 hr at room temperature.

B. Insolubilization of Human Serum Proteins

Human serum (10 ml) is first dialyzed against 0.15 M NaCl overnight and then mixed with either 1 ml of 1 M phosphate buffer, pH 7.4, or 1 ml of 1 M sodium acetate, pH 5.0. To this solution 2.5% glutaraldehyde solution (3 ml) is added and the gel, usually formed after 20 min, is allowed to stand for 3 hr at room temperature.

C. Insolubilization of the IgG Fraction

IgG (25 mg) is dialyzed against 0.1 M phosphate buffer, pH 7.4, and adjusted to a concentration of 50 mg/ml. Glutaraldehyde solution (2.5%, 0.1 ml) is added dropwise. Polymerization is almost instantaneous and the gel is left for 3 hr at room temperature to complete insolubilization.

Batchwise Procedure

The insolubilized proteins (24–400 mg) are dispersed in 0.2 M phosphate buffer (20–200 ml, respectively) and homogenized in a Potter homogenizer. The suspension is then centrifuged at 4°C (5000 rpm for 10 min) and the pellet is resuspended in phosphate buffer. This operation is repeated three times. The immunoadsorbent is subsequently suspended and washed twice with the eluting solution to be used (0.2 N acetic acid, 0.1 M glycine-HCl buffer, pH 2.5, or 3 M NH$_4$SCN) until the optical density of the supernatant solution reads less than 0.02 at 280 nm.

The immunoadsorbent is then suspended and washed in phosphate-buffered saline, pH 7.2, and is ready for adsorption of antibodies or antigens. Appropriate amounts of antisera or antigens to be isolated are mixed with the suspension and stirred at room temperature for 30 min. The unadsorbed material is removed by repeated washings with buffered saline, and the adsorbed proteins are finally eluted by suspending the immunoadsorbent in the eluting solutions. This step must be carried out using a small volume of eluting solution (4–20 ml) and repeated two or three times until no protein can be detected in the eluted solutions.

After use, the immunoadsorbent is washed several times with buffered saline and is stored at 4°C in the presence of 0.02% sodium azide.

The yield of antibodies eluted from insolubilized antigens is in the range of 60–90%, whereas the recovery of homologous antigens from insolubilized antibodies is only 30–85%. When isolation of antigens is sought, it should be borne in mind that a significant decrease in the adsorption capacity of the insolubilized antibodies or antisera after each use has been reported (Avrameas and Ternynck, 1969).

Such immunoadsorbents can also be used in columns; this procedure, however, is less satisfactory than the batchwise technique because it is difficult to maintain a constant flow rate, especially after a few regeneration cycles.

VIII. SEPARATION OF POLYPEPTIDE CHAINS

Heavy (H) and light (L) chains of Ig's are linked together by one interchain disulfide bridge, whereas the two H chains are bonded in the hinge region by one or several interchain disulfide bridges, according to the subclasses considered (Milstein and Pink, 1970). Their separation requires the reduction of all interchain disulfide bridges, which is brought about by the action of mercaptan followed by alkylation of the sulfhydryl groups produced and subsequent dissociation of the chains in the presence of 1 M acetic or propionic acid. The latter step is usually carried out by gel filtration chromatography on Sephadex G-100, which separates H from L chains, but the H-chain fraction is usually not free of the L chain (Fleischman *et al.*, 1962). For all animal species, dissociating agents stronger than 1 M acetic acid are preferable if pure H chains are desired, that is, a 6 M urea–1 M acetic acid mixture or 5 M guanidine hydrochloride adjusted to pH 3.5. The reduction of interchain disulfide bridges is called mild or partial since intrachain disulfide bonds are usually not split under the reducing conditions used (0.1 M 2-mercaptoethanol or 0.01 M dithiothreitol at pH 8.3 in the absence of denaturing media). Full reduction of Ig's, on the contrary, requires the presence of high concentrations of denaturing agents (10 M urea or 6–8 M guanidine-HCl) to break all inter- and intrachain disulfide bonds (Small and Lamm, 1966).

A. Partial Reduction with 2-Mercaptoethanol

The Ig preparation of any class or subclass (600 mg in a volume of 30 ml) is dialyzed against 200 vol of 0.4 M Tris–HCl buffer, pH 8.4, and 2-mercaptoethanol (0.36 ml, 0.15 M) is added. The stoppered tube is placed in a 37°C water bath for 60 to 90 min. The alkylation step is carried out by adding a slight molar excess of iodoacetamide over the mercaptan concentration (1.1 gm, 0.2 M) dissolved in 5 ml of 0.4 M Tris–HCl buffer, pH 8.3, and the tube is placed in ice for 30 min. When alkylation with iodoacetic acid is to be used, the latter must first be neutralized with NaOH or 1 M Tris–HCl, pH 8.3. It is very important to maintain the pH value at 8.3 during the alkylation reaction for quantitative results. If this precaution is not taken, iodoacetic acid will cause the pH to drop to the acidic range and methionine residues may become alkylated as well (Wilkinson, 1969). Iodoacetamide and iodoacetic acid should be recrystallized twice to remove traces of free iodine prior to use.

B. Reduction with Dithiothreitol

Partial reduction can also be achieved under the same conditions as described above except that reduction is conducted in the presence of dithiothreitol (10 mM) for 2 hr at room temperature followed by alkylation with 22 mM iodoacetamide for 30 min at 0°C.

Chain Separation

The partially reduced and alkylated IgG fraction is subsequently dialyzed overnight against 1 M acetic acid (or 1 M propionic acid). The protein solution (600 mg in about 35 ml) is then loaded on top of a Sephadex G-100 column (5 × 150 cm) equilibrated in 1 M acetic acid (1 M propionic acid). H- and L-chain fractions are detected by adsorbance at 280 nm. The H chain is known to aggregate under these conditions and elutes as a large peak usually preceded by a shoulder of polymeric material. The L-chain peak is smaller and should be completely separated from the H-chain fractions.

For Ig belonging to the G class, the L chains should account for one-third of the total IgG preparation. In reality, the L-chain fraction accounts for 26–30% of all material absorbing at 280 nm eluted from the column. When the yield of L chain falls below 28%, a small amount of L chain is found under the aggregated H-chain peak, either because the reduction was not complete or because the L chain was not fully dissociated from the H chain in the presence of 1 M acetic acid. In that instance, strong dissociating agents should be used, for example, 1 M acetic acid containing 6 M urea or 5 M guanidine-HCl, under which conditions the recovery of L chain approaches the theoretical yield (33%).

The 1 M acetic acid H- and L-chain fractions are pooled separately and freeze-dried. When urea or guanidine is being used for elution, the protein eluates are first dialyzed against H_2O and lyophilized. The dried material is best stored at 4°C in a well-stoppered vial.

The solubility of the chains is good below pH 5 in acetate buffer but not above pH 7, particularly with respect to the H chain. Solubility of the H chain can be easily improved by polyalanylation of the preparation (Fuchs and Sela, 1965), a technique that does not alter the antigenic properties of the chain, as long as the degree of polyalanylation is moderate (Freedman and Sela, 1966a,b).

Separation of the mildly reduced chains of IgM molecules is generally carried out by filtration on Sephadex G-150 or G-200 in the presence of denaturing agents (Riesen and Jaton, 1976). For mouse IgM proteins, 6 M urea is added to the 1 M acetic acid solution for elution (Robinson et al., 1973).

The degree of purity of H and L chains is best tested by 5% SDS–polyacrylamide gel electrophoresis (Weber and Osborn, 1969) or by double immunodiffusion with specific anti-H-chain or anti-L-chain antiserum.

IX. USE OF PROTEIN A FROM *Staphylococcus aureus* AS AN IMMUNOADSORBENT FOR THE ISOLATION OF Ig's

Protein A is found covalently bound to the peptidoglycan moiety of the *Staphylococcus* cell wall and can be isolated from the cells by enzymatic digestion with lysostaphin (Sjöquist et al., 1972). Further purification steps including ion exchange chromatography and gel filtration yield pure protein A. This protein began to receive attention in 1970 because of its remarkable property of strongly reacting with the Fc protion of the IgG class of different species (Forsgren and Sjöquist, 1966; Sjöquist et al., 1967). Because of this, protein A can be isolated free of any other components by affinity chromatography on a column of IgG–Sepharose 4B (Hjelm et al., 1972). Protein A is eluted from the immunoadsorbent with 0.1 M glycine-HCl, pH 3.0. Conversely, protein A can be efficiently coupled to Sepharose 4B (Hjelm et al., 1972) and the resulting immunoadsorbent, which contains 4 mg of protein/ml of packed gel, can bind as much as 20 mg of IgG/ml of gel. The recovery of IgG is 95% after elution with 0.1 M glycine-HCl buffer, pH 3.0, and the protein is free of contamination with other Ig classes as detected by immunoelectrophoretic analysis. This technique is recommended for removing IgG from the serum of different species. The immunoadsorbent will also remove IgG from preparations of any other Ig classes. This greatly facilitates the preparation of IgA, IgM, IgD, and IgE, which do not react with protein A. Moreover, the human IgG_3 subclass does not bind to protein A (Kronvall and Williams, 1969), thus allowing the purification of this Ig from the other subclasses. Protein A can, of course, be used for removing Fc fragments from papain digests of IgG.

Application of Protein A to the Isolation and Characterization of Trace Amounts of Radiolabeled Ig's

All cell-associated Ig's, whether cell-surface Ig's or their intracellular precursors (or the precursors of Ig's destined for secretion), are difficult to isolate except after radiolabeling, which allows their detection in trace quantities. After radiolabeling, the cells are solubilized in detergent, and the lysates are treated with an anti-Ig antiserum raised in another species. This is usually followed by precipitation with a second antiserum directed against the Ig's of the first antiserum. The labeled cellular Ig's present in the precipitate are then examined by SDS–gel electrophoresis under reducing or nonreducing conditions (Laemmli, 1970). The labeled poly-peptide chains separated on the gel are then identified by counting the radioactivity present in various gel slices or by autoradiography after gel drying. This procedure has been improved by substituting the second antiserum for protein A-bearing staphylococci of the Cowan strain. This technique, introduced by Kessler (1975), avoids the necessity of an indirect immunoprecipitation. The protein A-bearing staphylococci bind immune complexes very rapidly via Fc moieties and are of high affinity, and the nonspecific uptake of other cell material is minimal (Kessler, 1975). Furthermore, very small amounts of anti-Ig's can be used, which considerably increases the sensitivity and the resolving power of the SDS–polyacrylamide gel electrophoresis method. The complex formed between labeled cellular Ig's–anti-Ig's (IgG fraction of the antiserum) and staphylococcal cells can be pelleted by centrifugation at low speed, and no loss of radioactive material is apparent upon repeated washing. This material is then directly analyzed by SDS–gel electrophoresis and sub-sequent autoradiography of the dried gel. The recoveries of mouse lymphocyte Ig's by this technique are reported to be significantly greater than those obtained by the conventional double-antibody method (Kessler, 1975).

The following method is presently used in our laboratory to identify and isolate membrane Ig's or any type of cell-associated Ig's. Proteins are made radioactive by biosynthetic labeling (incubation of cell suspensions in the presence of one or several radioactive amino acids) or by radioiodination of intact cells in the presence of lactoperoxidase, a procedure known to label surface proteins selectively (Marchalonis *et al.*, 1971) (see Chapter 10).

Radioiodination with lactoperoxidase is best performed in the presence of glucose oxidase and small amounts of glucose to generate peroxide, a procedure that appears to be much gentler than adding peroxide to the cell suspension (Hubbard and Cohn, 1972). About 0.5 mCi of carrier-free ^{125}I is used to label 3×10^7 lymphoid cells. After iodination, the cells are washed several times in phosphate-buffered saline containing 5 mM potassium iodide and lysed by gentle homogenization in the presence of 0.5% Nonidet P-40 (NP-40) in 0.05 M Tris–HCl buffer, pH 7.4, containing 0.05 M KCl and 0.005 M MgCl$_2$. The sedimentable particles (e.g., nuclei and ribosomes) contained in this lysate are removed by centrifugation for 30 min at 100,000–150,000 g, and the clear lysate is dialyzed for 18 hr against a large volume of PBS containing 0.02% NP-40. After dialysis, fractions of the lysate (containing about $0.5–1 \times 10^6$ cpm) are incubated for 30 min at 37°C with 10–20 μg of a 2% IgG fraction containing antibodies against the class of membrane Ig's to be isolated. A 10% suspension of staphylococcal cells (2–4 μl), prepared and washed according to Kessler (1975), is then added and incubated for 15 min at room temperature; after centrifugation (2–5 min, 1000–1500 g), the pellet is washed several times with PBS (0.2–0.5 ml) and finally suspended in 40 μl of SDS sample buffer with or without reducing agent and then boiled. After centrifugation, the supernatant is loaded on an SDS–polyacrylamide gel (Laemmli, 1970). Essentially the same procedure is used to isolate radioactive Ig's from biosynthetically labeled cells.

Figure 6 illustrates the results obtained with this technique. The autoradiographic pattern of ^{125}I-labeled Ig chains after SDS–polyacrylamide gel electrophoresis under reducing conditions indicates the presence of μ, δ-like, and L chains. "δ-like" chains are usually seen as a broad band (Fig. 6, gel A). Polypeptide chains (μ and L) can also be detected in a cell lysate from [^{35}S]methionine biosynthetically labeled spleen cells 3 days after intraperitoneal injection of *Escherichia coli* lipopolysaccharide (Fig. 6, gel B). The L chains exhibit several bands, a pattern commonly observed with polyclonal Ig's of mouse splenocytes. The band of intermediate mobility corresponds to the protein described as "membrane-associated immunoglobulin-detaining protein," or MAID (Premkumar *et al.*, 1975).

Gel C of Fig. 6 compares the electrophoretic mobility of intracellular μ chains (right) with that of secreted μ chains (left); note that intracellular μ chains run slightly faster than secreted μ chains, a pattern that is consistently observed (P. Vassalli and B. Lisowska-Bernstein, unpublished data).

In conclusion, the isolation of minute amounts of radiolabeled Ig chains by the formation of complexes with specific anti-Ig antibodies and

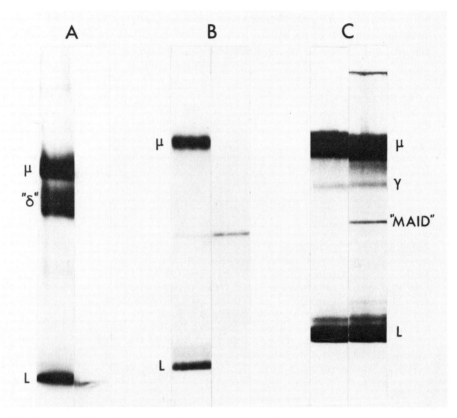

Fig. 6. Autoradiographic pattern of labeled Ig chains after SDS–polyacrylamide gel electrophoresis under reducing conditions. The immune complexes between labeled Ig's and IgG fractions of specific antisera were reacted with protein A-bearing staphylococcal cells (see the text for details). (A) ^{125}I-Labeled mouse spleen cells. The cell lysate (1.4×10^6 cpm) was precipitated with rabbit anti-mouse IgG (left) and control, normal rabbit IgG (right). The lysate was run in a 7.5% SDS–polyacrylamide gel. (B) [^{35}S]Methionine biosynthetically labeled mouse spleen cell populations rich in IgM plasma cells 3 days after an intraperitoneal injection of *E. coli* lipopolysaccharide. The cell lysate was run in a 17.5% polyacrylamide gel. The cell lysate (about 1×10^5 cpm) was precipitated with rabbit anti-mouse IgG (left) and control IgG (right; the same amount of normal rabbit IgG but four times the radioactivity). (C) [^{14}C]Leucine biosynthetically labeled mouse spleen cell populations rich in IgM plasma cells. (Left) Precipitate of rabbit IgG anti-mouse Ig's with the proteins released during the incubation (72,000 cpm) by the cells in the medium. μ, γ, and L chains are seen. (Right) Precipitate of the same antiserum with the corresponding cell lysate (160,000 cpm). In addition to the detection of Ig chains, membrane-associated immunoglobulin-detaining protein (MAID) is apparent.

Staphylococcus A and the analysis of these complexes by SDS–gel electrophoresis followed by autoradiography constitute a highly sensitive and accurate technique for the study of cell-associated Ig's.

ACKNOWLEDGMENTS

This work was supported in part by Grant No. 3.733.76 from the Swiss National Science Foundation.

Thanks are due to Dr. M. Lamm for helpful comments and criticisms of the manuscript and to Dr. B. Lisowska-Bernstein for making available parts of the material presented in Fig. 6.

REFERENCES

Aasted, B., Sogn, J. A., and Kindt, T. J. (1967). *J. Immunol.* **116**, 387.

Avrameas, S., and Ternynck, T. (1967). *Biochem. J.* **102**, 37c.

Avrameas, S., and Ternynck, T. (1969). *Immunochemistry* **6**, 53.

Axén, R., Porath, J., and Ernback, S. (1967). *Nature (London)* **214**, 1302.

Bazin, H., Beckers, A., and Quérinjean, P. (1974). *Eur. J. Immunol.* **4**, 44.

Bourgois, A., and Fougereau, M. (1970). *Eur. J. Biochem.* **12**, 558.

Braun, D. G., and Krause, R. M. (1968). *J. Exp. Med.* **128**, 969.

Capra, J. D., Tung, A. S., and Nisonoff, A. (1975). *J. Immunol.* **114**, 1548.

Chesebro, B., and Metzger, H. (1972). *Biochemistry* **11**, 767.

Cuatrecasas, P., and Anfinsen, C. B. (1971). *Annu. Rev. Biochem.* **40**, 259.

Curd, J., Smith, T. W., Jaton, J.-C., and Haber, E. (1971). *Proc. Natl. Acad. Sci. U.S.A.* **68**, 2401.

Dandliker, W. B., Alonso, R., de Saussure, V. A., Kierszenbaum, F., Levinson, S. A., and Shapiro, H. C. (1967). *Biochemistry* **6**, 1460.

Doellgast, G. I., and Plaut, A. G. (1976). *Immunochemistry* **13**, 135.

Eisen, H. N. (1973). *In* "Microbiology" (B. D. Davis *et al.*, eds.), p. 352. Harper, New York.

Fahey, J. L., and Horbett, A. P. (1959). *J. Biol. Chem.* **234**, 2645.

Fleischman, J. B., Pain, R., and Porter, R. R. (1962). *Arch. Biochem. Biophys., Suppl.* **1**, 174.

Forsgren, A., and Sjöquist, J. (1966). *J. Immunol.* **97**, 822.

Freedman, M. H., and Sela, M. (1966a). *J. Biol. Chem.* **241**, 2383.

Freedman, M. H., and Sela, M. (1966b). *J. Biol. Chem.* **241**, 5225.

Fuchs, S., and Sela, M. (1965). *J. Biol. Chem.* **240**, 3558.

Goebel, W. F., and Avery, O. T. (1931). *J. Exp. Med.* **54**, 431.

Goetzl, E. J., and Metzger, H. (1970). *Biochemistry* **9**, 1267.

Hjelm, H., Hjelm, K., and Sjóquist, J. (1972). *FEBS Lett.* **28**, 73.

Hubbard, A. L., and Cohn, Z. A. (1972). *J. Cell Biol.* **55**, 390.

Jaton, J.-C., Waterfield, M. D., Margolies, M. N., and Haber, E. (1970). *Proc. Natl. Acad. Sci. U.S.A.* **66**, 959.

Jaton, J.-C., Schweizer, M., and Knight, K. L. (1976). *Eur. J. Immunol.* **6**, 878.

Johansson, B. G. (1972). *Scand. J. Clin. Lab. Invest.* **29**, Suppl. 124, 7.

Keckwick, R. A. (1940). *Biochem. J.* **34**, 1248.

Kessler, S. W. (1975). *J. Immunol.* **115**, 1617.

Koshland, M. E. (1975). *Adv. Immunol.* **20**, 41.

Kronvall, G., and Williams, R. C., Jr. (1969). *J. Immunol.* **103**, 828.
Laemmli, U. K. (1970). *Nature (London)* **227**, 680.
Leslie, R. S. Q., and Cohen, S. (1970). *Biochem. J.* **120**, 787.
Levy, H. B., and Sober, H. A. (1960). *Proc. Soc. Exp. Biol. Med.* **103**, 250.
Little, J. R., and Eisen, H. N. (1966). *Biochemistry* **5**, 3385.
Lowry, O. H., and Hunter, T. H. (1945). *J. Biol. Chem.* **159**, 465.
Marchalonis, J. J., Cone, R. E., and Santer, V. (1971). *Biochem. J.* **124**, 921.
Milstein, C., and Pink, J. R. L. (1970). *Prog. Biophys. Mol. Biol.* **21**, 209.
Morrison, S. L., and Koshland, M. E. (1972). *Proc. Natl. Acad. Sci. U.S.A.* **69**, 124.
Müller-Eberhard, H. J., and Osterland, C. K. (1968). *Methods Immunol. Immunochem.* **2**, 57.
Oettgen, H. F., Binaghi, R. A., and Benacerraf, B. (1965). *Proc. Soc. Exp. Biol. Med.* **118**, 336.
Ollander, J., and Little, J. R. (1975). *Immunochemistry* **12**, 383.
Peterson, E. A., and Sober, H. A. (1956). *J. Am. Chem. Soc.* **78**, 751.
Pincus, J. H., Jaton, J.-C., Block, K. J., and Haber, E. (1970). *J. Immunol.* **104**, 1143.
Premkumar, E., Potter, M., Singer, P. A., and Sklar, M. D. (1975). *Cell* **6**, 149.
Riesen, W. F., and Jaton, J.-C. (1976). *Biochemistry* **15**, 3829.
Robinson, E. A., Appella, E., and McIntire, K. R. (1973). *J. Biol. Chem.* **248**, 7112.
Sjöquist, J., Forsgren, A., Gustafson, G. T., and Stalenheim, G. (1967). *Cold Spring Harbor Symp. Quant. Biol.* **32**, 577.
Sjöquist, J., Melon, B., and Hjelm, H. (1972). *Eur. J. Biochem.* **29**, 572.
Small, P. A., and Lamm, M. (1966). *Biochemistry* **5**, 259.
Sogn, J. A., Yarmush, M. L., and Kindt, T. J. (1976). *Ann. Immunol. (Paris)* **127c**, 397.
Tracey, D. E., Liu, S. H., and Cebra, J. J. (1976). *Biochemistry* **15**, 624.
Weber, K., and Osborn, M. (1969). *J. Biol. Chem.* **244**, 4406.
Wilde, C. E., and Koshland, M. E. (1973). *Biochemistry* **12**, 3218.
Wilkinson, J. M. (1969). *FEBS Lett.* **4**, 170.

3

Peptide Mapping at the Nanomole Level

B. A. Moss

I. OBJECTIVE

Conventional peptide mapping or fingerprinting on paper sheets (Ingram, 1963; Bennett, 1967; Canfield and Anfinson, 1963; Laver, 1969), while providing a powerful tool in protein structural studies, generally requires at least 50–100 nmoles of protein per analysis. Many proteins, however, may be available in microgram amounts only, demanding more sensitive peptide mapping techniques. This may be achieved simply by mapping on thin-layer plates of cellulose or silica gel and revealing the pattern of peptides by chromogenic (Burns and Turner, 1967; Bates *et al.*, 1975) or fluorescent reagents (Atherton and Thomson, 1969; Blitz and Fine, 1974; Vandekerckhove and van Montagu, 1974; Fey and Hirt, 1974; Schmer and Kreil, 1967; Zanetta *et al.*, 1970; Spivak *et al.*, 1971; Kremer and Ullrich,

IMMUNOLOGICAL METHODS

1971) or by autoradiography (Rice and Means, 1971; Bray and Brownlee, 1973; Waterson and Konigsberg, 1974; Gruenstein and Rich, 1975; Davison, 1976). We have adopted a technique involving two-dimensional chromatography of fluorescent dansyl peptides on thin layers of silica gel. The method operates satisfactorily on 1 nmole of protein and permits good resolution of the tryptic peptides.

II. PRINCIPLE OF THE METHOD

In the absence of complete sequence studies, the primary structures of similar proteins may be compared in terms of the homology of peptides cleaved from them by proteases or by chemical means. Trypsin is the enzyme preferred in such structural studies, due to its specificity: It cleaves only those peptide bonds that involve the carboxyl groups of lysine and arginine residues. The resultant tryptic peptides are then separated on thin layers of cellulose or silica gel by two-dimensional electrophoresis and chromatography.

This produces a characteristic peptide map for each protein and allows the definition of similarities and differences among proteins. The relative mobility of peptides in either dimension depends on their amino acid composition and, to a lesser extent, on their sequence.

The standard peptide mapping approach, however, usually fails to resolve a variable "core" of insoluble peptides and may not effectively separate electrophoretically neutral peptides. In either case, important differences in the primary structures of closely related proteins might be overlooked. These problems may be overcome to some extent by coupling the peptides with dansyl chloride.[1] This reagent covalently binds to free amino, phenol, imidazole, and sulfhydryl groups yielding intensely yellow to yellow–orange fluorescent derivatives, which not only permit detection of nanomole amounts of peptides, but also make them more hydrophobic, thus facilitating their separation by two-dimensional chromatography on silica gel plates with organic solvent systems.

III. MATERIALS

All reagents are of analytical grade or of the highest quality available. Ammonia-free water for making aqueous solutions: distilled water passed

---

[1] Abbreviations used: dansyl, 1-dimethylaminonaphthalene-5-sulfonyl; dans-OH, 1-dimethylaminonaphthalene-5-sulfonic acid; dans-NH$_2$, 1-dimethylaminonaphthalene-5-sulfonamide.

through a mixed-bed ion exchange resin and redistilled twice from a quartz-glass still

Denaturing buffer: 7 M guanidine hydrochloride–0.5 M Tris–2 mM EDTA, adjusted to pH 8.5 with glacial acetic acid

Iodoacetic acid (Koch-Light Laboratories, Colnbrook, Buckinghamshire, England) recrystallized from n-heptane

Trypsin–TPCK (Worthington Biochemical Corp., Freehold, New Jersey): 0.5 mg in 1 ml of 1 mM HCl, 2.5 mM CaCl$_2$

Sequanal grade dansyl chloride as a 10% (w/v) stock solution in dry acetone or as a crystalline solid: Dansyl amino acids, 2-mercaptoethanol, dithiothreitol, and guanidine hydrochloride are from Pierce Chemical Co. (Rockford, Illinois)

Dansyl chloride solution: 5.4 mg/ml (20 mM) in dry acetone, freshly prepared from the stock solution or the solid; the actual concentration of dansyl chloride may be checked by measuring the extinction at 369 nm ($E = 3.67 \times 10^3$) after dilution (Gray, 1964; Neuhoff, 1973)

Absolute ethanol (E. Merck, Darmstadt, G.F.R.) and 70% aqueous ethanol

Methyl acetate, isopropanol, and isobutanol (Merck), redistilled before use

Triethylamine (Merck) refluxed over phthalic anhydride (1 gm/liter, 1 hr) and ninhydrin (1 gm/liter, 1 hr) before distillation over ninhydrin (1 gm/liter)

Aqueous solutions of triethylamine (TEA): 0.1 M TEA and 0.2 M TEA–bicarbonate, pH 8.5; the latter solution is prepared by bubbling CO$_2$ through 0.2 M TEA until the desired pH is obtained

Thin-later chromatography tanks with ground-glass lids and thin-layer glass plates, 20 × 20 cm (e.g., those supplied by Desaga, Heidelberg, G.F.R.): The glass plates are washed in nonabrasive detergent (5% RBS 35 solution Pierce Chemical Co.) rinsed three times with distilled water, once with methanol, and dried with a soft linen towel; the dried plates are stored in a dust-free sealable plastic container

Pear-shaped distillation flasks (25 ml, Pyrex) and screw-cap Reactivials (3 ml, Pierce Chemical Co.), siliconized to prevent adsorption of the dansyl peptides to the glass: The vessels are washed, air-dried, exposed for at least 1 min to a 5% solution of triethylchlorosilane (Merck) in toluene, rinsed twice with distilled water and twice with acetone, air-dried, and finally dried overnight in a 105°C oven.

Chromatography columns (0.7-cm diameter × 10 cm) plugged with siliconized glass wool (e.g., Supelco Co., Bellefonte, Pennsylvania)

Dowex 50-X4, 200–400 mesh, H⁺ form (Bio-Rad Laboratories, Richmond, California): treated three times with a mixture of acetone and

25% ammonia (1:1, v/v), washed with water until neutral, and
equilibrated with 0.01 M acetic acid, pH 3.5

Silica gel (Kieselgel G nach Stahl type 60, Merck): Thin-layer glass plates
are coated with silica gel slurry to a thickness of 0.3 mm by means of a
Camag spreader (Muttenz, Switzerland)

Forced-air drying oven at 105°C

Ultraviolet light viewing box (e.g., Chromato-Vue, Ultra-Violet Products,
Inc., San Gabriel, California)

Mixer, such as a Whirlmix or Vortex Genie mixer

IV. PROCEDURE

Proteins to be compared are reduced and alkylated, digested, and mapped
at the same time and under the same conditions.

A. Reduction and Alkylation of Protein

Complete reduction and S-carboxymethylation of protein preparations
contained in 3-ml screw-capped Reactivials are performed in denaturing
buffer (7 M guanidine hydrochloride–0.5 M Tris-acetate–2 mM EDTA, pH
8.5). The protein (100–200 μg, or 2–4 nmoles of protein of molecular weight
50,000) in 75 μl is reduced under nitrogen for 1 hr at 50°C by adding
dithiothreitol dissolved in 25 μl of denaturing buffer. The concentration of
dithiothreitol is such that it gives a 50-fold molar excess over protein
sulfhydryl groups. The proteins are then alkylated under nitrogen at 25°C in
the dark, with neutralized iodoacetic acid in 25 μl of denaturing buffer. A
threefold molar excess of iodoacetic acid over the dithiothreitol
concentration is used. The alkylation is stopped after 1 hr by quenching
with an excess of 2-mercaptoethanol (10 μl). The protein is precipitated with
1 ml of cold (-20°C) absolute ethanol acidified with glacial acetic acid (10
μl). After at least 30 min at -20°C, the flocculent protein is sedimented by
centrifugation (1500 g for 10 min) and washed with cold (-20°C) 70%
ethanol to remove salts (3 × 1 ml). Excess ethanol is carefully withdrawn
with a fine Pasteur pipette, and the protein precipitate is dried with a stream
of nitrogen.

B. Digestion of Protein with Trypsin

For tryptic digestion, the reduced, S-carboxymethylated protein (100–200
μg) is suspended in distilled water (0.1 ml) and warmed for 2 min in a

boiling water bath. After cooling to room temperature, 0.1 ml of 0.2 M TEA–bicarbonate buffer, pH 8.5, is added. Trypsin–TPCK (1 μg in 2 μl of 1 mM HCl–2.5 mM CaCl$_2$) is added with gentle mixing, and the mixture is incubated under nitrogen at 37°C. The flocculent suspension usually clears within 1 hr. After 2 hr of digestion, an additional 2 μl of trypsin–TPCK solution is added, and the incubation is continued for 4 hr. The tryptic digest can be dansylated immediately.

C. Dansylation of Peptides

The technique of fingerprinting dansyl peptides on silica gel with organic solvent systems was introduced in 1967 by Schmer and Kreil. The procedure described here has been adapted from this original technique and from the methods of Zanetta *et al.* (1970) and Tamura *et al.* (1973).

Note: Because the dansyl fluorophore is subject to photochemical degradation (Zanetta *et al.*, 1970; Gray, 1967; Seiler, 1970), all operations are undertaken rapidly and as much as possible under dark conditions.

To the tryptic peptide mixture (amounting to 100–200 nmoles of total peptides) in 0.2 ml of 0.1 M TEA–bicarbonate buffer is added 0.8 ml of 0.1 M TEA, pH 12. The pH of the mixture at this stage should be 10.5–11, using a glass electrode. Then 1 ml of 20 mM dansyl chloride in acetone is added (100- to 200-fold molar excess). The vial, which is wrapped in aluminium foil to protect the contents from light, is flushed with nitrogen, tightly capped, and shaken on the Vortex mixer. (The apparent pH of this mixture should be 10–10.5.) Dansylation of the peptides is effected by incubation for 2 hr at 37°C, by which time the pH has dropped to 9–9.5. At the end of the reaction, 3 M KOH (10–25 μl) is added to ensure conversion of any excess dansyl chloride to dans-OH. The orange–yellow color of the original dansyl chloride solution should now be discharged to a pale yellow. The pH is then adjusted to about 3.5 by adding glacial acetic acid (50–150 μl). The pH may be checked by withdrawing 1 μl of the mixture and spotting on pH paper.

D. Separation of Dansyl Peptides from By-Products

After adjustment to pH 3.5, the reaction mixture is applied to a column of Dowex 50-X4 (resin bed, 0.7-cm diameter × 1 cm) equilibrated with 0.01 M acetic acid, pH 3.5. The vial is washed with 0.01 M acetic acid (2 × 1 ml) and the washings are transferred to the column. The blue–green fluorescence (dans-OH) and salts are washed from the column with 0.01 M acetic acid, pH 3.5 (75 ml), followed by acetone:0.01 M acetic acid (1:4, v/v; 2 × 0.5 ml) and the effluents are discarded.

The yellow fluorescent band of dansyl peptides is displaced from the resin with water:acetone:25% ammonia (0.85:1:0.15, v/v/v; 17.5 ml) into the siliconized pearshaped flask (25-ml capacity). The flask is sealed with Parafilm, which is then perforated, and the contents are frozen in a dry ice–alcohol bath. The flask is wrapped in aluminium foil, carefully placed inside a freeze-drying vessel protected from light, and lyophilized overnight. The residue of dansyl peptides is dissolved in acetone:water (1:1, v/v; 100–200 μl) for two-dimensional thin-layer chromatography. To minimize evaporation of acetone, it is advisable to keep the sample chilled in an ice bath.

E. Two-Dimensional Thin-Layer Chromatography of Dansyl Peptides

A slurry is prepared from 54 gm of silica gel G and 125 ml of distilled water in a closed 250-ml Büchner flask with vigorous swirling for 1 min while deaerating on a water aspirator pump. The homogeneous suspension is poured into the hopper of the spreader, with the slit width of the hopper set at 0.3 mm. The glass plates (20 × 20 cm) are quickly pushed through and coated. Coating of 8 to 10 plates should take about 1 min. The plates are air-dried on a horizontal surface until the coating is opaque. They can then be stored in a rack at room temperature. The thickness of the dry layer is about 0.2 mm.

The plates are activated in a forced-air oven at 105°C for 30 min and cooled for 10 min at room temperature before applying the sample. The plate is oriented such that the first dimension will be in the direction of spreading the silica gel, and the origin is in the lower left-hand corner 2 cm from the bottom and 2 cm in from the side (Zanetta *et al.*, 1970).

The dansyl peptide mixture (25–50 μl, equivalent to peptides derived from about 1 nmole of protein) is carefully spotted onto the plate with intermittent drying from a warm hair dryer. It is advisable to spot amounts of about 2.5 μl at a time, using a finely drawn out 10-μl capillary tube. The spot diameter should be kept less than 5 mm (about 2.5 mm) to ensure subsequent good resolution of the dansyl peptides. Before development, the plates are heated in the oven at 105°C for 5 min, followed by 5 min at room temperature (20°C) in a chromatography cabinet. Chromatography is undertaken in a nonsaturated chamber (Brenner and Niederwieser, 1967). Development in the first dimension (methyl acetate:isopropanol:25% ammonia, 9:6:4, v/v/v; 140 ml) is for 1.5 hr. By this time, the chromatography front is about 2 cm from the top of the plate. The plate is dried with warm air from the hair dryer until opaque, placed in the oven at 105°C for 5 min, and cooled in the chromatography cabinet for 10 min.

Development in the second dimension (isobutanol:acetic acid:water, 15:4:2, v/v/v; 140 ml) is for 3.5 hr or until the solvent front is about 2 cm from the top of the plate. The plate is then quickly dried in warm air from the hair dryer and viewed under long-wavelength ultraviolet light, and the fluorescent spots are rapidly outlined to avoid excessive photochemical degradation.

F. Controls

Control blanks are run with each experiment. They contain the same components, except for the protein under study, and undergo the same treatment as the protein sample. It is also desirable to subject a reference crystalline protein, such as hen egg lysozyme, to the same treatment as a check on the enzymatic digestion.

Marker dansyl amino acids can be applied prior to the chromatography (Zanetta *et al.*, 1970), but since it is preferable to utilize the maximum area of the plate to resolve the dansyl peptides, this is not essential. Traces of dans-OH and dans-NH$_2$, as well as some unknown side products, are carried through into the dansyl peptide fraction and serve as convenient markers in the comparison of different fingerprints (Schmer and Kreil, 1967; Zanetta *et al.*, 1970).

V. CRITICAL APPRAISAL

Fluorescent dansyl peptide mapping by two-dimensional thin-layer chromatography on silica gel G has been effectively used on a nanomole scale both in the comparative analysis of related proteins and in the partial determination of the primary structure of proteins (Schmer and Kreil, 1967; Zanetta *et al.*, 1970; Spivak *et al.*, 1971; Moss and Hamilton, 1974). Experiments with reference proteins such as bovine serum albumin, ribonuclease, hen egg lysozyme, and chicken globins established that 90% or more of the expected tryptic peptides could be accounted for on the maps.

It should be possible to compare the structural similarities and differences of any homogeneous proteins available in amounts of about 100 μg. However, several points of the technique should be considered. Although dansyl chloride is one of the best reagents available at present for labeling amino acids and peptides, the reaction depends on a number of factors that are difficult to control, especially when quantitative analysis is desired. These factors have been studied in detail in several laboratories (Spivak *et al.*, 1971; Neuhoff, 1973; Gros and Labouesse, 1969; Gray, 1972). It has been found that the optimum labeling conditions for most amino acids and peptides are a pH of between 9.5 and 10.5 and a severalfold excess of dansyl chloride. Since the reagent is hydrolyzed to dans-OH by water and by hydroxyl ion, the reactive groups are labeled as a function of their ability to compete for the reagent under the conditions chosen. The relatively high concentrations of dansyl chloride produce large amounts of dans-OH during the reaction; since this interferes with the thin-layer chromatography, it must be removed.

Dansylation of peptides without reactive amino acid side chain groups generally presents no problem, but peptides containing lysyl, tyrosyl, and histidyl residues, and N-terminal glutamyl peptides, can yield multiple products due to varying reactivities of their side chains and to varying stabilities of the dansylated functional group. These problems can largely be overcome by using conditions similar to those recommended by Tamura *et al.* (1973). The dansylation is carried out in aqueous triethylamine to avoid interfering buffer salts and make it more compatible with thin-layer chromatography. The dansylation mixture in 50% acetone has an apparent pH of about 10.5 and the concentration of dansyl chloride is 10 mM, which, in terms of total reactive groups, represents about a 50-fold molar excess. These conditions promote the quantitative dansylation of the ϵ-amino group of lysine and the tyrosine hydroxyl group and prevent conversion of dansylglutamic acid and dansylglutamine to dansylpyroglutamic acid. Unstable imidazole–dansylhistidine is hydrolyzed by the alkaline conditions encountered during removal of dans-OH. We have obtained identical fingerprints after dansylation of peptides for 16 hr at 8°C, as suggested by Tamura *et al.* (1973), and 2 hr at 37°C, as described here. Peptides containing methionine and S-carboxymethyl cysteine can also generate extra products due to oxidation during chromatography. To minimize this problem, 2-mercaptoethanol (5 mM) should be included in the solvent systems.

Dansyl amino acids and peptides are unstable on silica gel thin-layer plates and undergo photochemical degradation into nonfluorescent yellowish compounds within a few hours. The dansyl derivatives, O-dansyl-tyrosine and imidazole–dansylhistidine, are readily decomposed by a short exposure to ultraviolet light, or to sunlight, into bluish-green fluorescent compounds. Decomposition is not prevented by storage of the chromatographed plates in the dark. This property of the dansyl derivatives makes quantitation based on fluorescence a difficult proposition (Pouchan and Passeron, 1975) and underlines the importance of working rapidly and without light.

Zanetta *et al.* (1970) established that thin-layer chromatography of the dansyl peptides on silica gel was preferable to polyamide layers because of the low capacity and the difficulty of elution from the latter. Peptide mapping was difficult to reproduce, and many of the spots trailed on the polyamide layers. Ready-made commercial silica gel thin-layer plates could be used, in principle, provided quantitation is not required, but low capacity and poor reproducibility speak against their use. The laboratory-made plates with silica gel G, in conjunction with solvents of dielectric constants of the order of 20–25, as proposed by Zanetta et al. (1970), permit good resolution of dansyl peptides even for proteins of high molecular weight. It is possible to obtain reliable maps from as little as 0.1 nmole of protein, but the optimum range for a protein of molecular weight of, say, 50,000 is 0.5–1.5 nmoles.

As with all tryptic peptide mapping procedures, the theoretical number of peptides may not be resolved. Deviations may occur as a result of incomplete cleavage of the lysine and arginine bonds, so that daughter peptides and uncleaved parent peptides appear simultaneously. Nonspecific lysis may also occur. Using dansyl peptide mapping, as with other fluorescent methods, makes it difficult to assign exact numbers to peptides, since the intensity of fluorescence is not proportional to the amount of peptide per spot (Fey and Hirt, 1974; Schmer and Kreil, 1967; Zanetta et al., 1970; Spivak et al., 1971). One way these problems can be overcome is by subsequent analysis of the peptides by appropriate means (Zanetta et al., 1970; Spivak et al., 1971; Neuhoff, 1973; Brown and Perham, 1973). Comparative mapping may also be limited by the low mobility of some large dansyl peptides on supports with high adsorption capacity, such as silica gel. However, these peptides may be separately evaluated by other proteolytic or chemical hydrolysis.

No fingerprinting technique is absolutely reproducible, and the dansyl method is no exception. Although the same overall pattern is obtained from different experiments with dansylated tryptic digests, detailed comparisons should only be made when the proteins under study are analyzed in parallel. Mixing of the different dansylated tryptic digests and cochromatography are mandatory controls for chromatographic anomalies and help to identify peptides with chemical differences.

VI. AN EXAMPLE OF THE APPLICATION OF THE METHOD TO ANTIGENIC VARIANTS OF INFLUENZA-A VIRUS HEMAGGLUTININ

An influenza virus (NT60) and its single-step antigenic mutant, 29C (Fazekas de St.Groth and Hannoun, 1973; Fazekas de St.Groth, 1978), were purified and the antigenic protein (HA) was removed by controlled digestion with bromelain, reduced, and S-carboxymethylated, and the large

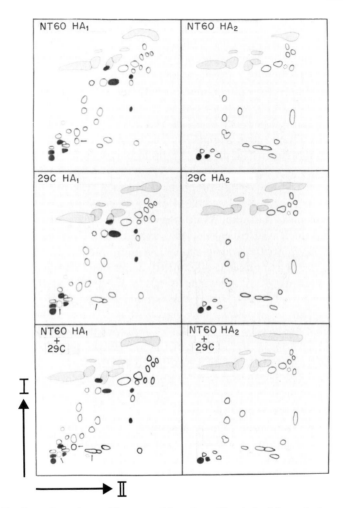

Fig. 1. Tracings of tryptic peptide maps of dansyl peptides derived from the hemagglutinin subunits, HA₁ and HA₂, of virus strains NT60 and 29C. Reduced and S-carboxymethylated hemagglutinin subunits were digested with trypsin–TPCK and dansylated. The dansyl peptides (from 1 nmole of protein) were separated by two-dimensional thin-layer chromatography on silica gel G. Chromatography in the first dimension (I, methyl acetate:isopropanol:25% ammonia, 9:6:4, v/v/v) was for 1.5 hr followed by development in the second dimension (II, isobutanol:acetic acid:water, 15:4:2, v/v/v) for 3.5 hr. Each solvent system was rendered 5 mM in 2-mercaptoethanol. The shaded areas indicate dans-OH, dans-NH₂, and unknown side products resulting from the reagents used. The corresponding subunits from both strains were also mixed in equal amounts (NT60 and 29C) and subjected to cochromatography. Peptides apparently different are indicated by arrows. The black areas represent spots containing [¹⁴C]carboxymethyl cysteine. The areas indicated by dashed lines represent weakly fluorescent spots. (From Moss and Underwood, 1978, by permission of Springer-Verlag.)

(HA$_1$) and small (HA$_2$) subunits were separated (Moss and Underwood, 1978).

The proteins were analyzed in parallel, and Fig. 1 illustrates the peptide maps obtained. Maps of HA$_2$ appeared to be identical and this was confirmed in the mixing experiment (NT60 and 29C) by comigration of the corresponding dansyl peptides from each virus. Maps of HA$_1$, on the other hand, were identical except for one major and one minor variable spot, as indicated by the arrows. HA$_1$ from both NT60 and 29C showed 36 major diagnostic spots and a few minor spots, while HA$_2$ showed 22 major diagnostic spots and some minor ones. The expected number of tryptic peptides based on the lysine plus arginine content (Moss and Underwood, 1978) is 37 for HA$_1$ and 24 for HA$_2$. Therefore, it seems likely that virtually all of the tryptic peptides are represented. The results of the comparative peptide mapping data are consistent with at least one amino acid substitution in the hemagglutinin molecule, confined to the larger subunit, HA$_1$ (which happens to carry the antigenic specificity of the molecule).

REFERENCES

Atherton, R. S., and Thomson, A. R. (1969). *Biochem. J.* **111,** 797.
Bates, D. L., Perham, R. N., and Coggins, J. R. (1975). *Anal. Biochem.* **68,** 175.
Bennett, J. C. (1967). *In* "Methods in Enzymology" (C. H. W. Hirs, ed.), Vol. 11, p. 330. Academic Press, New York.
Blitz, A. L., and Fine, R. E. (1974). *Proc. Natl. Acad. Sci. U.S.A.* **71,** 175.
Bray, D., and Brownlee, S. M. (1973). *Anal. Biochem.* **55,** 213.
Brenner, M., and Niederwieser, A. (1967). *In* "Methods in Enzymology" (C. H. W. Hirs, ed.) Vol. 11, p. 39. Academic Press, New York.
Brown, J. P., and Perham, R. N. (1973). *Eur. J. Biochem.* **39,** 69.
Burns, D. J. W., and Turner, N. A. (1967). *J. Chromatogr.* **30,** 469.
Canfield, R. E., and Anfinson, C. B. (1963). *In* "The Proteins" (H. Neurath, ed.), 2nd ed., Vol. 1, p. 311. Academic Press, New York.
Davison, P. F. (1976). *Anal. Biochem.* **75,** 129.
Fazekas de St.Groth, S. (1978). *In* "Topics in Infectious Diseases" (W. G. Laver, H. Bachmayer, and R. Weil, eds.), Vol. 3, p. 25. Springer-Verlag, Wien and New York.
Fazekas de St.Groth, S., and Hannoun, C. (1973). *R. Hebd. Seances Acad. Sci., Ser. D* **276,** 1917.
Fey, G., and Hirt, B. (1974). *Cold Spring Harbor Symp. Quant. Biol.* **39,** 235.
Gray, W. R. (1964). Ph.D. Thesis, University of Cambridge.
Gray, W. R. (1967). *In* "Methods in Enzymology" (C. H. W. Hirs, ed.), Vol. 11, p. 139. Academic Press, New York.
Gray, W. R. (1972). *In* "Methods in Enzymology" (C. H. W. Hirs and S. N. Timasheff, eds.), Vol. 25, p. 121. Academic Press, New York.
Gros, C., and Labouesse, B. (1969). *Eur. J. Biochem.* **7,** 463.
Gruenstein, E., and Rich, A. (1975). *Biochem. Biophys. Res. Commun.* **64,** 472.

Ingram, V. M. (1963). *In* "Methods in Enzymology" (S. P. Colowick and N. O. Kaplan, eds.), Vol. 6, p. 831. Academic Press, New York.

Kremer, B., and Ullrich, J. (1971). *Hoppe-Seyler's Z. Physiol. Chem.* **352,** 189.

Laver, W. G. (1969). *In* "Fundamental Techniques in Virology" (K. Habel and N. P. Salzman, eds.), p. 371, Academic Press, New York.

Moss, B. A., and Hamilton, E. A. (1974). *Biochim. Biophys. Acta* **371,** 379.

Moss, B. A., and Underwood, P. A. (1978). *In* "Topics in Infectious Diseases" (W. G. Laver, H. Bachmayer, and R. Weil, eds.), Vol. 3, p. 145. Springer-Verlag, Wien and New York.

Neuhoff, V. (1973). *In* "Micromethods in Molecular Biology" (V. Neuhoff, ed.), p. 85. Chapman & Hall, London.

Pouchan, M. I., and Passeron, E. J. (1975). *Anal. Biochem.* **63,** 585.

Rice, R. H., and Means, G. E. (1971). *J. Biol. Chem.* **246,** 831.

Schmer, G., and Kreil, G. (1967). *J. Chromatogr.* **28,** 458.

Seiler, N. (1970). *Methods Biochem. Anal.* **18,** 259.

Spivak, V. A., Levjant, M. I., Katrukha, S. P., and Varshavsky, J. M. (1971). *Anal. Biochem.* **44,** 503.

Tamura, Z., Nakajima, T., Nakayama, T., Pisano, J. J., and Udenfriend, S. (1973). *Anal. Biochem.* **52,** 595.

Vandekerckhove, J., and van Montagu, M. (1974). *Eur. J. Biochem.* **44,** 279.

Waterson, R. M., and Konigsberg, W. H. (1974). *Proc. Natl. Acad. Sci. U.S.A.* **71,** 376.

Zanetta, J. P., Vincendon, G., Mandel, P., and Gombos, G. (1970). *J. Chromatogr.* **51,** 441.

4

Electrophoresis of Proteins in Polyacrylamide Slab Gels

Béla Takács

I. INTRODUCTION

Since 1959, when Ornstein (1964) and Davis (1964) first described disc electrophoresis, this method has become perhaps the most commonly used analytical tool for the fractionation of proteins, polypeptides, and nucleic acids.

The use of polyacrylamide gel as a stabilizing medium as compared to liquid or granular medium lies in its favorable properties. Polyacrylamide is

IMMUNOLOGICAL METHODS

chemically stable and inert, is insoluble in most solvents, may be used at widely varying pH, ionic strength, and temperature differences, can easily be prepared with varying pore sizes, is transparent, is available in highly pure analytical grade, and can be prepared with good reproducibility.

Polyacrylamide gel is formed by the polymerization of acrylamide monomer (CH_2=CH—$CONH_2$) in the presence of a small amount of a bifunctional cross-linker, usually N,N-methylenebisacrylamide (Bis, CH_2=CH—$CONH$—CH_2—$HNCO$—CH=CH_2). The meshwork formed provides a pore size, therefore resistance to the passage of macromolecules. The weight ratios of acrylamide to Bis are critical because the relative amount of Bis cross-linker determines the stiffness and brittleness of the gel. In general, an increase in acrylamide concentration should be accompanied by a decrease in Bis concentration to produce elastic gels.

The term "disc electrophoresis" denotes a discontinuous separating electrophoretic system (Ornstein, 1964). As opposed to the continuous system, in which the same buffer system is present in the gel and in both electrode chambers, disc electrophorsis employs buffers with different pH values, resulting in discontinuous voltage and pH gradients. The system employs a stacking gel of large pore size and low pH on top of the separating gel of small pore size and high pH. Polypeptides migrate through the stacking gel quickly and concentrate at the surface of the lower or separating gel. This permits the use of relatively large volumes of dilute protein solutions without much loss of resolution.

A large number of multiphasic buffer systems are available to separate protein mixtures at any pH. In fact, a computer program has been developed and used to generate 4269 different multiphasic systems in the cathodic or anodic direction, at 0° or 25°C, at 0.5 pH intervals across the pH scale (Jovin, 1973).

This chapter will mention only a few of the most successful buffer systems employing either low or high pH in the presence of SDS or urea as the dissociating agent. For an extensive review of polyacrylamide gel electrophoresis, Maurer (1971) and Gordon (1975) should be consulted.

II. PROCEDURES FOR POLYACRYLAMIDE GEL ELECTROPHORESIS

A. Reagents

1. Acrylamide and Bis

As commercially obtained, they are sufficiently pure to be used directly in most investigations. However, when it is desirable to reconstitute the electrophoretically separated components or when the ultraviolet-absorbing impurities must be removed for direct ultraviolet scanning of the gels, acrylamide and Bis can easily be recrystallized from chloroform and acetone, respectively (Loening, 1967). One hundred grams of acrylamide is dissolved in 1 liter of chloroform at 50°C. Ten grams of Bis is dissolved in 1 liter of acetone at 50°C. Both solutions are then filtered while hot through Whatman No. 1 filter paper without suction. The solutions are then left overnight at $-20°C$ and the crystals are recovered and briefly washed with the respective cold solvents by vacuum filtration.

Acrylamide and Bis can also be purified by column chromatography through a mixed-bed ion exchange resin (Duesberg and Rueckert, 1965). It is a good idea to store acrylamide solutions over mixed-bed resin so as to continuously remove hydrolytic products (e.g., NH_3 and acrylic acid) that could cause a drop in the electrophoretic migration velocity (Raymond and Nakamichi, 1962). Because both of these compounds are neurotoxins (Allen *et al.*, 1965; Fullerton and Barnes, 1966), inhalation or contact with the skin should be avoided. The acute lethal dose (LD_{50}) for mice is 170 mg/kg.

The purity of acrylamide and Bis may differ considerably, depending on their origins. Acrylamide and Bis from Serva (Heidelberg, West Germany) give satisfactory results even without further purification.

2. *Sodium Dodecyl Sulfate (SDS)*

Unless specially pure stocks of SDS are used (for example, BDH Chemicals Ltd., Poole, England), it will be necessary to further purify SDS by recrystallization from 95% ethanol. A 10% solution of SDS should be clear and colorless.

3. *TEMED*

This compound (N,N,N',N'-tetramethylethylenediamine) is used to catalyze polymerization. It can be used without further purification and is stable at 4°C as an undiluted liquid.

4. *Ammonium Persulfate*

This is used, in combination with TEMED, to furnish free radicals for the chemical polymerization of acrylamide monomers. An aqueous solution (10%) of ammonium persulfate decomposes rapidly at room temperature and should, therefore, be prepared fresh daily.

5. *2-Mercaptoethanol*

This compound is stable at 4°C in a tightly closed container. It is used for the reduction of disulfide bonds of proteins.

B. Sample Preparation

SDS is one of the most effective detergents for dissolving protein aggregates not linked by covalent bonds. In combination with heat (100°C for 1 min) and a reducing agent (2-mercaptoethanol), SDS causes the denaturation of all proteins to their individual polypeptide chains. Since 1 mg of protein binds 1.4 mg of SDS (Reynolds and Tanford, 1970b), care should be taken to add enough of the detergent to achieve complete solubilization (usually a five-fold excess of SDS by weight).

Precipitated, lyophilized, or particulate protein samples are dissolved or dispersed in a 50 mM $NaHCO_3$ solution. SDS (5 mg/mg of protein) is added and the sample is incubated in a boiling water bath for 1 min. 2-Mercaptoethanol, 5% by volume, is added and the incubation is continued for 2 min longer. Samples are cooled and dialyzed against the "sample buffer" (see Table I) before electrophoresis. If the protein samples are relatively free of ionic solutes (especially K^+ and Ca^{2+}), they may be directly dissolved at a concentration of 0.05–1.0 mg of protein/ml in sample buffer by incubation in a boiling water bath for 3 min.

When protein samples are available as a solution, it is sometimes more convenient to add an equal volume of a double-concentrated sample buffer or one-half volume of a triple-concentrated sample buffer.

Difficulties in solubilizing dry samples or large pellets (e.g., immune precipitates) are sometimes encountered due to the formation of a gel-like layer of SDS around the precipitate. These problems can be overcome by dispersing the precipitate in a small volume of distilled water or $NaHCO_3$ solution before adding the sample buffer (see Table I).

Sample Concentration

If the samples are too dilute for direct analysis, they may be concentrated in a variety of ways. Lyophilization is suitable; however, after re-

Table I

Sample Buffer Composition

	1×	2×	3×
1 M Tris–HCl, pH 6.8	6.25 ml	12.5 ml	18.75 ml
2-Mercaptoethanol	5 ml	10 ml	15 ml
Glycerol	10 ml	20 ml	30 ml
SDS	2.3 gm	4.6 gm	6.9 gm
0.1% Bromphenol blue	1 ml	2 ml	3 ml
Distilled H_2O		to 100 ml	

Table II

Recipe for Discontinuous SDS Separating Gels of Various Porosities[a]

Solution	Final concentration of acrylamide[b] (%)						
	5	7.5	10	12.5	15	17.5	20
30% Acrylamide	5.0	7.5	10	12.5	15	17.5	20
1% Bisacrylamide	7.8	5.2	3.9	3.1	2.6	2.2	2.0
1.5 M Tris–HCl, pH 8.7	7.5	7.5	7.5	7.5	7.5	7.5	7.5
Distilled water	9.3	8.8	8.2	6.5	4.5	2.4	0.1
10% Ammonium persulfate	0.1	0.1	0.1	0.1	0.1	0.1	0.1
10% SDS[c]	0.3	0.3	0.3	0.3	0.3	0.3	0.3
TEMED	0.01	0.01	0.01	0.01	0.01	0.01	0.01

[a] From the Cold Spring Harbor Methods Manual.

[b] The columns represent amounts (in milliliters) of the various solutions necessary to make 30 ml of gel solution.

[c] Before adding SDS and TEMED, the solution is degassed.

constitution, salts (greater than 50 mM) must be removed by dialysis against the sample buffer. Vacuum dialysis may also be employed. This has the advantage of concentrating the sample and removing the excess salts simultaneously. Samples in dialysis bags may also be immersed in dry Sephadex G-100 or G-200 powder or in other large molecular weight hydrophilic materials (e.g., polyethelene glycol 6000). The most commonly used method to concentrate dilute samples is probably precipitation with TCA, ammonium sulfate, acetone, or alcohol. Proteins are precipitated with 10% TCA, pelleted, and washed with cold acetone to remove excess acid. When only very dilute protein solutions are available, for example, after elution of protein bands from gel strips, proteins may be coprecipitated with carbonate–bicarbonate using 9 parts of acetone (Weiner *et al.*, 1972).

C. Gel Solutions

The standard discontinuous gel system described below consists of an Ornstein (1964) and Davis (1964) stacking system with SDS added as modified by Laemmli (1970).

The convenient recipe shown in Table II has appeared in the Cold Spring Harbor Methods Manual.

For the preparation of the stacking gel, the following formula is used: 30% acrylamide, 1.0 ml; 1.0% bisacrylamide, 1.0 ml; 0.5 M Tris–HCl, pH 6.8, 2.5 ml; distilled water, 5.35 ml; 10% ammonium persulfate, 0.05 ml; 10% SDS, 0.1 ml; TEMED, 0.005 ml.

D. Apparatus and Gel Preparation

Because there are numerous advantages to using rectangular gel slabs rather than cylindrical gel columns, an apparatus for electrophoresis in slab gels will be described, although the same solutions can also be used for casting of tube gels. In a single gel slab, one can make a better direct comparison of samples under identical conditions of pH, temperature, current, and voltage gradient. An example is shown in Fig. 1, in which the kinetics of synthesis of bacteriophage T4-coded proteins in *Escherichia coli* B is studied. Here, identical conditions are especially important because of the rapidly changing polypeptide patterns and because of the small molecular size difference between some of the phage-coded proteins. Another example is shown in Fig. 2, in which small differences in molecular size of secreted IgD-like immunoglobulin molecules are revealed by eight clones of a human lymphoblastoid cell line.

Slab gels are thin enough to dry quickly for autoradiography, eliminating the need for slicing. When samples containing more than one isotope are run, sectioning of the gel slab with a simple device (see Fig. 7) can easily be accomplished prior to solubilization and counting.

The apparatus used in this laboratory was first described by Reid and Bieleski (1968) and was modified by Studier (1973). The gel slab is prepared between two glass plates (Fig. 3A). One of the glass plates is a rectangle, measuring 14 × 18 cm. The second is the same size but with a notch 2 cm deep and 14 cm long, cut out from one of the long edges. The two plates are placed together, with the notch at the top and three 5-mm-wide Plexiglas spacers between them along the two sides and along the bottom edge. The thickness of the spacers determines the thickness of the gel. In this laboratory, we have been using spacers with a thickness of 0.8–1.0 mm. The plates are clamped together using ordinary foldback office clips and made liquid-tight by running melted 1.5% agar around the outside edges. It helps if a small amount of vacuum grease is placed at the junction of the two short Plexiglas spacers with the long spacer at the bottom.

The acrylamide solution is poured between the plates to a level of about 2 cm from the notch. It is then gently overlayered with butanol that has been saturated with water. The plates are then lowered into a water bath at 35°C and the gel is allowed to polymerize for 1 hr. The purpose of this step is to accelerate polymerization but also to dissipate the heat produced during polymerization. The clips at the bottoms of the plates should be sufficient to hold the unit in an upright position during polymerization. The water level in the water bath should be at least to the level of the gel solution between the plates to assure even polymerization. After 1 hr, the unit is removed

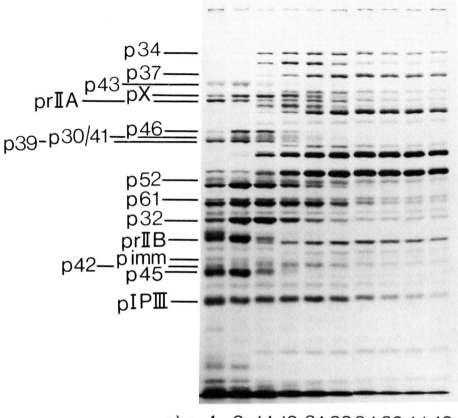

Fig. 1. Kinetics of synthesis of bacteriophage-coded proteins in *E. coli* B. Autoradiograph of SDS–polyacrylamide slab gel electrophoresis of infected and labeled cell lysates. (a) Time (minutes) of initiation of labeling after infection; (b) termination of labeling. Cells were cultured in M-9 medium (Bolle *et al.*, 1968) at 30°C. Infection (at a multiplicity of 5) was performed when bacteria had reached a density of 4×10^8 cells/ml, using the amber mutant of bacteriophage T4, HL-626. Radioactive labeling with ^{14}C-amino acids (1 μCi/ml of culture) was initiated in parallel cultures every 4 min after infection. A large excess of casamino acids (1% final concentration) was added 4 min later. Samples were rapidly cooled and the cells were collected by centrifugation. Pellets were dissolved in sample buffer and incubated at 100°C for 3 min before application to the gel. (10% acrylamide). Proteins identified as bands on the gel are referred to by the name of their structural gene preceded by a lowercase p, denoting product of gene 34, etc. For additional information, see Takács and Rosenbusch (1975).

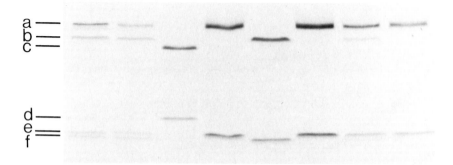

Fig. 2. Secretion of IgD-like immunoglobulins by eight clones derived from a spontaneous human lymphoblastoid cell line. Cultures, at a cell density of 2×10^6 cells/ml, were labeled biosynthetically with [^{14}C]leucine (1.5 μCi/ml) for 12 hr. Supernatants from each culture were incubated with rabbit anti-human δ-antiserum and with inactivated protein-A-bearing staphylococci overnight at 4°C. Bacteria were sedimented and washed three or four times with PBS by centrifugation (6000 g for 10 min). Pellets were dissolved in sample buffer and incubated at 100°C for 3 min before application to the gel. The polyacrylamide gel concentration was 12.5%. After electrophoresis (20 mA/slab) the gel was fixed, stained and destained, and dried onto filter paper. The dried gel was exposed on a Kodirex medical X-ray film. The apparent molecular weights of the resolved polypeptides are (a) 63,000, (b) 55,000, (c) 51,000, (d) 28,000, (e) 25,000, and (f) 24,000.

from the water bath and, if not used on the same day, may be left overnight at room temperature.

Before pouring the upper gel, the butanol and the unpolymerized gel layer are removed and the surface of the gel is rinsed with upper gel buffer. Excess liquid may be blotted off with a piece of chromatography paper, but care should be taken not to touch the surface of the gel. The comb is inserted (Fig. 3B) to a depth sufficient to leave a space of about 5 mm between the surface of the lower gel and the fingers of the comb. The solution to form the stacking gel is then poured in around the comb. The gel is allowed to polymerize for 30 min. A longer time will result in an equilibration of pH between stacking and separating gels, reducing the stacking efficiency of the upper gel. After the stacking gel has set, the bottom Plexiglas spacer is removed and the unit is attached to the electrophoresis apparatus so that the notch in the glass plate is next to and lines up with the notch on the upper buffer chamber (Fig. 4). A liquid-tight seal is provided by vacuum grease around the notch on the upper buffer chamber. Electrode buffer (0.025 M Tris, 0.192 M glycine, 0.1% SDS) is then placed in the lower buffer chamber to cover 3–4 cm of the bottom edge of the gel. To eliminate bubbles from the lower surface of the gel, the whole unit my be tilted while pouring in the running buffer. Alternatively, the lower buffer chamber may contain buffer before the gel sandwich is lowered into it at an angle to exclude trapped bubbles. Enough running buffer is then placed in the upper chamber to flow across the notch. The comb is then removed, leaving sample wells filled with running buffer. Samples (containing 10–15% glycerol) are then applied with Eppendorf pipettes. Up to 50 µl of a sample may be added to each well by allowing it to run down between the glass plates to the bottom of the sample well.

The electrodes are then connected to a power supply, with the anode to the lower chamber and the cathode to the upper chamber. Electrophoresis is run at constant current (20–30 mA for slabs of 0.8–1.5 mm thick) at room temperature until the marker dye, bromphenol blue, approaches the bottom of the gel, which takes about 3–4 hr.

Gradient Gel Electrophoresis

The use of gradient gels provides conditions of limiting pore size, which result in band sharpening during the run. In gradient gels, when constant voltage is applied, the mobilities of all proteins will decrease due to the

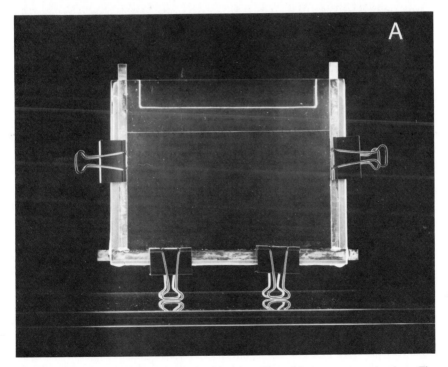

Fig. 3. Assembled glass plates with the Plexiglas side and bottom spacers in place. The polymerized separating gel is shown in A. B (*next page*) shows the gel sandwich with the comb inserted and the stacking gel polymerized.

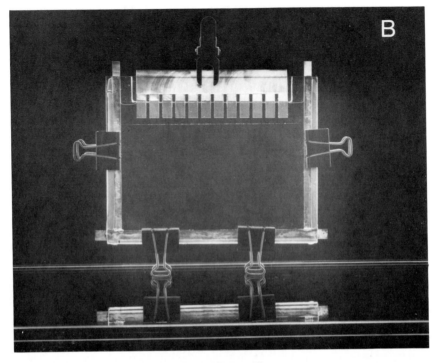

Fig. 3—*Continued*

progressively greater sieving. The fact that proteins will never come to a full stop at a particular region in the gel is probably due to the large variation in pore size at any region of the gel (Rodbard *et al.*, 1971).

An example of gradient slab gel electrophoresis is shown in Fig. 5. Exponentially growing cells of *E. coli* were infected with wild type and various amber mutants of bacteriophage T4 and labeled with ^{14}C-amino acids between 4 and 7 min postinfection. The stained and destained gel (Fig. 5A) was autoradiographed to reveal the distribution of the individual phage-coded proteins (Fig. 5B). Polypeptides with a molecular size difference of as little as 200–500 daltons can clearly be seen as individual bands.

Exponential or linear acrylamide gradients may be prepared using standard gradient mixers. In this laboratory, we have been using three channels of a multichannel peristaltic pump to prepare linear acrylamide gradient gels. To produce the gradient, an appropriate amount of the light solution, representing one-half of the volume needed to fill the gel compartment, is gently stirred magnetically. This solution is delivered by means of two channels of the peristaltic pump and long needles to the bottom of the slab gel compartment. Simultaneously, the heavy solution is transferred by means of a single channel to the mixing chamber. The higher concentration of acrylamide solution should contain glycerol (10%) to increase the stability of the gradient. The solutions should be kept cold (below 10°C) to avoid polymerization of the gel mixture during preparation. After removal of the needles, the gel is allowed to polymerize and is used as described for uniform gels.

Exponential gradients may be prepared in a similar way, but using only a single channel of the pump for the delivery of the mixed gel solution from the mixing chamber to the gel compartment.

The compositions of some of the most commonly used concentrations for preparing gradient gels are given in Table III. Other gel concentrations not listed in the table may, of course, be prepared.

For the preparation of gels with higher acrylamide concentrations, for example, 30 and 40%, the formula shown in Table IV has been used successfully in our laboratory.

For the preparation of stacking gel, the formula described in Section II,C is used.

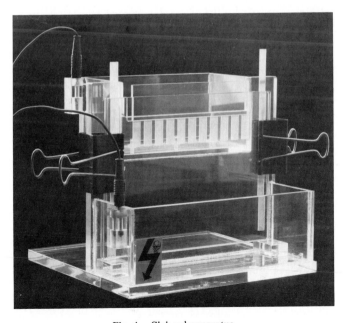

Fig. 4.   Slab gel apparatus.

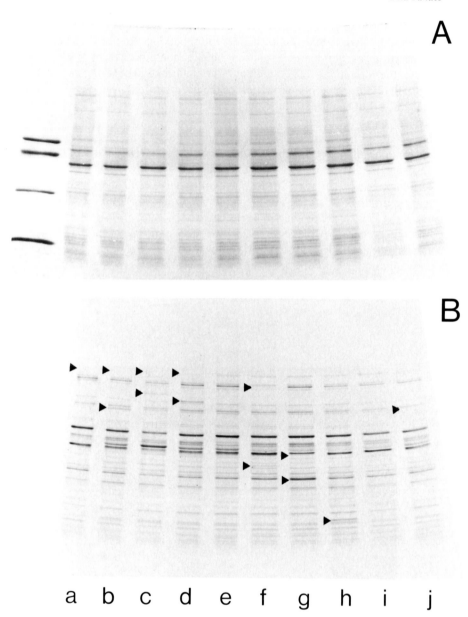

Fig. 5. Identification of prereplicative T4 proteins. *E. coli* B was infected with various mutants of bacteriophage T4. The infected cells were labeled 3 min after infection with ¹⁴C-

Table III

Recipe for the Preparation of Discontinuous SDS Gradient Gels

	Acrylamide concentration (%)				
Stock solutions	7.5	10	12.5	15	20
1.5 M Tris–HCl (pH 8.8)–0.4% SDS (ml)	7.5	7.5	7.5	7.5	7.5
30% Acrylamide–0.8% Bis (ml)	7.5	10	12.5	15	20
Distilled H_2O (ml)	14.9	12.4	6.9	4.4	—
10% Ammonium persulfate (ml)	0.1	0.1	0.1	0.1	0.1
Glycerol (ml)[a]	—	—	3	3	2.4
TEMED (ml)	0.01	0.01	0.01	0.01	0.01

[a] Glycerol should be added to the heavy solution only.

E. Staining Procedures

The textile dye, Coomassie brilliant blue R250, was first introduced by Fazekas *et al.* (1963) to stain proteins on cellulose acetate strips. The dye was subsequently used in methanol:acetic acid:distilled water (5:1:5, v/v/v) to visualize proteins in polyacrylamide gels (Meyer and Lamberts, 1965). Because of its high sensitivity and uniform protein binding, Coomassie brilliant blue is the most widely used dye employed in sample visualization after electrophoresis.

At the end of the run, the gel sandwich is removed from the electrophoresis apparatus. The two Plexiglas spacers are removed and the plates are gently pried apart with a spatula while running a stream of water between them. The gel is slid off the plate into an oversized petri dish (20 cm) containing the staining solution (0.25% Coomassie brilliant blue in methanol:acetic acid:distilled water, 5:1:5) prewarmed to 37°C. During staining (45–60 min) the dish is rotated slowly on a platform shaker in a

---

amino acids. Labeling was terminated 8 min after infection. Electrophoresis was performed as described in the legend to Fig. 1. Plate A represents the stained, fixed, and destained slab after drying. Plate B is the autoradiograph of the same slab. The gel was prepared from 7.5 and 20% acrylamide solutions to produce a linear gradient of acrylamide. For further details see the text (Section II, D—Gradient Gel Electrophoresis). The arrows indicate either the absence of a polypeptide band or the appearance of an amber fragment.

	a	b	c	d	e	f	g	h	i	j
Mutant	B22	A504	B263	B277	αgt-, βgt-	r88H	r196	HL618	D+	116
Gene	43	43	43	43	—	A	B	32	—	39

Table IV

Recipe for the Preparation of Gels with Higher Acrylamide Concentrations

Stock solutions	Acrylamide concentration (%)	
	30	40
1.5 M Tris–HCl (pH 8.8)–0.4% SDS (ml)	7.5	7.5
Acrylamide (gm)	6	8
Bis (gm)	0.12	0.16
Distilled H_2O	To 20 ml	
10% Ammonium persulfate (ml)	0.1	0.1
TEMED (ml)	0.01	0.01

37°C incubator. Alternatively, a gyrotory water bath shaker (New Brunswick, New Brunswick, New Jersey), containing enough water at 37°C so that the dish is not floating, may be employed.

An alternate method to stain protein zones in plyacrylamide gels, which uses dilute perchloric acid solutions of Coomassie brilliant blue R250, was introduced by Reisner *et al.* (1975). The technique makes use of the fact that the Coomassie brilliant blue exhibits a color change in perchloric acid that is reversed when the dye binds to protein. Since the dye produces only a pale orange background when it interacts with the gel, but stains proteins with an intense blue color, the technique requires no destaining. Furthermore, in this system, ampholytes do not bind the dye, which makes the system useful for staining the gels after isoelectric focusing.

Another quick visualization method involves the use of Remazol dyes (Griffith, 1972). According to this method, proteins are stained during solubilization, before analysis by SDS–polyacrylamide gel electrophoresis. The migration and separation of proteins during electrophoresis may be visually observed.

Staining of Glycoproteins

A number of procedures based on the use of periodic acid–Schiff reagent to visualize glycoproteins are available (Clarke, 1964; Caldwell and Pigman, 1965; Keyser, 1965). The procedure for staining glycoproteins in polyacrylamide gels according to Zacharius *et al.* (1969) is given in Table V.

F. Destaining

After staining, the dye is removed with a water aspirator and replaced with destaining solution (methanol:acetic acid:distilled water, 5:1:5). A spoonful of technical-grade anion exchange resin is added (obtainable from Lienberger AG, Zentweg 13, 3000 Bern 32, Switzerland; No. 3 AsI).

The resin eliminates the necessity of replacing the destaining solution. Destaining at 37°C with gentle shaking takes about 60 min.

G. Drying

When destaining is complete, the gel is washed free of resin with either destaining solution or water, transferred onto a plastic sheet (Saran Wrap or part of a clear plastic bag will do) and overlaid with a piece of wet chromatography paper (Whatman 3MM) somewhat larger than the gel itself. This sandwich is then transferred onto the drying apparatus with the paper side toward the porous plate (Fig. 6). The gel is dried by connecting the drying apparatus to a suitable vacuum source, such as a water aspirator pump. The drying time can be reduced by applying heat to the gel from an infrared lamp positioned about 50 cm above the sandwich. During drying, the gel slab is reduced to a thin, hard, smooth layer that remains attached to the filter paper.

H. Autoradiography

The dried gel may be stored in a notebook or otherwise kept under weight to prevent curling. Radioactive patterns are detected by superimposing the

Table V

Staining of Glycoproteins in Polyacrylamide Gels[a]

Step	Treatment	Time (min)
1	Immerse gel in 12.5% trichloroacetic acid	30
2	Rinse briefly with distilled water	0.5
3	Immerse in 1% periodic acid solution prepared in 3% acetic acid	60
4	Wash extensively (10 × 10 min) with distilled water until test for IO_3 with $AgNO_3$ is negative; should be done in the dark	100
5	Immerse in fuchsin–sulfite reagent in the dark (2% rosaniline in water is decolorized with SO_2, treated with charcoal, and diluted 20 times with water)	50
6	Wash gel (3 × 10 min) with freshly prepared 0.5% Na-metabisulfite	30
7	Wash extensively with frequent changes of distilled water by agitation	O.N.[b]
8	Store in 7% acetic acid	

[a] From Zacharius *et al.* (1969).
[b] O.N., overnight.

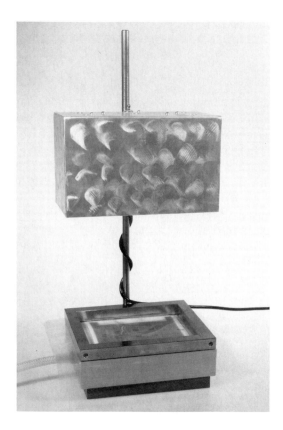

Fig. 6. The gel drying apparatus.

dried gel onto a medical X-ray film (Kodirex) and exposing it for a period best determined by trial. As a rough guide, the application of a complex sample of polypeptides, containing 50–100 resolvable bands and approximately 50,000 cpm, usually requires an exposure time of 24–36 hr. The exposed film is then processed using X-ray developer and fixer according to the manufacturer's instructions.

The radioactive patterns may be converted to graphical form using a recording densitometer. Exposure times should be chosen to yield linear responses of bands on the film and of the peak heights in the densitometer. Quantitation of the autoradiographs can be achieved by using a densitometer equipped with an integrator. Alternatively, the peak areas on the densitometer tracings may be determined by triangulation or by cutting out the individual peaks and weighing them.

Techniques to enhance the efficiency of detection of radioactive bands are available (Randerath, 1970; Bonner and Laskey, 1974). In fact, these methods allow the detection of ^{3}H-labeled polypeptides in polyacrylamide gels by autoradiography. The gel is dehydrated in dimethyl sulfoxide (DMSO) and then impregnated with the scintillant, PPO, prior to drying and exposing at $-70°C$. In this case, the grains of the film are not exposed by the β particles themselves, but by the light generated when β particles interact with PPO.

I. Slicing the Gel

The autoradiographic procedure is limited to relatively high-energy emitters such as ^{14}C, ^{35}S, ^{32}P, ^{125}I, and ^{131}I. When the gel contains ^{3}H or more than one isotope, quantitative analysis of radioactivity may best be done by slicing the gel and determining the radioactivity in each slice in a scintillation counter.

Gel slabs may be sliced with simple devices containing a parallel array of razor blades or thin wires. The gel is first cut with a razor blade into longitudinal strips, with the entire width of all the bands in the strip. Each strip is then cut to obtain approximately 1-mm slices with the device shown in Fig. 7. Each slice is then transferred, using fine forceps, to scintillation vials, and an aliquot of a suitable solubilizer is added to destroy the gel structure.

J. Gel Solubilization

Gel slices are dissolved in 0.5–1.0 ml of 30% H_2O_2 at 60°C overnight in capped scintillation vials. Ten milliliters of scintillation fluid (7 parts of toluene containing 4 gm of PPO and 0.2 gm of POPOP per liter and 6 parts of Triton X-100) is added prior to counting.

An alternate method involves the use of NCS solubilizer (Amersham/ Searle Corp., Arlington Heights, Illinois) to cause swelling of the gel slices and diffusion of the proteins into the scintillation fluid (Ames, 1974). To each gel slice 10 ml of scintillation mixture (143 ml of NCS solubilizer, 3.73 liters of toluene, 14 gm of PPO, and 0.21 gm of POPOP) is added, and the capped vials are incubated overnight at 37°C.

Solubilizable polyacrylamide gels may be obtained by replacing the Bis cross-linker with ethylene diacrylate (EDIA) (Choules and Zimm, 1965) or N,N'-diallyltartardiamide (DATD) (Anker, 1970). EDIA gel slices are solubilized for several hours at room temperature at alkaline pH, for example, in 0.5–1 ml of concentrated NH_4OH prior to the addition of the

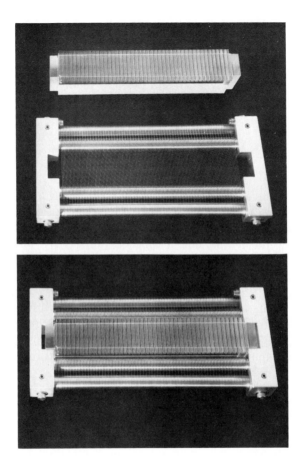

Fig. 7. Apparatus for slicing slab gel strips. The upper part of the figure illustrates the apparatus before assembly, the lower part after assembly.

water-miscible scintillation fluid. DATD gel slices may be dissolved in 0.5–1 ml of a 2% solution of periodic acid at room temperature for 30 min.

K. Elution of Protein Bands from Gel Fractions

After electrophoresis, but prior to fixation and staining, individual protein bands may be eluted from the sliced gel into a sufficient amount of 5 mM NaHCO$_3$ containing 0.1% SDS to cover each slice. Agitation at 37°C for 12 hr is usually sufficient to complete the elution. Part of each sample may be rerun on another gel, part used for scintillation counting, and part used for renaturation after removing the SDS (see Section II,M).

Recovered proteins may be injected, either directly or after SDS removal, into animals for antibody production.

The amount of protein in each band may be scaled up either by using thicker Plexiglas spacers (up to 0.5 cm) or by applying the sample on top of the entire width of the stacking gel. In the latter case, the stacking gel is prepared without the use of a comb.

L. Preparative Electrophoresis

There are two basic approaches to large-scale fractionation of protein mixtures on polyacrylamide gels. The first approach involves electrophoresis of the samples on larger and thicker slab gels and subsequent elution of the bands from the cut gel as described above. The second approach involves electrophoresis through short columns or slabs. As the samples emerge they are collected by a continuous stream of buffer across the lower face of the gel. An example for this second system is shown in Fig. 8. The apparatus shown is a modification of the standard analytical slab gel apparatus and was prepared in our own workshop. The most important feature of the apparatus is the elution cell made of Plexiglas (Fig. 8B), which fits tightly to the underside of the gel sandwich. A sheet of dialysis membrane stretched tightly over the elution cell provides a small

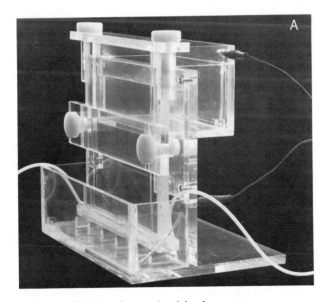

Fig. 8A. Preparative slab gel apparatus.

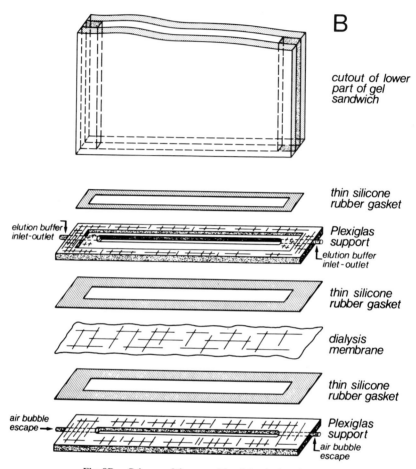

Fig. 8B. Schema of the assembly of the elution chamber.

elution chamber below the lower surface of the gel. Elution buffer is pumped into the chamber from one side and fractions are collected from the opposite side. The ionic strength of the elution buffer should be higher than that of the gel buffer to reduce adsorption of the emerging proteins to the membrane. The compositions of electrode and elution buffer solutions and of solutions for the separating and spacer gels according to Duesberg and Rueckert (1965) are given in Table VI. For the preparation of discontinuous preparative gels containing SDS, the solutions described in Section II,C may be used.

The difficulties encountered most often with preparative electrophoresis are heat dissipation problems, which can lead to curved bands and problems

Table VI

Stock Solutions for the Preparation of Acidic and Alkaline Separation and Spacer Gels[a]

Solution	Component	pH 9.9 system[b]	
		Separation gel	Stacking gel
A	10 N HCl (ml)	12	12
	Tris (gm)	80	72.6
	TEMED (ml)	5.8	11.5
	10 M Urea (ml)	800	800
B	Acrylamide (gm)	30	30
	Bis (gm)	0.8	0.8
	10 M Urea (ml)	80	80

Solution	Component	pH 4.5 system[b]	
		Separation gel	Stacking gel
C	CH_2COOK (gm)	30	30
	CH_3COOH (ml)	120	60
	TEMED (ml)	25	3
	10 M Urea (ml)	800	800
D	Acrylamide (gm)		10
	Bis (gm)		2.5
	10 M Urea (ml)		80
	Distilled H_2O (ml)		To 100
E	Riboflavin (mg)		40
	Distilled H_2O (ml)		To 100

[a] According to Duesberg and Rueckert (1965).

[b] For the preparation of alkaline separation gels, 16 ml of solution A, 9 ml of solution B, and 30 ml of 8 M urea are mixed and polymerized by the addition of a cold solution of 22.5 mg of ammonium persulfate in 15 ml of 8 M urea. The stacking gel is prepared from 1.8 ml of solution A, 1.8 ml of solution B, and 7.8 ml of 8 M urea and is polymerized with a solution of 4.5 mg of ammonium persulfate in 3 ml of 8 M urea. Both upper and lower electrode vessels are filled with Tris-glycine buffer (0.05 M Tris, 0.4 M glycine). The elution chamber is flushed with a solution prepared from 52 gm of Tris, 14 ml of acetic acid, and 800 ml of 10 M urea. For the preparation of acid gels, 3 ml of solution C, 6 ml of solution A, and 15 ml of 8 M urea are polymerized by the addition of 27.5 mg of ammonium persulfate in 24 ml of 8 M urea. The upper gel is formed by photopolymerization of 0.4 ml of solution C, 2 ml of solution D, and 5.6 ml of 8 M urea with 0.1 ml of solution E. Both upper and lower electrode vessels are filled with a solution prepared from 31.2 gm of β-alanine and 8 ml of acetic acid in a final volume of 1 liter. Samples are eluted with a solution prepared from 19 ml of acetic acid, 14 gm of ammonium acetate, and 800 ml of 10 M urea.

with sample dilution. High molecular weight proteins take a longer time to emerge, over a longer period of time than proteins of smaller size. Problems of heat dissipation can be overcome, at least partially, by using the preparative slab gel shown in Fig. 8. The gel in this system is not only thinner than most gels used in the column system but the whole sandwich may be lowered into a continuously cooled lower electrode buffer solution. The problem of sample dilution can be reduced either by programming the flow rate of elution buffer to decrease with time or by using gradient gels, which is more effective (see Section II,D—Gradient Gel Electrophoresis).

M. Removal of SDS

The excellent solubilizing properties of SDS very often make it the method of choice to dissociate complex biological samples. However, after separation of the protein–SDS complexes, it is often necessary to remove the bound SDS before further studies (e.g., isoelectric focusing and antigen–antibody reactions) can be undertaken. Simple dialysis might not be sufficient to remove the bound SDS (Weber and Kuter, 1971). However, two methods have been reported by which the quantitative removal of SDS from proteins is possible. Furthermore, the removal of SDS from a number of enzymes resulted in their renaturation and recovery of part of the enzymatic activity.

According to the method of Tuszynski and Warren (1975), protein–SDS complexes in 1 mM Tris–HCl buffer, pH 7.7, containing 1% mercapto-ethanol and 5 M urea are subjected to electrodialysis at a constant current of 20 mA. During 11 hr of electrophoretic dialysis, quantitative removal of SDS should be possible.

Another method for SDS removal involves ion exchange chromatography in 6 M urea (Weber and Kuter, 1971). Protein solutions containing SDS are made 6 M with respect to urea either by adding solid urea or by dialyzing against 50 mM Tris-acetate buffer, pH 7.8, containing 10 mM 2-mercaptoethanol and 6 M urea. The solution is then applied to a small Dowex 1-X2 column, equilibrated with the same buffer. One milliliter of Dowex 1-X2 resin can bind as much as 100 mg of SDS. The urea serves to keep the proteins soluble and to weaken the protein–SDS interactions. The removal of SDS may be monitored by adding a drop of concentrated KCl solution to an aliquot of the test sample. When present, SDS will form an insoluble precipitate with KCl. Urea may be removed by dialysis or by adsorbing the proteins onto a DEAE column followed by washing with urea-free buffer. In the latter case, the adsorbed proteins can be recovered from DEAE by standard procedures (e.g., elution with high salt).

N. Molecular Weight Determination

To obtain an estimate of the molecular size of the various protein bands after electrophoresis, protein standards with well-characterized polypeptide chain molecular weights should routinely be run on the same slab gel. However, the use of proteolytic enzymes (e.g., trypsin and chymotrypsin) should be avoided since these proteins are active even after boiling in 2% SDS. When autoradiography is routinely used, it might be convenient to prepare labeled protein molecular weight markers. This can be done with [^{14}C]iodoacetate or [^{14}C]acetic anhydride.

The molecular weight of an unknown protein may be estimated by comparing its mobility to the mobilities of known standards run on the same gel.

Studies of the hydrodynamic properties of protein–SDS complexes indicate that these are rodlike particles, with the length of the rod varying uniquely with the molecular weight (Reynolds and Tanford, 1970a; Fish et al., 1970). Since in the SDS–polyacrylamide gel system the apparent free mobilities of protein–SDS complexes are nearly constant, the molecular size of such complexes, over a specified range, may be determined from plots of relative mobility versus the logarithm of molecular weight. On a single slab gel, proteins are exposed to identical conditions of pH, temperture, current, and voltage gradient, so that direct comparison of molecular sizes is possible. The distance of each molecular weight standard from the top of the gel is measured and plotted, on semilog paper, against its respective molecular weight (Fig. 9). The molecular weight of an unknown protein is then extrapolated from its migration distance.

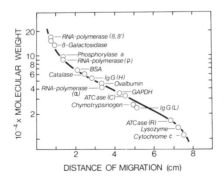

Fig. 9. Calibration curve of molecular weights for polyacrylamide slab gel electrophoresis. BSA, bovine serum albumin; IgG (H and L), heavy and light chains of immunoglobulins; ATCase (C and R), catalytic and regulatory polypeptide chains of aspartate transcarbamylase from *E. coli*; GAPDH, glyceraldehyde-3-phosphate dehydrogenase from yeast. The polyacrylamide gel concentration was 10%.

From Fig. 9 it is clear that the log molecular weight versus migration distance is sigmoidal in nature. Nevertheless, an almost linear relationship exists in the molecular weight range between 15,000 and 100,000. Estimation of molecular size outside these limits is, of course, possible if well-characterized molecular weight markers are available.

III. CONCLUSION

The use of polyacrylamide gel electrophoresis to analyze and to separate complex mixtures of proteins and nucleic acids has greatly enhanced our understanding of many cellular and viral systems. The simplicity of the equipment and its ease of operation, as well as the good reproducibility of the results, make the method preferable to many other techniques of analysis. In combination with two-dimensional techniques and isoelectric focusing, polyacrylamide gel electrophoresis may prove to be the method of choice not only at the analytical level but also for preparative operations.

REFERENCES

Allen, R. C., Popp, R. A., and Moore, D. J. (1965). *Histochem. Cytochem.* **13,** 249.
Ames, G. F. (1974). *J. Biol. Chem.* **249,** 634.
Anker, H. S. (1970). *FEBS Lett.* **7,** 293.
Bolle, A., Epstein, R. H., Salser, W., and Guiduschek, E. P. (1968). *J. Mol. Biol.* **31,** 325.
Bonner, W. M., and Laskey, R. A. (1974). *Eur. J. Biochem.* **46,** 83.
Caldwell, R., and Pigman, W. (1965). *Arch. Biochem. Biophys.* **110,** 91.
Choules, G. L., and Zimm, B. H. (1965). *Anal. Biochem.* **13,** 336.
Clarke, J. T. (1964). *Ann. N.Y. Acad. Sci.* **121,** 428.
Davis, B. J. (1964). *Ann. N.Y. Acad. Sci.* **121,** 404.
Duesberg, P. H., and Rueckert, R. R. (1965). *Anal. Biochem.* **11,** 342.
Fazekas de St.Groth, S., Webster, R. G., and Datyner, A. (1963). *Biochim. Biophys. Acta* **71,** 377.
Fish, W. W., Reynolds, J. A., and Tanford, C. (1970). *J. Biol. Chem.* **245,** 5116.
Fullerton, P. M., and Barnes, J. M. (1966). *Br. J. Ind. Med.* **23,** 210.
Gordon, A. H. (1975). *In* "Laboratory Techniques in Biochemistry and Molecular Biology. Electrophoresis of Proteins in Polyacrylamide and Starch Gels" (T. S. Work and E. Work, eds.), Vol. 1, Part I. North-Holland, Amsterdam.
Griffith, I. P. (1972). *Anal. Biochem.* **46,** 402.
Jovin, T. M. (1973). *Ann. N.Y. Acad. Sci.* **209,** 477.
Keyser, J. W. (1965). *Anal. Biochem.* **9,** 249.
Laemmli, U. K. (1970). *Nature (London)* **277,** 680.
Loening, U. E. (1967). *Biochem. J.* **102,** 251.
Maurer, H. R. (1971). *In* "Disc Electrophoresis and Related Techniques of Polyacrylamide Gel Electrophoresis" (K. Fishbeck, ed.), De Gruyter, Berlin.
Meyer, T. S., and Lamberts, B. L. (1965). *Biochim. Biophys. Acta* **107,** 144.

Ornstein, L. (1964). *Ann. N.Y. Acad. Sci.* **121,** 321.

Randerath, K. (1970). *Anal. Biochem.* **34,** 188.

Raymond, S., and Nakamichi, M. (1962). *Anal. Biochem.* **3,** 23.

Reid, M. S., and Bieleski, R. L. (1968). *Anal. Biochem.* **22,** 374.

Reisner, A. H., Nemes, P., and Bucholtz, C. (1975). *Anal. Biochem.* **64,** 509.

Reynolds, J. A., and Tanford, C. (1970a). *J. Biol. Chem.* **245,** 5151.

Reynolds, J. A., and Tanford, C. (1970b). *Proc. Natl. Acad. Sci. U.S.A.* **66,** 1002.

Rodbard, D., Kapadia, G., and Chrambach, A. (1971). *Anal. Biochem.* **40,** 135.

Studier, F. W., (1973). *J. Mol. Biol.* **79,** 237.

Takács, B. J., and Rosenbusch, J. P. (1975). *J. Biol. Chem.* **250,** 2339.

Tuszynski, G. P., and Warren, L. (1975). *Anal. Biochem.* **67,** 55.

Weber, K., and Kuter, D. J. (1971). *J. Biol. Chem.* **246,** 4504.

Weiner, A. M., Platt, T., and Weber, K. (1972). *J. Biol. Chem.* **247,** 3242.

Zacharius, R. M., Zell, T. E., Morrison, J. H., and Woodlock, J. J. (1969). *Anal. Biochem.* **30,** 148.

5

Resolution of Immunoglobulin Patterns by Analytical Isoelectric Focusing

Dietmar G. Braun, Kerstin Hild, and Andreas Ziegler

I. INTRODUCTION

Isoelectric focusing (IEF) in polyacrylamide slab gels has become a frequently used method to study the heterogeneity of antibody responses and to screen genetically defined populations of laboratory animals for the pattern of specific antibodies (Williamson *et al.*, 1973; Williamson, 1971; Kreth and Williamson, 1973; Pink and Askonas, 1974; Braun *et al.*, 1973; Cramer and Braun, 1974; Wabl and Du Pasquier, 1976). IEF has also been used to screen human sera for the occurrence of naturally acquired antibodies to the streptococcal group polysaccharide antigens (Riesen *et al.*,

107

IMMUNOLOGICAL METHODS
Copyright © 1979 by Academic Press, Inc.
All rights of reproduction in any form reserved.
ISBN 0-12-442750-2

1976). If the IEF method is performed in polyacrylamide gels, large molecules (such as IgM) cannot be analyzed because they do not enter the gel. This difficulty has been overcome by the use of polymerizable thin layers containing Sephadex as an anticonvective medium (Ziegler and Köhler, 1976). The amount of specific antibodies required can be further reduced by several orders of magnitude if isotope-labeled antigens are used to develop the IEF patterns. Therefore, this method is applicable for screening complex mixtures of biological material (e.g., sera, ascites fluid, urine, and spinal cord fluid).

II. PRINCIPLE OF THE METHOD

IEF is a high-resolution separation method. It separates ampholytes such as amino acids and oligo- and polypeptides as well as protein molecules according to their isoelectric points (pI) in ion-free media. However, IEF became a practical method for the fractionation of macromolecular ampholytes only when natural pH gradients and suitable carrier ampholytes were introduced (Svensson, 1961, 1962a,b; Vesterberg and Svensson, 1966). In liquid media, shallow pH gradients formed by low molecular weight ampholytes and stabilized by sucrose density gradients (Svensson, 1962b) first served to study the heterogeneity of myoglobulins, cytochrome *c*, lactoperoxidase, and many other proteins (Vesterberg and Svensson, 1966; Vesterberg, 1967; Flatmark and Vesterberg, 1966; Haglund, 1967). For the fractionation of immunoglobulins, the column approach is used mainly for preparative work; polyacrylamide gels (which have better stabilizing properties) have the capacity to highly resolve, and therefore identify, the product of a single lymphocyte clone (clonotype) in a mixture of other proteins and antibodies (Williamson, 1971; Braun *et al.*, 1973; Askonas *et al.*, 1970; Eichmann, 1972). This latter technique will be described in detail with two modifications: the polyacrylamide slab gel and the gel using polymerizable thin layers containing Sephadex.

III. MATERIALS

Glass plates (220 × 170 × 3 mm) siliconized with Repelcote (Hopkin and Williams, Chadwell Health, Essex, England)
Ilford (Essex, England) gelatin-coated glass plates (21.6 × 16.8 cm)
Silicone tubing: inside diameter, 2 mm; outside diameter 1.2 mm
Metal clamps: foldback 1413 (Myers, Birmingham, England; six clamps for preparing one gel; see Fig. 1B)

Focusing box (33 × 23 × 10 cm) with a sealing lid made of Plexiglas and containing two rod-shaped graphite electrodes (19 × 1 cm) with safety plugs (see Fig. 1A)

Power supply (constant voltage)

Flat membrane electrode (Ingold, Zürich, Switzerland) and pH meter

Solutions (to be kept at 4°C in the dark)

  A. 1.0 ml of N,N,N',N'-tetramethylethylenediamine (TEMED) in 150 ml of triple-distilled or freshly deionized water

  B. 100 gm of acrylamide (recrystallized) and 2.7 gm of N,N'-bismethylacrylamide made to a volume of 300 ml with triple-distilled or freshly deionized water

  C. 2 mg of riboflavin in 100 ml of triple-distilled or freshly deionized water

  D. 5% ethylenediamine in deionized water

  E. 5% phosphoric acid in deionized water

Ampholine from LKB Producer AB (Stockholm; a series of Ampholines is available); appropriate mixtures of Ampholines can be used to establish a number of different pH gradients, the widest range being between pH 2.5–11

IV. PROCEDURES

A. Assembling the Gel Chamber

Place the Ilford plate with the coated side against the siliconized glass plate. Separate both plates by silicon tubing (outside diameter 1.2 mm) positioned on three sides to form a rectangular chamber (volume ~ 30 ml) with one side open (Fig. 1). Clamp both plates together by squeezing the tubing between the foldback metal clamps. Bring the chamber to a vertical position and then fill it with the solution of polyacrylamide gel.

B. Preparing the 5% Polyacrylamide Gels

Place the mixture (solution A, 1.5 ml; solution B, 6.0 ml; Ampholine, 2.0 ml; and triple-distilled H_2O, 26.5 ml) in a 250-ml suction flask under vacuum (water pump) for approximately 2 min while stirring with a magnet. This step prevents the occurrence of air bubbles in the gel. Add, at this point only, 4.0 ml of solution C, mix well, and pipette the mixture immediately into the prepared gel chamber, avoiding air bubbles. Place triple-distilled water on top of the gel solution with a Pasteur pipette (to a depth of 0.5

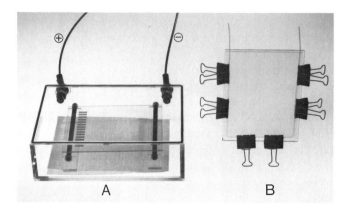

Fig. 1. (A). Isoelectric focusing box (the closing lid is not shown) made of Plexiglas with a plate in the focusing position. The polyacrylamide gel layer rests on two graphite electrodes. The gel is supported above by the gelatin-coated Ilford glass plate. Sample application filter papers are on the surface of the gel. (B). Chamber for pouring the polyacrylamide gel. This chamber is constructed of a siliconized plate and an Ilford glass plate, which are separated by silicone tubing and held together by foldback clamps.

cm). For polymerization, place the gel in front of a fluorescent light for 4–12 hr.

For isoelectric focusing of specific antibodies from hyperimmune sera, it is advisable to add to the gels 2 *M* urea (freshly deionized) (Cramer and Braun, 1974). To achieve deionization a 10 *M* stock solution of urea is stirred in Amberlite monobed resin MB-1, analytical grade (BDH laboratory reagents, manufactured by The Rohm & Haas Co., Philadelphia, Pennsylvania), for 30 min, and the Amberlite is then removed by filtration through a glass-sintered filter. Under these conditions, weak aggregates of antibodies or antigen–antibody complexes are disrupted; however, subsequent antigen binding using a focused antibody is not impaired.

C. Loading the Gel with Samples

After the gel has solidified, the clamps and silicon tubing are carefully removed with the Ilford plate facing down. The siliconized glass plate is removed slowly starting at one end. The gel should adhere to the Ilford plate.

Place the plate with the polyacrylamide side facing up on millimeter paper and apply the samples at one end. The anodal end is preferred for separating antibodies; in principle, this should not matter, but experience shows that resolution and band formation are optimal under these conditions. Application of the samples (2–50 μl) is achieved using high-voltage electrophoresis filter papers (5 × 10 to 20 mm). The filter paper remains on the gel during isoelectric focusing.

D. Focusing Procedure

Isoelectric focusing (Awdeh et al., 1968) is performed at 4°C in a humidified box (Fig. 1). The electrodes are made dust- and particle-free by wiping. The upper circumference of the anode is wetted slightly with 5% phosphoric acid, whereas 5% ethylenediamine is used for the cathode. The plate prepared for focusing and loaded with samples is then placed with the gel side on the electrodes (sample side is anodal), without contact of the samples and the anode (Fig. 1). The mobile electrodes should be parallel to the short sides of the gel ends.

Focusing is then started with a current below 6.5 mA/plate. To reach the final 450 V/plate (the voltage at which the plates are subsequently run for 20 hr), the voltage is increased stepwise to approach 6.5 mA every 30 min for about 2 hr. After 20 hr, the voltage is increased to 600 V for 2–3 hr, at which time 1–2 mA/plate is reached.

For termination of a run, the voltage is disconnected from the box, the filter paper strips are carefully removed, and the plate is then processed further.

E. Determining the pH Gradient

The pH gradient established under focusing conditions is measured with a flat membrane electrode (Ingold, Zürich, Switzerland) and recorded on millimeter paper. This part should be performed quickly to avoid diffusion of the sample in the gel. An example will be given in Section IV,F for developing isoelectric focusing gels containing specific antibodies with isotope-labeled antigen. These conditions may be modified to optimize different antigen–antibody systems.

F. Antigen Binding and Autoradiography

Originally the technique was based on overlaying the gel at 37°C in a moist chamber for 45 min with phosphate-buffered saline, pH 7.2, containing 10 μCi of ^{131}I-labeled polysaccharide antigen (Williamson, 1971; Cramer and Braun, 1974; Askonas et al., 1970). We describe here, in detail, the method developed by Keck et al. (1973) and later used with slight modifications by Cramer et al. (1976), which we prefer because it results in gels of much higher quality.

Immerse the gel at room temperature in 400 ml of 18% buffered Na_2SO_4 (w/v) for 1 hr; change for fresh Na_2SO_4 three times. This step, like all subsequent steps, is carried out under constant slow rocking; the urea and Ampholines are washed out, and the immunoglobulins are precipitated.

Transfer the gel for an additional hour into 400 ml of 18% buffered Na_2SO_4 containing 0.05% glutaraldehyde (v/v). This step causes a mild cross-linking and thus insolubilizes the protein. Excess glutaraldehyde is then reduced by 10 $\mu g/ml$ of $NaBH_4$ in 400 ml of borate-buffered saline (BBS is 0.01 M borate, 0.15 M NaCl), pH 8.1, for 2 hr (three changes) with continued rocking.

The gel is washed for 30 min in BBS and then prepared for the addition of the isotope-labeled antigen. For this purpose, the Ilford plate with the gel is clamped to another glass plate, this time using a second type of silicone spacer tubing (i.d., 0.4 mm; o.d., 2.4 mm) to obtain a chamber with a free volume of about 30–35 ml between the gel and the second glass plate. The procedure for obtaining this chamber is the same as described above. The chamber, held in a vertical position, is slowly filled with BBS containing 10 μCi of iodinated antigen (specific activity, 0.5–2 $\mu Ci/\mu g$) and incubated for 16–18 hr at room temperature. The excess radioactive material is then poured off, the second glass plate is removed, and the gel is washed with constant slow rocking with three changes of BBS for 2 hr. It is then air-dried and autoradiographed.

Gels are autoradiographed on either Kodak RP Royal X-Omat RP/R-54 X-ray films or Agfa–Gevaert Osray M3-DW X-ray films for 12–72 hr for ^{131}I-labeled antigens. ^{125}I-Labeled antigens are less convenient because the exposure times may vary between 2 and 15 days.

G. Staining of Protein Patterns

The banding patterns of focused immunoglobulins are generally revealed by staining with either Coomassie brilliant blue dye or bromphenol blue dye.

For staining with Coomassie brilliant blue dye, the plates are first washed in 10% TCA for several hours to remove the Ampholines. Staining is carried out in 0.25% (w/v) Coomassie brilliant blue in methanol:distilled water:acetic acid (5:5:1) for 1 hr; destaining is achieved by keeping the plate in 7.5% acetic acid and 5% methanol (Awdeh et al., 1968).

For staining with bromphenol blue dye (pH 3.0–4.6), the gels are first treated (30 min) in a destaining solution (30% ethanol, 5% acetic acid, and 65% distilled water; 400 ml) to remove Ampholines and urea, followed by treatment with 0.1% bromphenol blue dye (w/v) in 40% ethanol, 5% acetic acid, and 55% distilled water for 60 min. Excess dye is subsequently removed with a destaining solution.

H. Preparing ^{131}I-Labeled Polysaccharide Antigen

Labeling the streptococcal group polysaccharide antigens with ^{131}I requires first its modification by introducing covalently bound tyramine that can function as an acceptor for the isotope. To achieve this, the polysaccharide is activated with cyanogen bromide and then reacted with tyramine.

Procedure

Ten milligrams of the purified group polysaccharides (Cramer and Braun, 1974), approximately 10^{-6} mole, is solubilized in distilled water. The pH is adjusted to 10.5–11 by adding 0.01 N NaOH. Two milligrams of cyanogen bromide (Fluka, Buchs, Switzerland) is added to this with constant stirring and the pH is adjusted by further addition of 0.01 M NaOH. After 6 min, the pH is reduced to 8.5 by adding 2 M NaHCO$_3$. Tyramine (13.7 mg, 10^{-4} mole; Fluka, Buchs, Switzerland) is dissolved in 1.0 ml of 1 M NaHCO$_3$ and added to the activated polysaccharide; this mixture is stirred at room temperature for 4–5 hr. The mixture is then dialyzed overnight against distilled water at 4°C. The ultraviolet spectrum (220–350 nm) of the polysaccharide is determined before and after tyramination.

The chloramine-T procedure is used for isotope labeling. Chloramine-T (2 mg/ml) and Na$_2$S$_2$O$_5$ (2.5 mg/ml) solutions are freshly prepared for iodination. One-tenth milliliter of 0.3 M sodium phosphate buffer, pH 7.5, is pipetted into a 3-ml plastic tube. To this 0.5 ml (2 mg/ml) of the tyraminated polysaccharide is added, followed by 0.1 ml of the chloramine-T solution. After 1 min, 1 mCi of carrier-free ^{131}I as sodium salt (Radiochemical Centre, Amersham, England) is added, mixed well, and reacted for 1 min. The reaction is stopped by adding a solution of Na$_2$S$_2$O$_5$. The reaction mixture is then placed into a small dialysis casing or run over a Sephadex G-25 column (0.5 × 2 cm) to remove unbound iodine (see Chapter 33), an aliquot is counted, and the specific activity of the polysaccharide is determined. The reagent prepared in this way is ready for use.

I. Isoelectric Focusing in Polymerizable Thin-Layer Sephadex Gels

This technique has the advantage that it is also applicable to IgM (Ziegler and Köhler, 1976; A. Ziegler and W. F. Riesen, unpublished).

Fifteen grams of Sephadex G-75 superfine (Pharmacia, Uppsala, Sweden) is stirred overnight at room temperature in 280 ml of solution containing 4% (w/v) acrylamide, 0.13% (w/v) N,N'-methylenebisacrylamide, and 2.8%

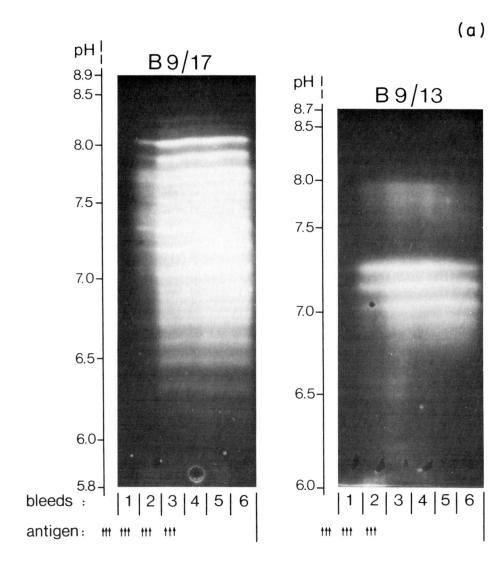

Fig. 2. Autoradiographs of isoelectric focusing patterns in 5% polyacrylamide slab gels developed by ^{125}I-labeled polysaccharide showing oligoclonal and multiclonal antibody produced *in vivo* and *in vitro*. pH scale is indicated. (a) Two mouse anti-streptococcal group A polysaccharide antisera, 15 μl, demonstrating pattern development and persistence after antigen administration (arrows). Bleeds are given in weeks after immunization was begun. Mouse B9/17 shows a heterogeneous response, and mouse B9/13 shows an oligoclonal response. (From Cramer and Braun, 1975.) (b) Patterns of 5 μl of antiserum (rabbit K27-293) to the streptococcal group A-variant polysaccharide and of pools from microculture

K 27- 293 (b)

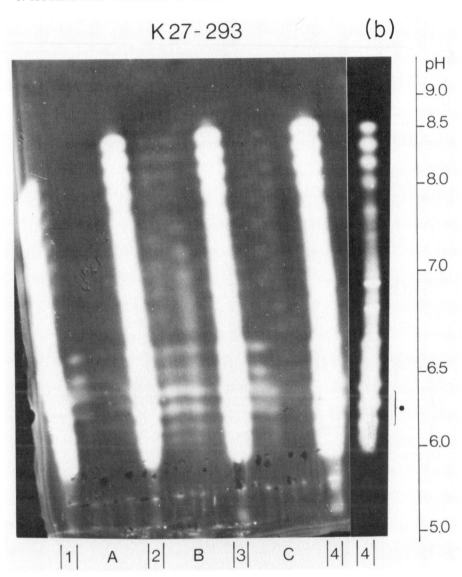

supernatants of blood lymphocytes from K27-293 stimulated by streptococcal A-variant vaccine (A–C). An asterisk marks the position of the dominant clonotype (14.5 mg of antibody/ml) in the antiserum. (From Braun et al., 1976.) (c, next page) Patterns of 30 µl of serum from patients with various acute streptococcal infections developed with iodinated group A polysaccharide with the exception of position 15': This pattern was developed with iodinated group A-variant polysaccharide (note the dominant cross-reactive clonotype). Normal human control serum (C) containing a single clonotype can also be seen. (From Riesen et al., 1976.)

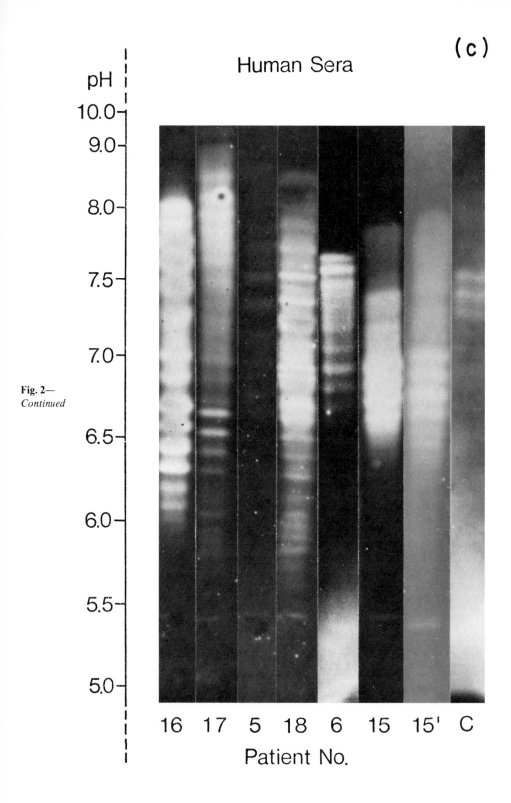

Fig. 2— *Continued*

(w/v) carrier ampholytes of the desired pH ranges. Ilford gelatin-coated glass plates are coated with the Sephadex gel to a thickness of 1 mm by means of a thin-layer spreader (DESAGA, Heidelberg, Germany). The coated plates are left at room temperature for 30 min prior to use. Application of the sample and isoelectric focusing are performed as described above, except that the electrodes are placed on the plate with the Sephadex layer and focusing is carried out for 18 hr, adjusting the initial voltage slowly to 150 V; 15 hr later the gels are run for an additional 3 hr at 500 V, the power never exceeding 1 W.

After completion of the run, the pH gradient is measured as described in Section IV,E and the Sephadex is then polymerized by spraying about 3 ml of a polymerization-inducing solution [1 M phosphate adjusted to pH 6.15 with Tris, 1% (v/v) TEMED, and 10% (w/v) ammonium persulfate] on the gel, followed by incubation of the plate under nitrogen. Polymerization is complete after 2 min provided the spraying solution is less than 1 week old. If milder conditions of polymerization are required, the following spray can be used: 1.6 mg of riboflavin and 0.4 ml of TEMED dissolved in 100 ml of distilled water or buffer. The plate is kept for 30 min under nitrogen and fluorescent light.

Staining of protein and identification of specific antibody by ^{131}I-labeled polysaccharide antigen are done as described above.

If intact 19 S IgM's are to be run, the Sephadex layer must also contain 8 M urea and 0.5% Nonidet P-40. Because immunoglobulins are denatured under these conditions, techniques of overlaying radioactive antigens cannot be employed.

V. APPLICATION, SENSITIVITY, AND REPRODUCIBILITY OF IEF

Analytical IEF has a wide range of applications for the detection of small differences in isoelectric points of various molecules and macromolecules (Righetti and Drysdale, 1974). Polyacrylamide gels exclude very large molecules (e.g., IgM) from separation, a difficulty that has been overcome by the use of polymerizable thin layers of Sephadex gels (Ziegler and Köhler, 1976). Focused proteins can be identified by a variety of techniques (Righetti and Drysdale, 1974); for example, enzymes can be identified by an overlay with substrate-impregnated paper (Delincée and Radola, 1971) and specific antibodies can be identified either by a hemolytic assay (Philips and Dresser, 1973) or by binding of isotope-labeled antigens and subsequent autoradiography (Williamson *et al.*, 1973; Williamson, 1971; Kreth and

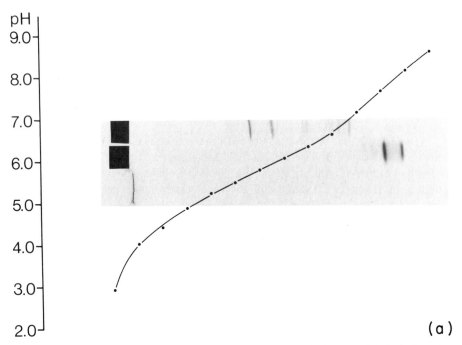

(a)

Fig. 3. Isoelectric focusing in 2.8% Ampholine containing Sephadex gels with the indicated pH gradients. (a) Patterns of 200 μg of Bence Jones protein Whi (top gel), 100 μg of sperm whale myoglobin (middle gel) and 50 μg of tomato bushy stunt virus (bottom gel) are shown. Stained with bromphenol blue. (From Ziegler and Köhler, 1976.) (b) Autoradiographs of two rabbit anti-streptococcal group A-variant antisera developed with the iodinated A-variant polysaccharide. (From Ziegler and Köhler, 1976.)

Williamson, 1973; Pink and Askonas, 1974; Braun *et al.*, 1973; Cramer and Braun, 1974; Wabl and Du Pasquier, 1976; Riesen *et al.*, 1976).

For detecting specific antibodies, the method has such high resolution power and sensitivity that several micrograms of clonally defined antibodies can be detected either in immune sera or in culture supernatants containing the products of specific lymphocyte clones secreted by several hundred cells (Braun *et al.*, 1976).

Analytical IEF is of particular usefulness in approaching the heterogeneity problem of specific antibodies (Williamson, 1971; Kreth and Williamson, 1973; Cramer and Bruan, 1974; Braun and Jaton, 1974). It has

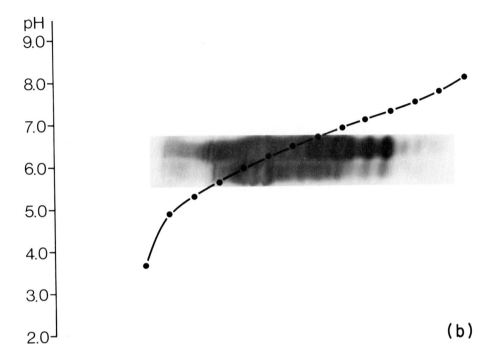

Fig. 3—*Continued*

a resolving power similar to anti-idiotypic antisera. In fact in well-documented cases of idiotypic identity of clonotypes, the IEF patterns were overlapping (Eichmann, 1972; Braun and Kelus, 1973). Since idiotypy and analytical IEF reveal different properties, there may be cases where more information is obtained by one or the other method. However, these cases have yet to be identified.

It is our experience that analytical IEF is a fast and reliable method for the genetic analysis of antibody responses at the clonotype level. The method may be regarded as being superior to idiotypic analysis when studying the expression of a number of clonotypes in the course of an immune response, since up to five to seven clonotypes may be identified within a single comparative run.

Examples of IEF under different conditions and with materials of different sources are provided in Figs. 2, 3, and 4. From Fig. 4 it is obvious that the overlay technique (Williamson, 1971; Cramer and Braun, 1974;

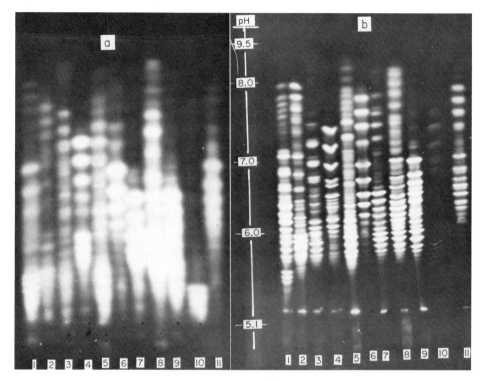

Fig. 4. Comparison of isoelectric focusing patterns of rabbit hyperimmune sera Nos. 1–11 with specificity for the streptococcal group A-variant polysaccharide (a) developed by the overlay technique (Williamson, 1971; Cramer and Braun, 1974; Askonas *et al.*, 1970) and (b) developed by the method of Keck *et al.* (1973).

Askonas *et al.*, 1970) is inferior to the method using slight cross-linking of the focused antibodies with glutaraldehyde followed by binding of isotope-labeled antigen (Keck, *et al.*, 1973; Cramer *et al.*, 1976).

REFERENCES

Askonas, B. A., Williamson, A. R., and Wright, B. E. G. (1970). *Proc. Natl. Acad. Sci. U.S.A.* **67,** 1398.

Awdeh, Z. L., Williamson, A. R., and Askonas, B. A. (1968). *Nature (London)* **219,** 66.

Braun, D. G., and Jaton, J.-C. (1974). *Curr. Top. Microbiol. Immunol.* **66,** 29.

Braun, D. G., and Kelus, A. S. (1973). *J. Exp. Med.* **138,** 1248.

Braun, D. G., Kjems, E., and Cramer, M. (1973). *J. Exp. Med.* **138,** 645.

Braun, D. G., Quintáns, J., Luzzati, A. L., Lefkovits, I., and Read, S. E. (1976). *J. Exp. Med.* **143,** 360.

Cramer, M., and Braun, D. G. (1974). *J. Exp. Med.* **139**, 1513.

Cramer, M., and Braun, D. G. (1975). *Scand. J. Immunol.* **4**, 63.

Cramer, M., Schwartz, M., Mozes, E., and Sela, M. (1976). *Eur. J. Immunol.* **6**, 618.

Delincée, H., and Radiola, B. J. (1971). *Protides Biol. Fluids, Proc. Colloq.* **18**, 493.

Eichmann, K. (1972). *Eur. J. Immunol.* **2**, 301.

Flatmark, T., and Vesterberg, O. (1966). *Acta Chem. Scand.* **20**, 1497.

Haglund, H. (1967). *Sci. Tools* **14**, 18.

Keck, K., Grossberg, A. L., and Pressman, D. (1973). *Eur. J. Immunol.* **3**, 99.

Kreth, H. W., and Williamson, A. R. (1973). *Eur. J. Immunol.* **3**, 141.

Philipps, J. M., and Dresser, D. W. (1973). *Eur. J. Immunol.* **3**, 524.

Pink, J. R. L., and Askonas, B. A. (1974). *Eur. J. Immunol.* **4**, 426.

Riesen, W. F., Skvaril, F., and Braun, D. G. (1976). *Scand. J. Immunol.* **5**, 383.

Righetti, P. G., and Drysdale, J. W. (1974). *J. Chromatogr.* **98**, 271.

Svensson, H. (1961). *Acta Chem. Scand.* **15**, 325.

Svensson, H. (1962a). *Acta Chem. Scand.* **16**, 456.

Svensson, H. (1962b). *Arch. Biochem. Biophys.*, *Suppl.* **1**, 132.

Vesterberg, O. (1967). *Acta Chem. Scand.* **21**, 206.

Vesterberg, O., and Svensson, H. (1966). *Acta Chem. Scand.* **20**, 820.

Wabl, M., and Du Pasquier, L. (1976). *Nature (London)* **264**, 642.

Williamson, A. R. (1971). *Eur. J. Immunol.* **1**, 390.

Williamson, A. R., Salaman, M. R., and Kreth, H. R. (1973). *Ann. N.Y. Acad. Sci.* **209**, 210.

Ziegler, A., and Köhler, G. (1976). *FEBS Lett.* **64**, 48.

6

Isolation of Monoclonal Antibody by Preparative Isoelectric Focusing in Horizontal Layers of Sephadex G-75

Wolfgang Schalch and Dietmar G. Braun

I. INTRODUCTION

Homogeneous antibodies are needed for the determination of the amino acid sequence, three-dimensional structure, and the production of anti-idiotypic antibodies in order to understand structure–function relationships in the immune system.

Homogeneous antibodies have been obtained mainly from myelomas (Eisen *et al.*, 1968). These antibodies, when tested by analytical isoelectric

IMMUNOLOGICAL METHODS
Copyright © 1979 by Academic Press, Inc.
All rights of reproduction in any form reserved.
ISBN 0-12-442750-2

focusing (IEF), generally consist of three to five bands (Askonas *et al.*, 1970). There is evidence that this microheterogeneity originates from minor modifications during and/or after secretion of the antibody (Awdeh *et al.*, 1970). Therefore, even with myeloma proteins, an additional purification step is necessary. This chapter discusses the application of preparative IEF for the isolation of rabbit monoclonal IgG starting with material of polyclonal origin.

II. PRINCIPLE OF THE METHOD

The general problem in preparative IEF is preventing convection and the concomitant remixing of separated zones.

The classical approach to preparative IEF (Vesterberg and Svensson, 1966) uses vertical columns filled with a sucrose gradient to stabilize the separation medium. Limitations of this method include the perturbance of zones caused by precipitating proteins during focusing and the partial remixing of focused proteins during emptying of the column. Effective separation, however, has been achieved in some cases (Hoffman *et al.*, 1972; Schalch and Bode, 1975). Both drawbacks are bypassed by IEF in a horizontal rather than a vertical plane. In this case, proteins eventually precipitating during the run do not interfere with adjacent zones. In addition to this, the free accessibility to the separation medium during all stages of the experiment makes it possible to apply the sample at any desired position as well as to limit diffusion immediately after focusing by partitioning defined areas of the separation medium.

Two methods have been proposed for horizontal preparative IEF. In the self-stabilizing zone convection electrophoresis described by Valmet (1969), a rather complicated apparatus is used in which focusing is carried out without added sucrose or the equivalent. The focused proteins themselves serve as the stabilizing medium.

On the other hand, a very simple apparatus is available for preparative IEF in horizontal layers in which granulated gels are used for the stabilization of the separation medium. This method was originally proposed by Radola (1974). Sephadex G-75, free from charged contaminants that would interfere with pH gradient formation, serves as the separation medium. The gel is prepared from a thin gel slurry by evaporation of water until a defined degree of gel consistency is reached.

The sample can, depending on its volume, be initially included into the gel or applied as a narrow zone at any desired position within the electrofocusing tray. Immediately after the run, a fractionating grid is pressed into the gel (in this way limiting diffusion), and the pH gradient is measured. The corresponding fractions are then scraped out and the protein is eluted from the gel with small amounts of suitable buffer. Every fraction is tested for purity by analytical IEF, and corresponding fractions are pooled. The protein is separated from ampholytes by gel filtration through a Sephadex G-50 column.

For the preparative IEF experiments described here we used LKB Multiphor equipment (LKB Produkter AB, Stockholm, Sweden) for electrophoresis in connection with the LKB Ampholine electrofocusing kit for granulated gels. By using the described technique, we were able to isolate single bands from rabbit IgG showing the usual multiband pattern.

III. MATERIAL

Multiphor, basic unit (LKB 2117)
Ampholine electrofocusing kit for granulated gels (LKB 2117-501) consisting of one 24.4 × 11.0 × 0.6-cm tray (Fig. 1a), one sample applicator (Fig. 1b), and one fractionating grid (Fig. 1c)
Electrode strips, 10.5 × 0.65 cm
Whatman No. 3 filter paper

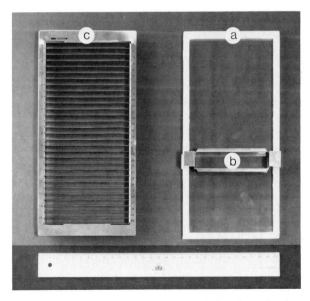

Fig. 1. Basic equipment for preparative IEF consisting of the gel tray (a), the sample applicator (b), and the fractionating grid (c).

Power supply (0–1000 V, 0–200 mA)
Ultrodex, that is, specially treated Sephadex G-75 superfine (available from LKB)
Small fan
40% Ampholine solution of desired pH range
30 Disposable syringes
pH meter with a flat-bed electrode (Ingold, Zürich, Switzerland)
1 *M* Orthophosphoric acid (anodic site)
1 *M* Sodium hydroxide (cathodic site)
Triple-distilled water, used for all solutions

IV. PROCEDURE

The procedure follows the LKB instruction manual (LKB application note 198) with minor modifications.

A. Sample

Dialyze the antibody solution or antiserum thoroughly against a 1% glycine solution. The maximum sample volume is 95 ml.

B. Preparation of the Gel Bed

Place on each end of the tray (Fig. 1a) three layers of electrode strips, which have been thoroughly soaked in a 2% (v/v) Ampholine solution. If the sample volume exceeds 3 ml, add 5 ml of a 40% Ampholine solution and make up to 100 ml with triple-distilled water in a 150-ml beaker. Add 4 gm of Ultrodex powder slowly, stirring slightly. When the mixture is homogenized, weigh the beaker, pour the gel suspension carefully on the tray, and determine the exact weight of the gel suspension delivered by reweighing the beaker. Mount a small fan above the tray and start evaporation with a light stream of air, taking care not to cause waves on the gel surface. The water loss is checked by occasionally weighing the tray. Stop evaporation when the water loss reaches the evaporation limit, which ranges, depending on the batch of Ultrodex, from 25 to 35% of the initial weight of the gel suspension. The useful value of the evaporation limit for each batch of Ultrodex is indicated on the Ultrodex bottle. The evaporation usually takes 100–150 min. The gel then has the proper consistency for starting the IEF experiment. If the sample volume is less than or equal to 3 ml, it can be applied as a narrow zone by using the sample applicator (Fig.

1b). In this case, adjust the Ampholine concentration of the sample to 2% (v/v), press the sample applicator at the desired position into the gel bed (already properly evaporated), add the sample, and mix thoroughly into the gel suspension within the applicator. Now remove the sample applicator and let the gel hydrostatically equilibrate for 2–3 min.

C. Focusing

Transfer the tray onto the cooling plate (5°C) of the Multiphor with a film of a 0.1% (w/v) aqueous SDS solution in between. Place one electrode strip soaked in 1 *M* phosphoric acid at the anode and another strip soaked in 1 *M* sodium hydroxide at the cathode each on top of the strips already in the tray. Connect the power lines and switch on the power supply, adjusting the voltage and current to yield a power of 7–8 W.

Under these conditions, the separation of IgG will be complete after approximately 24 hr.

D. pH Measurement

Immediately after switching off the power supply, press the fractionating grid (Fig. 1c) into the gel bed. In this way, the gel bed is sectioned into 30 partitions. Now measure the pH value in every compartment using a surface glass electrode (see Chapter 5). If a surface glass electrode of the proper size is not available, the pH can be measured with comparable precision after suspending the gel fractions in distilled water.

E. Elution of Fractions

The gel in each compartment of the fractionating grid is transferred with a spatula to a small column about 5 cm long, with a diameter of about 1 cm. These columns can easily be made using 5- or 10-ml disposable syringes with a piece of glass wool in the tip. The gel is then suspended in 2.5 ml of suitable buffer (usually PBS) or, if the pH measurement has not yet been performed, in distilled water. When the gel has settled and all of the solution has entered the gel, terminate elution by adding about 2.0 ml of buffer. The eluates are collected in small reagent tubings.

F. Analysis of Fractions

For the preliminary inspection of the separation, we did not use a print technique of the gel surface as suggested by LKB because of substantial loss of material. After complete elution, the volumes are equalized and the optical density is measured at 280 nm. A detailed picture of the separation, however, is obtained by direct analysis of all fractions by analytical IEF. In this way also, more exact information is gained as to what fractions can be pooled. Naturally, a protein determination according to Lowry *et al.* (1951) is not possible at this stage because of the presence of the ampholytes.

G. Separation of Protein and Ampholytes

After pooling the fractions, the volume is reduced by ultrafiltration or lyophilization to a sufficiently small size. Gel filtration on Sephadex G-50 (fine) equilibrated with a suitable buffer is then carried out. A column 20 cm long with a diameter of 2.5 cm can desalt samples of up to a volume of 6 ml.

V. APPLICATIONS

Figure 2 shows the analytical IEF pattern of successive fractions of a preparative IEF run. The analytical IEF was evaluated by the technique described in Chapter 5, that is, overlaying with ^{131}I-labeled antigen (A-variant streptococcal carbohydrate). The material applied was the main fraction from a preparative agarose block electrophoresis run (Braun and Krause, 1968; see also Chapter 2) of a single rabbit antiserum. In the example shown, 150 mg of IgG antibody was applied for the preparative run. The total amount of protein that can be applied depends on the heterogeneity of the sample and the range of the pH gradient chosen. The maximum amount of protein in a single-focused zone varies from about 5 mg for wide-range pH gradients (about pH 3.5–10) to about 40–50 mg for narrow-range between 60 and 70% of the starting material.

VI. LIMITATIONS

Preparative IEF of whole sera is limited by the total amount of serum albumin in the sample; its total amount per run should not exceed 10–20 mg for wide-range pH gradients and 80–100 mg for narrow-range pH gradients. Therefore, it is always advantageous to prepurify the antibody from the serum by ammonium sulfate precipitation, preparative agarose block electrophoresis, affinity chromatography, or a suitable combination of these methods (see Chapter 2).

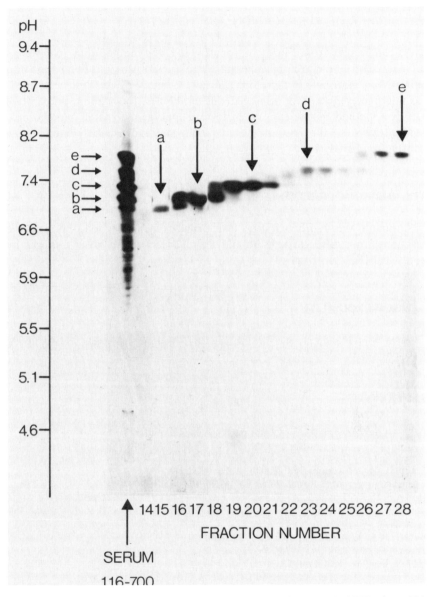

Fig. 2. ^{131}I-Labeled A-variant carbohydrate autoradiograph of an analytical IEF gel on which successive fractions of a preparative IEF experiment were applied. The preparative run was carried out with 150 mg of prepurified IgG from serum 116-700. pH gradient, 6–8; focusing time, 20 hr. The letters correlate the purified preparations to the bands present in the original antiserum, which was obtained from a rabbit hyperimmunized with A-variant streptococcal vaccine.

VII. DEGREE OF PURIFICATION AND SENSITIVITY

As can be seen from Fig. 2, preparative IEF is a method that achieves an efficient subfractionation of coherent clonotypes of three to five bands into single-band material. It therefore also allows study of the molecular basis for microheterogeneity of homogeneous antibodies. In addition, preparative IEF is a method that selectively enriches clonotype-associated bands of low concentration in the immune serum. This material escapes detection by conventional analysis.

VIII. REPRODUCIBILITY

Although the reproducibility from run to run is good, pooling the fractions from different runs should only be carried out after analysis by analytical IEF.

ACKNOWLEDGMENT

W. S. was the recipient of a EMBO long-term fellowship and thanks EMBO for the financial support.

REFERENCES

Askonas B. A., Williamson, A. R., and Wright, B. E. G. (1970). *Proc. Natl. Acad. Sci. U.S.A.* **67,** 1398.

Awdeh, Z. L., Williamson, A. R., and Askonas, B. A. (1970). *Biochem. J.* **116,** 241.

Braun, D. G., and Krause, R. M. (1968). *J. Exp. Med.* **128,** 969.

Eisen, H. N., Simms, E. S., and Potter, M. (1968). *Biochemistry* **7,** 4026.

Hoffman, D. R., Grossberg, A. L., and Pressman, D. (1972). *J. Immunol.* **108,** 18.

Lowry, O. H., Rosebrough, N. J., Farr, A. L., and Randall, R. J. (1951). *J. Biol. Chem.* **193,** 265.

Radola, B. J. (1974). *Biochim. Biophys. Acta* **386,** 181.

Schalch, W., and Bode, W. (1975). *Biochim. Biophys. Acta* **405,** 292.

Valmet, E. (1969). *Sci. Tools.* **16,** 8.

Vesterberg, O., and Svensson, H. (1966). *Acta Chem. Scand.* **20,** 820.

7

Isotachophoresis of Immunoglobulins

Andreas Ziegler and Georges Köhler

1. INTRODUCTION

Immunoglobulins of one class (e.g., IgG) are closely related molecules, and, if different binding or antigenic properties cannot be exploited, the only discriminative characteristic for analytical work is their isoelectric point. This characteristic has been widely employed since the original demonstration that isoelectric focusing (IEF) in polyacrylamide gels may be used to distinguish between IgG species (Awdeh et al., 1968).

One of the drawbacks of IEF in polyacrylamide slab gels is the size restriction exerted on very large molecules, but this problem has recently been solved by the use of polymerizable thin layers containing Sephadex as an anticonvective medium (Ziegler and Köhler, 1976a; see also Chapter 5). Other, more serious, disadvantages are the sensitivity of many proteins to low ionic strength in the medium in which focusing is carried out and the tendency of these molecules to precipitate during the focusing procedure.

These problems can, at least in the cases we have studied, be overcome by using isotachophoresis (ITP), an electrophoretic method based on Kohlrausch's (1897) "regulating function." In this procedure, ions are separated according to their different electrophoretic mobilities so that they align in order of descending mobility between two appropriately chosen ions, one of which (the "leading ion") has a higher mobility than the other (the "terminating ion"). Since the regulating function is valid for both small and large ionic species, proteins can be analyzed without difficulty provided certain requirements are met.

IMMUNOLOGICAL METHODS
Copyright © 1979 by Academic Press, Inc.
All rights of reproduction in any form reserved.
ISBN 0-12-442750-2

These requirements are as follows.

1. The medium in which ITP is carried out must not restrict the molecules sterically.
2. Leading and terminating ions must be chosen so that the ions to be discriminated have an electrophoretic mobility intermediate between the leading and terminating ions.
3. The type and amount of spacer molecules must be chosen very carefully (spacers are ions that are able to increase the separation between sample molecules with different mobilities because of their intermediate mobility).

With these three requirements in mind, it is possible to exploit the two most attractive features of analytical ITP (Ornstein, 1964; Haglund, 1970; Routs, 1971; Jovin, 1973); that is, the ionic strength in the system can be regulated over a wide range, and the sample ions carry a net charge. Thus, precipitation of proteins at or near their isoelectric points is avoided.

We describe a procedure for ITP in polyacrylamide slab gels found to be suitable for the analysis of radioactivity labeled murine IgG species secreted by cell lines in culture (Ziegler and Köhler, 1976b).

II. PROCEDURE

A slab gel apparatus as described by Studier (1973) is used, but we employ gels with a thickness of 0.1 cm. The following stock solutions are required.

Solution A: Phosphate, 1 *M*, adjusted to pH 6.5 with tris(hydroxymethyl)aminomethane (Tris)

Solution B: Acrylamide (32%, w/v)/*N,N'*-diallyltartardiamide (DATD) (5.7%, w/v) (both from Serva, Heidelberg, West Germany) in distilled water

Solution C: *N,N,N'N'*-Tetramethylethylenediamine (TEMED)

Solution D: Ammonium persulfate (15 mg/ml) (should be freshly prepared)

The leading buffer is 0.05 *M* phosphate adjusted to pH 6.5 with Tris; the terminating buffer is 0.3 *M* 6-aminocaproic acid adjusted to pH 9.1 with Tris. Carrier ampholytes (Ampholine, LKB Produkter AB, Stockholm, Sweden) of pH 3.5–10 are used as spacers. Bromphenol blue (BPB) serves at the tracking dye.

The two glass plates and the three spacers are clamped together as described by Studier (1973) and sealed by pouring 2% (w/v) agarose along the edges. Solution A, 2 ml, solution B, 5 ml, and 31 ml of water are mixed and degassed for 5 min with a water suction pump; 0.03 ml of solution C and 2 ml of solution D are then added, the mixture is poured between the glass plates, and a slot-former (10–25 shots) is inserted (for details of this procedure, see Chapter 4).

When the gel has set, the spacer at the bottom of the gel and the slot-former are removed. The slab gel is attached to the electrophoresis apparatus, the lower chamber is filled with leading buffer, and air bubbles are removed from the lower edge of the gel. The terminating buffer is

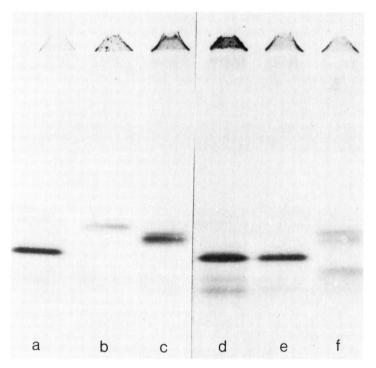

Fig. 1. Isotachophoresis of six different [^{14}C]lysine-labeled immunoglobulin G-containing culture supernatants. The run was performed in the presence of Ampholine spacers in a DATD-cross-linked polyacrylamide slab gel. Samples were made up as described in Section II; each contained 20 μl of pH 3.5–10 Ampholine. The electrophoresis was carried out for 18 hr; the cathode is on top. (a) P3-X63 Ag8 (a myeloma line, secreting an IgG containing γ_1 and κ chains. (b) Sp2/HL (γ_{2b}; κ)—*Note:* Sp–lines are cloned sublines from myeloma × spleen cell fusions (Köhler and Milstein, 1976); they secrete immunoglobulins whose heavy and light chains are named H and L when derived from the spleen cell and G and K (for γ and κ) when derived from the myeloma parent (here always P3-X63 Ag8). (c) Sp2/HK (γ_{2b};κ). (d) Sp3/HK (γ_1;κ). (e) Sp3/HLK (γ_1;κ). (f) PlBul (a myeloma line, γ_{2a};κ; expresses also free light chains). (From Ziegler and Köhler, 1976b.)

placed in the upper chamber, so that all slots are completely filled with liquid. (The buffer in the upper chamber cannot flow down between the glass plate and apparatus because Vaseline or silicone grease is first applied horizontally.)

Samples are made up by mixing a suitable amount of radioactively labeled cell culture supernatant (in our experiments, usually 50 μl) with 100 μl of 25% (w/v) sucrose/0.005% (w/v) BPB in water. Ampholine is added in varying amounts depending on the experiment, but samples of a given run should always contain the same amount of Ampholine.

The sample mixtures are applied, using a Hamilton syringe, to the individual gel slots. Anode and cathode are connected with the reservoirs containing the leading and terminating buffers, respectively. The gel is run at room temperature at a constant current of 5 mA for different periods of time, depending on the amount of Ampholine present. Typical experiments take 12–24 hr (0–50 μl of Ampholine per slot).

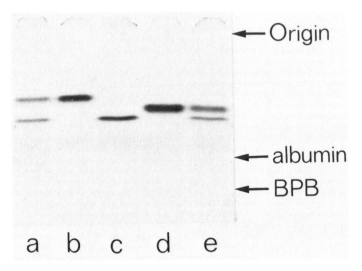

Fig. 2. Isotachophoresis of [^{14}C]lysine-labeled immunoglobulin G-containing culture supernatants in a DATD-cross-linked slab gel. The samples contained 20 μl of pH 3.5–10 Ampholine, sucrose, and BPB as described in Section II; conditions of electrophoresis were as in Fig. 1. The positions of sample application, serum albumin, and front marker are indicated. (a) 25 μl of W6/32 + 25 μl of P3-X63 Ag8 (mixture of fetal calf and horse serum)—*Note:* The W6– lines are cloned lines secreting antibody directed against human cell-surface antigens. They are derived from myeloma (P3-NSI/1-Ag4-1) × spleen cell fusions and are fully described in the article by Barnstable *et al.* (1978). (b) 50 μl of W6/32 (supernatant contains 10% fetal calf serum). (c) 50 μl of P3-X63 Ag8 (supernatant contains 10% horse serum). (d) 50 μl of W6/34 (supernatant contains 10% fetal calf serum). (e) 25 μl of W6/34 + 25 μl of P3-X63 Ag8 (mixture of fetal calf and horse sera).

The gel is then carefully removed and stained for 1.5 hr in 0.2% (w/v) BPB in ethanol:distilled water:acetic acid (100:85:15, v/v/v); destaining is achieved by treating for 6 hr in ethanol:distilled water:acetic acid (6:13:1, v/v/v). The stained gel is then placed on wet cellophane and covered by a slightly larger piece of wet Whatman 3MM paper. The sandwich is placed, cellophane side up, on a drying block. The cellophane is pressed on the block with a heavy frame. The gel is then dried by a combination of negative pressure and heat. A simpler procedure is to use one of the commercially available gel slab dryers; we have had good experience with Model 224 from Bio-Rad Laboratories, Richmond, California. The gel is finally auto-radiographed (for example, on Kodak RP Royal X-Omat films).

Two typical examples of an isotachophoretic separation of radioactive immunoglobulins are presented in Figs. 1 and 2; the immunoglobulins depicted in slots b and c of the gel in Fig. 1 and slots b and d of the gel in Fig. 2 do not give detectable patterns after IEF because they precipitate at low ionic strength.

III. DISCUSSION

The procedure of analytical ITP in polyacrylamide slab gels has been shown to be suitable for proteins that precipate in low ionic strength solutions, for example, under the conditions of IEF (Ziegler and Köhler, 1976b). IgG species differing only in the variable part of their light chains could be discriminated (Fig. 1, slot b versus slot c).

This method has also been successfully applied to other immunoglobulins with similar properties (Barnstable et al., 1978; A. Ziegler, unpublished observations). However, comparisons of different immunoglobulins by ITP have an important limitation: Since all negatively charged ionic species in a sample add to the spacing effect of the Ampholine, it is impossible to compare side-by-side samples (such as sera) containing widely varying amounts of individual ionic species, a property that does not affect IEF. On the other hand, identity or nonidentity of components in two different samples might be determined by mixing the two samples. This drawback has been avoided in our experiments because all samples contained identical amounts of unlabeled ionic species (10% horse or fetal calf serum) in vast excess over the radioactive IgG to be analyzed. Another limitation of ITP as compared to IEF in polymerizable Sephadex gels (Ziegler and Köhler, 1976a) is the steric hindrance exerted on large molecules (for example, IgM) by conventional polyacrylamide gels. Among the advantages of our method, mentioned above, are the possibility of running proteins that cannot be focused because of their solubility properties, the use of a standard apparatus for gel electrophoresis, and the low costs of an experiment.

REFERENCES

Awdeh, A. L., Williamson, A. R., and Askonas, B. A. (1968). *Nature (London)* **219**, 66.
Barnstable, C. J., Bodmer, W. F., Brown, G., Galfrè, G., Milstein, C., Williams, A. F., and Ziegler, A. (1978). *Cell* **14**, 9.
Haglund, H. (1970). *Sci. Tools* **17**, 2.
Jovin, T. M. (1973). *Biochemistry* **12**, 871.
Köhler, G., and Milstein, C. (1976). *Eur. J. Immunol.* **6**, 511.
Kohlrausch, F. (1897). *Ann. Phys. (Leipzig)* [3] **62**, 209.
Ornstein, L. (1964). *Ann. N.Y. Acad. Sci.* **121**, 321.
Routs, R. J.(1971). Ph.D. Dissertation, Eindhoven University of Technology, Eindhoven.
Studier, F. W. (1973). *J. Mol. Biol.* **79**, 237.
Ziegler, A., and Köhler, G. (1976a). *FEBS Lett.* **64**, 48.
Ziegler, A., and Köhler, G. (1976b). *FEBS Lett.* **71**, 142.

8

The Chemical Modification of Proteins, Haptens, and Solid Supports

Hansruedi Kiefer

I. INTRODUCTION

The preparation of antigens or derivatized solid supports often causes considerable problems to nonchemists. Therefore, I will discuss some of the basic reaction mechanisms. With this knowledge, it should be easier to apply established procedures to new systems. All of the methods described in this chapter are of general use and can easily be adapted to a variety of different molecules or supports. However, it is absolutely essential to make certain that the following conditions are met before starting on a new synthesis.

1. The solvents must be compatible with the reagents.
2. The pH and temperature requirements must be considered.
3. The stability of the reagents (especially proteins) must be preserved under the above conditions.

4. Unwanted side reactions (e.g., cross-linking) should be excluded.
5. If different rates of reaction are expected, the reaction time or temperature must be adjusted.

II. THEORETICAL BACKGROUND

A. Haptens—Macromolecules

1. *Proteins and Poly(Amino Acids)*

To avoid cross-linking of proteins, it is advantageous to activate the hapten, rather than some functional groups of the protein molecule. Two reaction mechanisms are important: (a) nucleophilic substitution and (b) azo coupling. While nucleophilic reactions with proteins involve primarily the ϵ-amino group of lysine, azo coupling occurs predominantly on tyrosine and histidine.

Examples of nucleophilic substitution are given in Reactions (1)–(3). An example of azo coupling is shown in Reaction (4).

It is important to note that the rates of all these reactions are pH dependent (pH 8–9) and that nucleophilic substitution on aromatic rings requires at least two NO_2 substituents (in the ortho or para position) in order to proceed at reasonable rates. The —SO_3H group can also be replaced by —F or —Cl (e.g., 2,4-dinitrofluorobenzene or picryl chloride).

The optimal rate for the coupling of diazonium salts to tyrosine lies at approximately pH 8, but the reaction can also be carried out at lower pH. The pH optimum for coupling to aromatic amines, however, is about 6.

2. Carbohydrates

For soluble as well as insoluble carbohydrates, cyanogen bromide or chloroacetate activation is usually the method of choice. An example of activation is shown in Reaction (5); examples of coupling are seen in Reactions (6)–(8).

$$\begin{array}{c}
\overset{|}{HC}-OH \\
\overset{|}{HC}-OH \\
\overset{|}{}
\end{array}
\quad \xrightarrow[-HBr]{CNBr} \quad
\left[\begin{array}{c}
\overset{|}{HC}-OH \\
\overset{|}{HC}-O-C\equiv N \\
\overset{|}{}
\end{array}\right]_{H_2O}$$

(5)

Reactive

$$\begin{array}{c}
\overset{|}{HC}-O \\
\overset{|}{HC}-O
\end{array}\!\!\!\bigg\rangle C=NH$$

Nonreactive

$$\begin{array}{c}
\overset{|}{HC}-OH \\
\overset{|}{HC}-O-\underset{\underset{O}{\|}}{C}-NH_2 \\
\overset{|}{}
\end{array}$$

Isourea

$$\begin{array}{c}
\overset{NH}{\overset{\|}{}} \\
\overset{|}{HC}-O-C-NH-R \\
\overset{|}{HC}-OH \\
\overset{|}{}
\end{array}$$

N-Substituted imidocarbonate

$$\begin{array}{c}
\overset{|}{HC}-O \\
\overset{|}{HC}-O
\end{array}\!\!\!\bigg\rangle C=N-R$$

N-Substituted carbamate

$$\begin{array}{c}
\overset{|}{HC}-O \\
\overset{|}{HC}-O
\end{array}\!\!\!\bigg\rangle C=NH \;+\; NH_2-R \longrightarrow$$

(6)

$$\begin{array}{c}
\overset{O}{\overset{\|}{}} \\
\overset{|}{HC}-O-C-NH-R \\
\overset{|}{HC}-OH \\
\overset{|}{}
\end{array}$$

$$\begin{array}{c}
\overset{|}{HC}-OH \\
\overset{|}{HO}-CH \\
\overset{|}{}
\end{array}
\;+\;
\begin{array}{c}
Cl \\
\overset{|}{CH_2}-COO^- \, Na^+
\end{array}
\longrightarrow
\begin{array}{c}
\overset{|}{HC}-O-CH_2-COO^- \, Na^+ \\
\overset{|}{HO}-CH \\
\overset{|}{}
\end{array}
\;+\; HCl$$

(7)

$$HC-O-CH_2-C\overset{O}{\underset{OH}{\|}} + \overset{N}{\underset{N}{\|}}\overset{R_1}{C}\overset{R_1}{\underset{R_2}{}} \xrightarrow{EDC} HC-O-CH_2-C\overset{O}{\|}-O-C\overset{HN^{R_1}}{\underset{N_{R_2}}{\|}}$$

(8)

$$HC-O-CH_2-C\overset{O}{\|}-O-C\overset{HN^{R_1}}{\underset{NH_2}{\|}} \xrightarrow{EDA} \begin{array}{l} HC-O-CH_2-C\overset{O}{\|}-NH-CH_2-CH_2-NH_2 \\ + \\ R_1-NH-C\overset{O}{\|}-NH-R_2 \end{array}$$

Cyanogen bromide activation requires a high pH (10.5–11.5), but the coupling reaction of an amine to the activated polysaccharide proceeds easily in 0.1 M NaHCO$_3$. This method is essentially that used for the preparation of affinity chromatography columns (Cuatrecasas, 1970).

The first step in the chloroacetate procedure used by Inman (1975) for the preparation of derivatized Ficoll antigens is also carried out at very high pH (1 N NaOH). At this point, it is appropriate to discuss the mechanism of the widely used carbodiimide method, which is the second step in this activation reaction.

The reaction of an amine with a carboxylic acid leads to amide formation, provided the carboxyl group is activated. Activation in this case means formation of an intermediate O-acylisourea. This intermediate cannot be isolated because it is unstable in aqueous solutions. However, it reacts in the presence of amines to form the desired amide. The first part of this two-step mechanism is catalyzed by protonation of one of the imide nitrogens and therefore requires slightly acidic conditions, whereas the second step involves a free amine. Under these conditions, it is not surprising that the reaction proceeds with optimal rates over a fairly large pH range (4.5–7). It should be remembered that carbodiimide coupling to proteins will always result in some degree of protein cross-linking, since both reaction partners are present on the same molecule. Carbodiimides react not only with carboxylic acids, but also with water, phenols, sulfhydryls, amines, and alcohols, often leading to rather stable intermediates.

An interesting new method of activating Sephadex has recently been published by Wilson and Nakane (1976). The method involves periodate oxidation for activation, followed by NaBH$_4$ reduction of a Schiff base. An example of this type of activation is shown in Reaction (9). A coupling reaction is shown in Reaction (10).

(9)

(10)

B. Haptens—Solid Supports

Solid supports have been used primarily in immunology to bind specific antibodies, antigens, or cells for purification purposes. They come in various forms, such as fibers, tubes, dishes, or beads. Our list shall be restricted to the following materials: (a) polysaccharide beads, (b) polystyrene beads and dishes, and (c) nylon fibers.

1. Polysaccharide Beads

Affinity chromatography on hapten-derivatized polysaccharide beads (e.g., Sepharose) is widely used for the purification of specific antibodies. The cyanogen bromide-activated beads are commercially available (Pharmacia, Uppsala, Sweden) and can be derivatized readily with any amine. Spacers can be introduced by using diamines of the type $H_2N(CH_2)_nNH_2$. The reactions involved have been described in Section II,A,2.

2. Polystyrene Tubes, Dishes, or Beads (Latex)

Polystyrene is often copolymerized with divinylbenzene or acrylic acid, the latter introducing aliphatic carboxyl groups, which can be derivatized (carboxyl latexes). These polymers always contain varying amounts of ionic or nonionic detergents, the hydrophilic groups of which are exposed on the surface and, aside from carboxyl groups, produce a net surface charge. These surface charges, incidentally, prevent latex beads from self-agglutination.

One method of introducing functional groups into polystyrene, which works for tubes, dishes, and beads, is nitration followed by reduction of the nitro group to yield aromatic amines [Reaction (11)].

$$(11)$$

The aromatic amines have the advantage of providing a number of useful coupling possibilities. The reaction with carbodiimide-activated carboxylic acids has been discussed (Section II,A,2). Another reaction involves the preparation of diazonium salts and subsequent azo coupling [Reaction (12)].

$$(12)$$

It is also possible to produce light-sensitive aromatic azides used to make covalent bonds in photoaffinity labeling (Layer *et al.*, 1976) [Reactions (13) and (14)].

$$(13)$$

$$(14)$$

It should be remembered that most polystyrenes are soluble in organic solvents, such as ethers and acetone.

3. Nylon

Nylon (6–6) is a copolymer of hexamethylenediamine and adipic acid [Reaction (15)] and is used to make molded articles, as well as fibers.

$$\text{HOOC}-(CH_2)_4-\text{COOH} \quad + \quad H_2N-(CH_2)_6-NH_2$$

$$\downarrow 280° \tag{15}$$

$$\left[\begin{matrix} O & O \\ \| & \| \\ -C(CH_2)_4-C-NH-(CH_2)_6-NH- \end{matrix} \right]_n \quad + \quad H_2O$$

Suspension polymerization does not yield beads, as is the case with styrene, but results in vesicle formation ["Artificial Cells" (Chang, 1972)]. For modification, terminal amino and carboxyl groups are available. The number of these functional groups at the surface can be increased by mild acid hydrolysis (3 N HCl). Unlike polystyrenes, nylon is insoluble in most organic solvents. The range of chemical reactions for modification is, therefore, much wider. A reaction sequence introducing a cleavable spacer molecule is shown by Reaction (16).

The terminal amino group can now be used for coupling to haptens or antigens, for examples, with carbodiimide.

Woodward K reagent

Activation

(17)

Coupling

Activation of carboxyl groups on nylon fibers in aqueous solution is best accomplished by Reaction (17).

C. Proteins—Solid Supports

The main contribution to this type of coupling reaction certainly comes from the field of immobilized enzymes. Basically, the same methods can be applied as for haptens, provided the support is activated. As mentioned before, activation of proteins often leads to unwanted cross-linking of the macromolecules. In addition to the reactions shown in the previous sections, there are a number of useful bifunctional reagents for coupling, some of which are listed below.

4,4'-Difluoro-3,3'-dinitro-
phenylsulfone (water insoluble)
(MacLeod and Hill, 1968)

Dimethyl adipimidate

(Dutton *et al.*, 1966)

$$N_2^+ - \langle\bigcirc\rangle - \langle\bigcirc\rangle - N_2^+ \qquad S=C=N-\langle\bigcirc\rangle-N=C=S$$

Bisdiazobenzidine
(Silman and Katchalski, 1966)

Phenyl-1, 4-diisothiocyanate
(Laursen et al., 1972)

Except for bisdiazobenzidine, these reagents react with nucleophiles ($-NH_2$).

III. EXPERIMENTATION

A. Haptens—Macromolecules

1. TNP-KLH [Reaction (1)]

At room temperature, 500 mg of KLH (Calbiochem, La Jolla, California) and 500 mg of K_2CO_3 in 25 ml of distilled water were stirred overnight. The cloudy solution was centrifuged for 20 min at 27,000 g in a Sorvall centrifuge and the supernatant was added to 500 mg of TNP-sulfonate in 25 ml of a 0.1 M K_2CO_3 solution. The reaction mixture was stirred overnight at room temperature and then dialyzed exhaustively against 0.01 M $NaHCO_3$ and twice against PBS and again centrifuged, if necessary.

The TNP content was measured in an ultraviolet spectrophotometer at 348 nm (E_m = 15,400). From the protein concentration, measured by the method of Lowry, a TNP content of 23 moles/protein molecular weight of 100,000 was calculated.

This procedure has successfully been used for BSA, ovalbumin, and GLT (copolymer L-Glu:L-Lys:L-Tyr, 62:34:4).

2. DNP-Ficoll (Inman, 1975)

a. Preparation of Carboxymethylated Ficoll (CM_{83}-Ficoll) [Reaction (7)]. A stock solution of 1.35 M sodium chloroacetate was prepared as follows: 64.4 gm of Chloroacetic acid was dissolved in a mixture of 300 ml of distilled water and 135 ml of 5.0 N NaOH. The solution was cooled to 25°C, adjusted to pH 6.8–7.2 with either 5 N NaOH or 10% (w/v) chloroacetic acid, and made up to 500 ml with distilled water.

The components of this reaction mixture were preheated to 40°C. Ficoll (13.3 gm) was dissolved in 185 ml of 1.35 M sodium chloroacetate. Fifty milliliters of 10.0 N NaOH was added with mixing (zero time), and the volume was made up to 250 ml with distilled water. Thus, the reaction mixture was initially 1.0 *M* in chloroacetate and 2.0 *M* in NaOH. The mixture was placed in a 40°C constant-temperature bath. After 30 min, 10 ml of 2.0 *M* NaH$_2$PO$_4$ was added and the whole batch was adjusted to pH 7 with 5 *N* HCl. The neutral solutions were dialyzed in the cold (4°C) against one or two daily changes of toluene-saturated distilled water for 4 or 5 days. One milliliter of toluene was shaken with each 2 liters of dialysis water in order to retard or prevent microbial growth.

The dialyzed solution was either used directly in the next reaction step or lyophilized for storage.

b. Preparation of N-(2-aminoethyl)carbamylmethylated Ficoll (AECM-Ficoll) [Reaction (8)]. The volume of dialyzed solution from a preparation of CM$_{83}$-Ficoll was measured. Ethylenediamine dihydrochloride (Eastman Organic Chemicals, Rochester, New York) was added and dissolved to the extent of 14.3 gm/100 ml of dialysate. The pH was adjusted to 4.7 with 1 *N* NaOH, and EDC·HCl (1.25 gm/100 ml of dialysate) was added with stirring over a 10-min period. During this time and for the next 3.5 hr, the pH was kept near 4.7 by adding 1 *N* HCl (or 1 *N* NaOH) as required. The solution was dialyzed in the cold against two daily changes of toluene-saturated 0.5 *M* NaCl for 2 days and against daily changes of toluene-saturated distilled water for 4 more days. The AECM-Ficoll was recovered by lyophilization.

c. Preparation of 2,4-Dinitrophenylated AECM-Ficoll (DNP–AECM-Ficoll). AECM-Ficoll was dinitrophenylated to different degrees with either (1) 1-fluoro-2,4-dinitrobenzene (FDNB) or (2) NaDNBS as follows.

1. A buffer was prepared having the composition 0.20 *M* Bicine [*N,N*-bis(2-hydroxyethyl)glycine] and 0.10 *M* NaOH (pH 8.35). Into 3.0 ml of this buffer was dissolved 180 mg of AECM-Ficoll (previously prepared from CM^{83}-Ficoll). Three milliliters of ethanol and 21 μl (for other volumes, see Table I) of 1.0 *M* FDNB (Eastman Organic Chemicals) in ethanol were added. The mixture was allowed to stand in the dark at room temperature for 2.5 hr, dialyzed in the cold against toluene-saturated distilled water for 3 days, clarified by centrifugation, and lyophilized.

2. AECM$_{83}$-Ficoll (636 mg, 1.5 μmoles) was dissolved in 10 ml of carbonate buffer (0.946 *M* Na$_2$CO$_3$, 0.054 *M* NaHCO$_3$, pH 10.6). Dissolution was achieved by stirring and manipulating with a glass rod for about 15 min. Na-DNBS was added and dissolved. The amounts used in several experiments are shown in Table II. The mixture was shaken with several drops of toluene and allowed to stand in the dark

TABLE I

Reaction of AECM-Ficoll with FDNB[a]

FDNB added[b] (μmoles)	FDNB added per mole of Ficoll (moles)	DNP bound per mole of Ficoll[c] (moles)	Percentage of FDNB bound
21	49	48	98
30	71	58	82
42	99	66	67

[a] From Inman (1975).

[b] This number of microliters of 1.0 M FDNB (in ethanol) was added to 180 mg (0.425 μmole) of $AECM_{83}$-Ficoll in aqueous Bicine and ethanol buffer, pH 8.35.

[c] The value, n, is determined spectrophotometrically. The term used, mole of Ficoll, refers to 4×10^5 gm of Ficoll not including the weight of added groups. Thus, n is actually an epitope density based on a calculated dry weight and is not dependent on the actual molecular weight, which is somewhat uncertain. However, a useful idea of the average number of haptenic groups per molecular unit is conveyed by this figure.

at room temperature for 2.7 days. The deep yellow solution was then dialyzed for 2 days in the cold against 0.2 M NaCl and for 3 days against distilled water, clarified by centrifugation, and lyophilized.

B. Haptens—Solid Supports

1. DNP-Lys-Sepharose

a. Sepharose Activation (Givol et al., 1970) [Reaction (5)]. For activation, 4.5 gm (wet weight) of washed Sepharose 4B (Pharmacia) was suspended in

TABLE II

Reaction of AECM-Ficoll with Na-DNBS at pH 10.6[a]

Na-DNBS added[b] (mg)	Na-DNBS added per mole of Ficoll (moles)	DNP bound per mole of Ficoll[c] (moles)	Percentage of Na-DNBS bound
36.5	90	10	11
142	350	39	11
365	900	56	6

[a] From Inman (1975).

[b] Added to 636 mg (1.5 μmoles) of $AECM_{83}$-Ficoll dissolved in 10 ml of 1 M carbonate buffer, pH 10.6.

[c] See footnote c, Table I.

15 ml of distilled water and 0.5 gm of CNBr (Eastman Kodak, Rochester, New York) was added. The pH of the suspension was adjusted to pH 11.0 and was kept at this pH for 8 min by adding 2 N NaOH. The reaction was terminated by filtration and the Sepharose was washed three times with cold distilled water (100 ml).

b. Coupling of DNP–Lysine (Givol et al., 1970) [Reaction (6)]. The activated Sepharose was suspended in 30 ml of 0.1 M NaHCO$_2$ containing 200 mg of DNP–lysine (Sigma Chemical Co., St. Louis, Missouri). After stirring overnight at 4°C the suspension was filtered and washed several times until the absorbance at 280 nm was less than 0.01.

2. Nitration and Reduction of Polystyrene

This method is applicable to latex, tubes, or dishes.

a. Derivatization of Polystyrene Latex [Reaction (11)]. To a cold (0°C) stirred mixture of concentrated H$_2$SO$_4$ and concentrated HNO$_3$ (2:1, v/v) was added 2.5 ml of Dow latex (available from Serva and from Feinbiochemica, Heidelberg, Germany) (bead diameter, 5.7 μm); stirring was continued for 10 min. The mixture was then centrifuged at 2500 g for 5 min, the acid was removed, and the beads were washed twice with cold distilled water by centrifugation. For the reduction, 11 gm of SnCl$_2$ (Merck, analytical grade) was dissolved in 10 ml of concentrated HCl and added to the washed nitrated latex. After 1 hr of stirring at room temperature, the latex was centrifuged, washed successively with 0.1 N HCl, distilled water, 0.1 N NaOH, and distilled water again, and resuspended in the original volume of buffer used for the coupling of proteins.

b. KLH–Latex. Four milliliters of nitrated and reduced latex (10% solid) was mixed with 8 mg of KLH and 40 mg of N-cyclohexyl-N'-[β-(N-methylmorpholino)-ethyl]carbodiimid-p-toluenesulfonate (CMC) (Merck-Schuchardt, 8011 Hohenbrunn, Germany) in 4 ml of PBS (pH 7.0) and stirred at room temperature for 2 hr. The latex was then washed five times with PBS and resuspended in 70% ethanol for storage.

3. Activation of Nylon Fibers (Edelman et al., 1971, Kiefer, 1973, 1975) [see Reaction (16)]

DNP Disks. The surface of the nylon mesh disks was hydrolyzed in 3 N HCl at room temperature as described by Edelman *et al.* (1971).

In the first step, the disks were treated for 10 min at reflux temperature with a saturated solution of succinic anhydride in benzene and washed successively with benzene, ether, 1 N NaOH, distilled water, 0.1 N HCl, distilled water, and absolute ethanol. Free carboxyl groups were then reacted with a 0.1 M solution of 1,2-diaminoethane in distilled water adjusted to pH 7.0 with trichloroacetic acid and containing 2 gm of CMC/50 ml. After 2 hr at room temperature, the disks were washed with distilled water, 0.1 N NaOH, distilled water, and ethanol.

The disks were then treated with 4 mg of PCl_5/ml of dry benzene at 60°C for 5 min, transferred directly into a solution of 5% (v/v) 1,2-diaminoethane in benzene, and stirred for 5 min. Next the disks were washed successively with benzene, ether, 1 N NaOH, Ethanol, and tetrahydrofuran (THF). Immediately after washing, they were stirred in a solution of 20 mg of DTNB-chloride/ml of dry THF for 2 hr at room temperature, washed three times with THF, and then quickly transferred into a solution of 5% 1,2-diaminoethane in THF and stirred for another hour until the disks were almost colorless. After washing with ethanol and distilled water, haptens or antigens were coupled to the disks with carbodiimide (CMC) as described previously (Kiefer, 1973).

The amount of hapten covalently bound to the disk can be measured by determining the absorption at 420 nm at two different pH values.

ϵDTNB, cleaved with ME (mercaptoethanol)	pH 9.0	= 17,000 at 420 nm
ϵDTNB, cleaved with ME	pH 1.0	= 0 at 420 nm
ϵTNP-caproic acid	pH 9.0	= 6600 at 420 nm
ϵTNP-caproic acid	pH 1.0	= 6600 at 420 nm
ϵDNP-caproic acid	pH 9.0	= 6600 at 420 nm
ϵDNP-caproic acid	pH 1.0	= 6600 at 420 nm

The measurements were done in 0.05 M $NaHCO_3$ adjusted to pH 9 with NaOH or to pH 1 with HCl.

In this way, it is possible to measure the amount of cleavable hapten as well as the amount of directly bound hapten, the latter by hydrolyzing the cleaved disks in concentrated HCl. On the average, we find 10^{-5} mmoles/disk of cleavable hapten, which corresponds to a density of 3.8×10^6 molecules of hapten/μm^2.

C. Coupling of Erythrocytes to Nylon Mesh Disks Activated with Woodward K Reagent [Reaction (17)]

The nylon disk was washed in pentane and carbon tetrachloride. It was hydrolyzed for 1 hr in 3 N HCl and washed thoroughly in distilled water and then in 0.1 N NaOH and again in distilled water until the pH of the water was neutral. The disk was then dried in ethanol and ether. Ten milligrams of Woodward K (Woodward and Olofson, 1961) (Fluka, Buchs, Switzerland) reagent was dissolved in 10 ml of distilled water at 4°C, and 10 ml of 0.2 M PBS (pH 7.0), precooled at 4°C, was added. The nylon disk was immersed in this solution and washed 45 min later with 0.1 M PBS. *Xenopus* blood, colleced in PBS that contained heparin (1 U/ml), was washed three times. Blood cells (diluted to 1/100 of whole blood) were reacted with the grid for 1 hr at room temperature in a beaker placed on an agitator (70 rpm). The cells were carefully resuspended intermittently.

SUGGESTED READING

Means, G. E., and Feeney, R. E. (1971). "Chemical Modification of Proteins." Holden-Day, San Francisco, California.
Weetall, H. H. (1972). Insolubilized antigens and antibodies. *In* "The Chemistry of Biosurfaces" (M. L. Hair, ed.) Vol. 2, pp. 598–610.
Zaborsky, O. R. (1973). "Immobilized Enzymes." CRC Press, Cleveland, Ohio.

REFERENCES

Chang, T. M. S. (1972). "Artificial Cells." Thomas, Springfield, Illinois.
Cuatrecasas, P. (1970). *J. Biol. Chem.* **245**, 3059.
Dutton, A., Adams, M., and Singer, S. J. (1966). *Biochem. Biophys. Res. Commun.* **23**, 730.
Edelman, G. M., Rutishauser, U., and Milette, C. F. (1971). *Proc. Natl. Acad. Sci. U.S.A.* **68**, 2153.
Givol, D., Weinstein, Y., Gorecki, M., and Wilchek, M. (1970). *Biochem. Biophys. Res. Commun.* **38**, 825.
Inman, J. K. (1975). *J. Immunol.* **114**, 704.
Kiefer, H. (1973). *Eur. J. Immunol.* **3**, 181.
Kiefer, H. (1975). *Eur. J. Immunol.* **5**, 624.
Laursen, R. A., Horn, M. J., and Bonner, A. G. (1972). *FEBS Lett.* **21**, 67.
Layer, P., Kiefer, H. R., and Hucho, F. (1976). *Mol. Pharmacol.* **12**, 958.
MacLeod, R. M., and Hill, R. J. (1968). *Fed. Proc. Fed. Am. Soc. Exp. Biol.* **27**, 521.
Silman, H. I., and Katchalski, E. (1966). *Annu. Rev. Biochem.* **35**, 873.
Wilson, M. B., and Nakane, P. K. (1976). *J. Immunol. Methods* **12**, 171.
Woodward, R. B., and Olofson, R. A. (1961). *J. Am. Chem. Soc.* **83**, 1007, 1010.

9

Reagents for Immunofluorescence and Their Use for Studying Lymphoid Cell Products

Luciana Forni

I. INTRODUCTION

Immunofluorescence entered cell biology in the early 1940s when Coons *et al.* (1941) first described the possibility of coupling fluorescent dyes to

IMMUNOLOGICAL METHODS
Copyright © 1979 by Academic Press, Inc.
All rights of reproduction in any form reserved.
ISBN 0-12-442750-2

immunoglobulin molecules without impairment of antibody activity and the use of such fluorescent reagents for a sensitive and specific detection of particulate as well as soluble antigens in animal tissues. The work done by Coons and associates in the next fifteen years provided, for the first time, standardization of a technique that had been successfully used by many research workers for several years. The potential of immunofluorescence became more apparent when Coons *et al.* (1955) applied the technique to detecting, in tissues, antibodies of a given specificity for which corresponding soluble antigens were available. The "indirect" method described by Mellors *et al.* (1955, 1959) provided an even more widespread application of the technique.

When fluorescent dyes became commercially available and fully equipped fluorescence microscopes were introduced to the market, immunofluorescence became accessible to less specialized laboratories, allowing the technique to be widely used in virology, microbiology, and pathology, as well as for diagnostic purposes. In basic immunology, some important problems concerning the differentiation of immunocytes have been elucidated by immunofluorescence (Pernis, 1967). The technique has been found to be a powerful tool for the study of cell membrane antigens and for physiological research (Möller, 1961; Pernis *et al.*, 1970; Frye and Edidin, 1970).

One of the critical points of the technique since its inception has been the possibility of nonspecific staining of the conjugates that Coons and Kaplan (1950) found empirically were removed by absorption on tissue powders. Later, Courtain (1958) observed that this nonspecific staining was due to the net charge of heavily coupled molecules and that these molecules could be removed from the conjugation mixture by electrophoresis or, even better, by anion exchange chromatography (Courtain, 1961; Riggs *et al.*, 1960; Goldstein *et al.*, 1961).

The availability of fluorescent reagents of high activity and specificity is obviously a crucial requirement for reliable results. Many reagents of widespread use, such as anti-human immunoglobulin reagents, are now commercially available; but the choice is, of course, very limited. This chapter will deal with the preparation, purification, and control of fluorochrome-labeled antibodies and with their use for the detection of membrane antigens of living cells as well as of internal antigens of fixed cells. It is not intended to be a complete review of immunofluorescence methods, but only a practical aid to anyone who wishes to use this type of approach.

All problems concerning theory and quantitation of fluorescence, principles of fluorescence microscopy, and the many possible applications of the fluorescent antibody technique have been dealt with in the last few years in many conferences and books, some of which are given in the Suggested Reading list at the end of the chapter.

The preparation of antisera and purified antibodies will not be considered in this chapter. The variety of antisera of different specificity that may be needed for all possible studies requiring the use of fluorescent antibodies is obviously such that it is impossible to even list them. Even the preparation of anti-immunoglobulin reagents and purified antibodies has as a prerequisite the preparation of highly purified antigens.

Many of the techniques of purification of antigens and antibodies, controls for activity and specificity of the antisera, as well as the preparation of some special antisera are described elsewhere in this volume. Basic immunochemical techniques can be found in the handbooks in the Suggested Reading list at the end of this chapter.

II. REAGENTS FOR IMMUNOFLUORESCENCE

A. Purification of Immunoglobulins

The immunoglobulin fraction of the antiserum is prepared by ammonium sulfate precipitation followed by anion exchange chromatography. The procedure is based on the method described by Cebra and Goldstein (1965). The aim is to obtain immunoglobulin fractions as homogeneous as possible as to isoelectric point (see Chapter 2). The conjugation of such fractions with fluorochromes results in a better yield of suitable conjugates, that is, preparations with high specific activity and negligible nonspecific staining.

The antiserum is diluted with an equal volume of phosphate-buffered saline (PBS)[1] and cooled in an ice bath. A volume of 3.2 M ammonium sulfate equal to the volume of the diluted serum is added dropwise with stirring; the final concentration will be 1.6 M (corresponding to 33% saturation in the cold). The mixture is automatically stirred gently for 30 min and then centrifuged in the cold (4°C) at 5000 g for 20 min. The pellet is dissolved in PBS to the original volume of the serum, and the procedure is repeated once more under the same conditions. Finally, the precipitate is dissolved in PBS, about one-half the original volume, and dialyzed against PBS in the cold to remove sulfate ions. Before chromatography, the crude immunoglobulin solution is dialyzed overnight in the cold against 100 vol of 0.01 M phosphate buffer, pH 7.5. The precipitate formed after dialysis is removed by centrifugation before applying the solution to the anion exchange cellulose column.

[1] 0.15 M NaCl, 0.01 M sodium phosphate, pH 7.2.

Diethylaminoethyl cellulose (DEAE),[2] 0.6–0.7 mEq/gm, is washed twice with 0.01 M phosphate buffer, pH 7.5, and the resulting sediment is packed into a column. The amount of cellulose to be used is 1 gm dry weight per 2 ml of original antiserum.

The dialyzed protein solution is applied to the column and allowed to enter the cellulose. Elution is then started with the same buffer used for the equilibration, and fractions of about one-half the volume of the protein solution applied to the column are collected. The availability of a fraction collector equipped with an ultraviolet recorder is helpful, but not absolutely necessary. After elution of the first peak of proteins, which represents the more basic IgG globulin fraction, a solution of 0.01 M phosphate and 0.05 M NaCl (pH 7.5) is applied to the column, and a second peak, containing "acidic" IgG, is collected.

The two fractions are made isotonic by either dialysis or the addition of an appropriate volume of $10\times$ PBS, concentrated to 5–10 mg/ml, and stored at $-20°$C.

Comments

1. In most antisera directed against protein antigens, the relevant antibody is almost equally distributed in both IgG fractions. This is not always the case for anti-hapten antibodies, which are often more restricted and can be exclusively present in one or the other of the two chromatographic fractions. Therefore, it is advisable, before conjugation, to check the antibody content of the preparations by the agar double-diffusion test.

2. There are individual differences among antisera in the concentration of basic versus acidic IgG present. Differences are also observed in the chromatographic behavior of antisera from different species. When separated on DEAE-cellulose under the conditions previously discussed, human and rabbit sera give one single peak of basic IgG eluted with the starting buffer, whereas sheep antisera usually give two peaks, one eluted with the void volume and a second that is slightly delayed. In our experience, those two peaks can be pooled for conjugation. Chromatography on DEAE-cellulose of mouse immunoglobulins often results in a very poor yield of purified material.

B. Preparation of Immunoglobulin Fragments

When the presence of the Fc portion of the immunoglobulin molecule might interfere with the detection of membrane antigens, for some special purposes it is necessary to use divalent antibody fragments obtained by

---

[2] Supplied by Serva (DEAE-SS), Whatman, Bio-Rad, and others.

enzymatic digestion. The procedure described below is basically that of Nisonoff (1964), with minor modifications.

The purified immunoglobulin preparation of the antisera is dialyzed against 0.1 M acetate buffer at pH 4.3. Crystalline pepsin,[3] at a globulin-to-pepsin ratio fo 50:1, is added to the solution, and, if necessary, pH is adjusted to 4.3 with 1 M acetic acid. The mixture is left to react in a 37°C water bath for 8–14 hr and is then cooled in an ice bath. It is then centrifuged to remove any precipitate that may have formed during the reaction, and the pH is adjusted to 8.0 with 1 M NaOH; at this pH pepsin is inactivated. The preparation is either dialyzed against large volumes of PBS to remove small peptides or made 2.4 M with ammonium sulfate, spun for 30 min at 5000 g, dissolved in PBS, and dialyzed to remove sulfate ions. At this point, the preparation is checked for purity either by agar-gel immunodiffusion, when the anti-Fab and anti-Fc antisera are available, or by the more sensitive technique of SDS–polyacrylamide gel electrophoresis (see Chapter 4) of the native as well as of the reduced and alkylated sample. If the digestion has not been complete, and intact IgG molecules are still present in considerable amounts in the preparation, the sample is purified by gel filtration on Sephadex G-150.[4]

Comments

The yield of pepsin $F(ab')_2$ fragment differs from one species of immunoglobulin to another. Rabbit immunoglobulin under the pH conditions discussed above is completely digested to $F(ab')_2$, whereas sheep immunoglobulin is to some extent resistant to pepsin digestion, even when the pH is decreased to 3.9. Mouse immunoglobulins are unique in that their sensitivity to pepsin digestion is very different for different subclasses, at least as observed on purified myeloma proteins (L. Forni, unpublished observations). For this reason, one may obtain not only a very low yield, but also material from a given subclass that might be a disadvantage if, as is often the case, the relevant antibody activity is not equally distributed throughout all the IgG subclasses.

Monovalent $F(ab')$ fragments of antibodies can be obtained from pepsin fragments prepared as described above by reduction and alkylation. The pepsin $F(ab')_2$ preparation is dialyzed against 0.1 M sodium acetate buffer, pH 5.0, and a reducing agent, such as mercaptoethanolamine-HCl or dithiothreitol,[5] is added to reach a final concentration of 0.01–0.015 M. The mixture is incubated in stoppered tubes in a 37°C water bath for 1–2 hr, and

---

[3] Pepsin, 2× crystallized, is supplied by Sigma.

[4] Produced by Pharmacia (Uppsala, Sweden).

[5] Mercaptoethanolamine-HCl is supplied by Sigma; dithiothreitol (Cleland's reagent) is supplied by Calbiochem.

the reaction is stopped by adding iodoacetamide[6] to a final concentration of 0.022–0.036 M. The mixture is then dialyzed against PBS.

This procedure results in complete reduction of divalent fragments. The yield is very close to the theoretical yield. These monovalent fragments have the advantage of being more soluble than monovalent Fab prepared by papain digestion.

C. Conjugation Procedures

The procedure described below is based on the methods described by Cebra and Goldstein (1965), Amante and Giuriani (1969), and Amante *et al.* (1972) with some modification. The procedure of conjugation and purification of conjugates is completed in 1 day and does not require much actual bench work. In our experience, it is therefore advisable to conjugate small amounts of antibody at a time (of the order of 10 mg of purified immunoglobulins), since conjugates often lose activity during storage.

The protein concentration with which we have obtained the best results, as yield of suitable conjugate, is around 4–5 mg/ml. With this range of protein concentration, the following amounts of fluorochrome per milligram of protein are used: fluorescein isothiocyanate (FITC) and crystalline tetramethylrhodamine isothiocyanate (TRITC),[7] 12.5 μg; amorphous tetramethylrhodamine isothiocyanate, 15 μg. When lower protein concentrations must be used, as with purified antibodies, is it advisable to decrease the relative amount of fluorochromes to avoid formation of hyperconjugated molecules and the resultant loss of antibody activity. Divalent and monovalent fragments of immunoglobulins must be conjugated at low fluorochrome concentrations, not exceeding 10 μg/mg of protein.

The required amount of fluorochrome is weighed in a tared bottle and dissolved in 50–100 μl of either 0.1 M Na_2CO_3 or dimethyl sulfoxide immediately before use. The protein solution (2.5 ml) is equilibrated in an ice bath, brought to pH 9.0 by adding 0.1 M Na_2CO_3, and added to the fluorochrome solution with gentle stirring. The conjugation mixture is kept as close as possible to pH 9.0 by adding, when necessary, 0.05 M sodium carbonate or bicarbonate. This procedure is carried out at ice bath temperature. If the pH of the mixture does not change after 15 min, the bottle is stoppered and the mixture is left to react in the cold, with gentle

---

[6] Iodoacetamide is supplied by BDH and other suppliers.

[7] Fluorescein isothiocyanate, isomer I, is supplied by Baltimore Biological Laboratories, Maryland. Tetramethylrhodamine isothiocyanate is supplied by Baltimore Biological Laboratories, Maryland, and by Nordic Immunology, Tilburg, The Netherlands.

stirring and protected from light, for 18 hr. For crystalline tetramethylrhodamine, the conjugation procedure is completed in 4 hr; longer reaction times often lead to a high proportion of hyperconjugated molecules. After completion of the reaction, the mixture is centrifuged to remove any precipitate that might have formed and is then processed for purification.

D. Purification of Conjugates

A column of 8- to 9-mm diameter and 60-cm length is packed with 4–5 gm of Sephadex G-50 (fine) washed two or three times with 0.01 M phosphate buffer pH 7.5 by spontaneous sedimentation to remove finest particles. The conjugation mixture is applied to the column, and after all the fluid has been absorbed in the gel, it is eluted with the same buffer used for the equilibration of the gel. The colored mixture soon divides into two fractions: the first and faster fraction representing the conjugated immunoglobulins, the second, the unreacted fluorochrome.

This gel filtration is often good enough for conjugates made with crystalline tetramethylrhodamine and for preparations of purified antibodies and immunoglobulin fragments. In both cases, the eluted samples are evaluated and processed as will be described in Sections II,E and II,F.

Usually, however, the gel filtration that removes the unbound fluorochrome is not sufficient to obtain conjugates devoid of nonspecific staining. Therefore, it is necessary to select, by anion exchange chromatography, the different components of the mixture with different net charges, which, being the original solution homogeneous with regard to isoelectric point, depend now almost exclusively on the number of molecules of fluorochrome bound per immunoglobulin molecule. This separation is performed by elution with a NaCl solution of increasing concentration.

A small column, or a glass syringe, is packed with 1.5 gm of DEAE-cellulose equilibrated with 0.01 M phosphate buffer, pH 7.5. The effluent from the Sephadex G-50 column is applied to the anion exchanger and eluted first with the same buffer and then with solutions, in the same buffer, which are 0.05, 0.1, 0.2, 0.3, and 0.4 M in NaCl. Each peak is collected separately and evaluated for protein concentration and the fluorochrome-to-protein ratio as described below.

For TRITC conjugates, fractions with a suitable degree of coupling are removed from the cellulose with 0.05 and 0.1 M NaCl. Fractions removed at higher salt concentrations are usually hyperconjugated.

For FITC conjugates, the fractions (if any) removed from the ion exchanger with low salt concentration are usually hypoconjugated, whereas fractions with a suitable degree of conjugation can be eluted with NaCl solutions as concentrated as 0.4 M.

E. Evaluation of Conjugates

The protein concentration and the fluorochrome-to-protein ratio of the conjugates are calculated on the basis of their optical density at 280 nm and at 495 nm, for FITC, 515 nm for amorphous TRITC and 555 nm for crystalline TRITC. The wavelengths in the visible spectrum are those at which the different conjugates give the maximum absorption (Cebra and Goldstein, 1965; Amante and Giuriani, 1969; Amante *et al.*, 1972). The calculations are made according to the following formulas, which take into account the absorption spectra of the different fluorochromes.

FITC

$$\frac{A_{280} - (0.35 \times A_{495})}{1.4} = \text{protein concentration (mg/ml)}$$

$$\frac{2.87 \times A_{495}}{A_{280} - (0.35 \times A_{496})} = \text{moles of FITC per mole of IgG}$$

TRITC (crystalline)

$$\frac{A_{280}}{1.4} = \text{protein concentration (mg/ml)}$$

$$\frac{6.6 \times A_{555}}{\text{mg/ml}} = \text{moles of TRITC per mole of IgG}$$

TRITC (amorphous)

$$\frac{A_{280} - (0.56 \times A_{515})}{1.4} = \text{protein concentration (mg/ml)}$$

For amorphous TRITC, it is not possible to calculate the number of fluorochrome groups per IgG molecule. In this case, a rough estimate of the degree of conjugation is given by the ratio A_{280}/A_{515}.

F. Storage of Conjugates

The conjugates are made isotonic by dialysis against PBS and adjusted to a protein concentration of 0.5 mg/ml. Preparation of purified antibodies can be used at much lower concentrations, of the order of 50 μg/ml.

The conjugates are sterilized by Millipore filtration, divided in small aliquots, and stored at 4°C in the dark.

G. Control of the Efficiency and Specificity of the Conjugates

1. Staining Efficiency

The staining efficiency of conjugates cannot be precisely predicted on the basis of molar ratio because, in practice, important variations exist, depending on the immunoglobulin species and the strength of the antisera.

As a rule, samples with molar ratios of less than 1 are poor reagents, although their antibody activity remains virtually intact because unlabeled molecules are present in the mixture, and these efficiently compete with the labeled molecules. On the other hand, conjugates with molar ratios of 2–3 give satisfactory results in general, with fluorescein, whereas nonspecific staining can result with rhodamine.

Antisera directed against the same antigens prepared from rabbit or goat can behave very differently when the efficiencies of conjugates with similar molar ratios are compared. Rabbit immunoglobulins cannot be labeled with more than two or three fluorescein molecules without loosing antibody activity, whereas sheep or goat immunoglobulins withstand heavier coupling (up to five to seven fluorescein molecules per IgG molecule) without impairment of staining efficiency.

Personal experience leads to the conclusion that the best way to check both the efficiency and the specificity of conjugates is by staining the cell samples, either on the membrane or in the cytoplasm. In fact, in many cases, the classic controls for specificity of staining, such as inhibition by preincubation with a large excess of unlabeled antibody or absorption of the antiserum with the corresponding antigen, cannot be performed for operational reasons. In these cases, staining the fixed smears of cells from any tissue and species can, if uniformly stained, give sufficient indications of the nonspecific characteristics of the conjugate.

2. Specificity of the Conjugated Antisera

Direct staining of cells is also the best control for specificity of the antisera. In fact, in many cases, antisera that are considered specific by immunodiffusion or hemagglutination can still contain contaminant antibodies detectable by immunofluorescence when indirect and more sensitive techniques are used.

Alloantisera, as anti-immunoglobulin allotypes, antihistocompatibility antigens, and any antiserum directed against polymorphic antigens, must be checked on postive as well as negative strains.

Anti-immunoglobulin antibodies with specificity for different classes or subclasses of immunoglobulins can be reliably checked by double staining of the cell samples with couples of antisera conjugated with different fluorochormes. Double stainings performed under conditions that allow the redistribution of molecules of one specificity at one pole of the cell ("capping") but not of the molecules of the other specificity (see Section III) are the most suitable for giving reliable and clear-cut results. Since it has been clearly established (see Rowe *et al.*, 1973; Knapp *et al.*, 1973) that different immunoglobulin molecules, when present on the membrane of the same cell, move independently, concomitant redistribution (double-stained caps) of two different immunoglobulins must be taken as an indication that at least one of the reagents is still not completely specific. In this latter case, the conjugates must be absorbed on solid immunoadsorbents and retested for both efficiency and specificity.

III. STAINING PROCEDURES

A. Detection of Membrane Antigens

Detection of membrane antigens is performed by staining living cells in suspension. The same procedure is applied to cells prepared either from fresh tissue or from culture. In both cases, the samples must be carefully and gently washed with balanced salt solutions containing protein [1% BSA or 10% fetal calf serum (FCS)] to remove any serum protein, or proteins secreted or released from the cells themselves in culture, which could interfere with the staining. A suitable cell density for the staining procedure is $10-20 \times 10^6$/ml. The staining is performed in small round-bottom tubes; either plastic or glass tubes may be used. However, it is advisable to use disposable ware since the possible presence of traces of detergent can drastically impair both the antigen structure of the cells and the antibody activity of the antisera, even when present in concentrations too low to induce cell lysis.

1. Direct Staining

Using this technique, 50–100 μl of the cell suspension ($1-2 \times 10^7$ cells) is mixed with an equal volume of the appropriate conjugated antiserum, gently resuspended, and kept in ice for 20–30 min. Then 3 ml of cold medium (BSS containing protein) is added and the tubes are spun in a refrigerated centrifuge for 10 min at 100 g. The pellet is resuspended and processed three times as above. In addition to carrying out the whole procedure in the cold, it is advisable to use medium containing 10–20 mM sodium azide to prevent unwanted redistribtuion of membrane antigens cross-linked by the relevant antibodies at one pole of the cell (capping) (Taylor *et al.*, 1971; Loor *et al.*, 1972).

Another procedure for removing the fluorescent reagent after staining in a gentler fashion, practical when the staining procedure has to be repeated more than once, is to pass the cell suspension over a large volume of fetal calf serum, either neat (undiluted) or in a discontinuous gradient made up with 6 ml of neat serum, 3 ml of 75% serum, and 2 ml of 50% serum. The staining mixture is diluted with medium to 1 ml and carefully layered over the serum, and the tube is spun for 15 min at 200 g in the cold. The supernatant is removed by suction and the pellet is resuspended in 50 μl of medium for further processing.

2. Double Staining

Double staining of the same cell suspension with two different antisera conjugated with different fluorochromes can be performed either in one step (as described in section III,A,1, by exposing the cells to a mixture of the two conjugates) or in two steps, by repeating the procedure twice. The latter procedure is used when there are possibilities of interference at the level of either the antisera or the membrane antigens.

Another double staining procedure may be used when the two antigens being studied are known or are expected to be present on the same cell. It has been shown by Taylor *et al.* (1971) and Loor *et al.* (1972) that membrane molecules of lymphocytes (as well as of other cells), when reacting with a ligand, undergo a redistribution with the molecules collecting at one pole of the cell. This "capping" phenomenon is energy and temperature dependent, and for this reason both low temperatures and inhibitors such as sodium azide are used in the usual staining procedure to prevent it. Sometimes, however, one can take advantage of this phenomenon to achieve better visualization of two antigens or to study possible physical relationships or physiological interactions between membrane molecules (see, for example, Forni and Pernis, 1975). The procedure is as follows.

First the cells are reacted with one fluorescent antiserum in an ice bath for 20 min as indicated above; then, after adding 0.5 ml of medium *without* sodium azide, the cell suspension is incubated for 10 min in a 37°C water bath. After this incubation, the cells are cooled by adding 3 ml of medium containing sodium azide and washed as indicated previously. A second staining is then performed using the second antiserum labeled with a different fluorochrome, this time strictly in the cold (4°C) and in the presence of sodium azide.

3. Indirect Staining

Indirect staining is performed either when the relevant antiserum is available in too small an amount to be processed for conjugation or when the antiserum has a very low antibody content, as can be the case for some alloantisera against membrane antigens and for antisera that are usually tested by complement-dependent cytotoxicity; the antibody content of these sera is often only a few micrograms per milliliter.

The staining procedure is the same as that for direct staining and should be repeated twice. The cells are first exposed to the relevant antiserum at the appropriate dilution and then, after washing, to a fluorescent antiserum to detect the first antibody as an antigen. With heteroantisera the detecting reagent of choice is, of course, an antiimmunoglobulin antiserum. With alloantisera, however, when working with cells such as lymphocytes, which could bear on the membrane endogenous immunoglobulins, anti-immunoglobulin antibodies cannot be used as a detecting reagent. In this case, a method that gives good results for sensitivity and specificity is the coupling of the alloantibodies with a hapten and the use of anti-hapten antibodies labeled with fluorochromes as the detecting reagent (Wofsy *et al.*, 1974).

Indirect staining is also used for detecting antigen-binding cells by immunofluorescence. To do this, cells are first incubated in ice for 30 min with the antigen solution at a concentration not exceeding 50 μg/ml. They are then washed thoroughly by centrifugation and stained with the corresponding antibody labeled with fluorochromes.

After staining, by whatever method has been used, for microscopical observation the cell pellet is resuspended in a few drops of phosphate-buffered glycerol.[8] One drop of the cell suspension is placed on a slide, covered with a coverslip, and sealed with nail polish.

Alternatively, when cell preparations need to be kept for a few days, cell smears can be prepared. In our experience, a suitable way to ensure a sufficient number of cells in a microscopic field is to resuspend the cell pellet in a minimal volume of 3% BSA in BSS or in 50% FCS. A drop of the cell suspension is placed with a Pasteur pipette on the point of a fountain pen, and lines are drawn on a microscope slide. The slides are dried in the air, fixed for 5 min in ethanol, rehydrated with two or three changes of PBS, and mounted in phosphate-buffered glycerol. These fixed preparations have the advantage of preventing any change of distribution of labeled molecules on the cell membrane that could take place during the observations if cells are kept at room temperature. In addition, in our experience, this method has been found to be very practical when rare cells, such as antigen-binding cells, need to be counted. In this case, it is obvious that it is important not to count the same cell twice, something easily prevented if the cells are arranged in lines.

[8] 60 ml of glycerol, 30 ml of distilled H_2O, 10 ml of 10 $\times$ PBS, and 1 ml of 1 M NaN$_3$ is a suitable reagent.

4. Comments

It is advantageous to discuss the misleading observations that may result from the properties of the fluorescent reagents. One, for example, is the staining of the lymphocyte membrane, not as a result of the presence of the relevant antigen, but by the reaction of the fluorescent antibody with special structures of the lymphocyte membrane—called Fc receptors because they react with the Fc portion of IgG. It has been found that many controversial results connected with the presence of IgG molecules on the membrane of B lymphocytes have been caused by such receptors (Winchester *et al.*, 1975). To prevent such unwanted staining, Winchester *et al.* suggest the use of pepsin fragments of antibodies in all work done with immunofluorescence on lymphoid cells.

However, since Fc receptors of lymphocytes react mainly, if not exclusively, with IgG molecules when aggregated my physical means or in the form of antigen–antibody complexes (Basten *et al.*, 1972), no picking up of fluorescent IgG molecules via Fc receptors has ever been observed in our experience, provided the antisera are absorbed with insolubilized antigens and freed from any aggregate larger than 40 S by ultracentrifugation for 1 hr at 100,000 *g*. In addition, we have observed that fluorescein and tetramethylrhodamine-labeled IgG's lose the ability to bind to Fc receptors (Forni and Pernis, 1975) or to protein A from *Staphylococcus aureus* (L. Forni, unpublished), just as they have been described by Trasher *et al.* (1975) to lose other Fc-dependent properties, such as complement fixation.

B. Detection of Intracytoplasmic Antigens

To detect intracytoplasmic antigens, the cells must be fixed with reagents that allow the fluorescent antibody to enter them by drastically modifying the structure of the membrane. A method is described below for intracytoplasmic detection of antigens of single cells.

The cells are suspended at a density of $1-4 \times 10^6$ cells/ml in a concentrated protein solution, such as 3% BSA in PBS or 50% FCS. The cell density varies according to the cells being studied. For instance, when immunoglobulin-containing plasma cells are studied in a cell suspension from spleen, lymph nodes, or any other lymphoid organs in which such cells account for only a small percentage of the total cell population, a cell suspension as dense as 4×10^6/ml may be used. On the other hand, when the percentage of immunoglobulin-containing cells is much higher, as in a suspension from a solid plasmocytoma, bone marrow from cases of multiple myeloma, lymphoblastoid lines, of stimulated cell cultures, the cell density should not exceed 10^6/ml.

Cell smears can be prepared with excellent results using a cytocentrifuge. These special centrifuges (available from Shandon, London) enable the experimenter to collect a monolayer of cells in a spot of about 5- to 7-mm diameter that can be stained easily with a small volume (10–20 μl) of conjugated antiserum.

The microscope slides placed in the cytocentrifuge are precoated with a thin film of protein by spinning with 100 μl of 3% BSA–PBS. Then, 100 μl of the cell suspension is placed in each well and spun for 15 min at 800–1000 rpm (a lower speed is advisable for more fragile cells such as myeloma cells or cells in culture). After spinning, a circle is drawn with a diamond pencil around the cell spot, which is not clearly visible when the slide is wet. The cell smears are fixed in ethanol or in ethanol–5% acetic acid for 10 min and washed three times for 10 min in PBS. The slides are then wiped with a fine paper tissue, all except the cell spot, on which a drop of 10–20 μl of conjugate is applied. The slides are incubated at room temperature in a humid box; drying of the conjugate on the cells will cause a high nonspecific background. After the incubation, the slides are washed three times in PBS and mounted in phosphate-buffered glycerol. The fixed cells can be stained indirectly by first incubating them with the relevant unlabeled antiserum and then, after thorough washings, with the detecting fluorescent reagent.

Using a similar procedure, cells producing antibodies of a given specificity can be detected. To do this, the samples are first incubated with the appropriate soluble antigen at a concentration not exceeding 50–100 μg/ml and then, after washings, with the specific antiserum labeled with a fluorochrome.

Double staining with two antisera labeled with different fluorochromes, as for cells in suspension, can be performed in a single step with a mixture of the two reagents or in two steps. Staining in a single step can be performed only with antisera that do not interfere with one another. Even more important, it can only be done with reagents that have been absorbed with insoluble antigens, since the presence in the conjugates of free antigen, or of antigen–antibody complexes in antigen excess, will result in the reciprocal inactivation of the reagents.

C. Detection of Membrane and Intracytoplasmic Antigens on the Same Cells

The procedure described above for staining surface and intracytoplasmic antigens can be combined. The cells are first stained for membrane antigens in suspension, usually with an antiserum labeled with tetramethyl-rhodamine. After washing, the cells are resuspended at the appropriate concentration in 3% BSA–PBS, and smears are prepared with a cytocentrifuge as described above, fixed for 10 min in ethanol, and processed for intracytoplasmic staining with a second antiserum labeled with fluorescein.

IV. GENERAL COMMENTS

A. Reproducibility of the Method of Conjugation

The reproducibility of the method of conjugation is quite good. As anticipated, however, there is substantial variation in efficiency depending on the species of immunoglobulin used.

More precisely, of the more widely used species of antisera, rabbit immunoglobulin labels poorly with fluorochromes in comparision to sheep and goat immunoglobulins. This results in advantages and disadvantages according to the fluorochrome used. In fact, when fluorescein is used, since a heavy labeling (two to five FITC groups per IgG molecule) is required for good staining efficiency, better results are obtained with sheep and goat immunoglobulin than with rabbit. On the other hand, since light labeling with TRITC (one TRITC group per IgG molecule) is necessary to produce conjugates lacking nonspecific staining, rabbit conjugates are usually better than sheep or goat. In general, whenever possible, it is advisable to label sheep and goat immunoglobulins with FITC and rabbit immunoglobulins with TRITC.

Personal limited experience indicates that human immunoglobulins, as well as horse immunoglobulins, can be labeled efficiently with both fluorescein and rhodamine. For human antibodies, conjugation of anti-HLA antibodies often results in a significant loss of activity, but this is probably due to the low antibody content. On the other hand, fluorochrome labeling of mouse immunoglobulins, even in the case of precipitating antisera such as anti-immunoglobulin allotypes, always gave us very unsatisfactory results.

B. Possible Discrepancy between Results Obtained with Immunofluorescence and with Cytotoxicity

With mouse alloantisera, usually tested by complement-dependent cytotoxicity, we have often observed significant discrepancies when the same sera were used for indirect immunofluorescence. In many cases, alloantisera, considered completely specific by all criteria (cytotoxicity and absorptions), were found to also stain cells from negative strains, even if in most cases only subpopulations of cells were involved. We have observed these types of discrepancies with three anti-Thy.1 antisera, some anti-H-2 antisera, and some anti-Ia antisera, all of which were of well-defined specificity. These discrepancies may be explained by assuming the presence of additional antibodies confined in immunoglobulin classes that do not fix complement, a possibility that is not unlikely.

SUGGESTED READING

Fifth International Conference on Immunofluorescence and Related Staining Techniques (*Ann. N.Y. Acad. Sci.* 1975, **254**).

Goldman, M. (1968). "Fluorescent Antibody Methods." Academic Press, New York.

Holborow, E. J., ed. (1970). "Standardization in Immunofluorescence." Blackwell, Oxford.

Kabat, E., and Mayer, H. H. (1971). "Experimental Immunochemistry." Thomas, Springfield, Illinois.

Kawamura, A., Jr. (1969). "Fluorescent Antibody Techniques and Their Applications." Univ. Park Press, Baltimore, Maryland.

Weir, D. M. (1973). "Handbook of Experimental Immunology," Vol. I. Blackwell, Oxford.

Williams, C. A., and Chase, M. W., eds. (1967). "Methods in Immunology and Immunochemistry," Vol. 1. Academic Press, New York.

Williams, C. A., and Chase, M. W., eds. (1967). "Methods in Immunology and Immunochemistry." Vol. 2. Academic Press, New York.

REFERENCES

Amante, L., and Giuriani, M. (1969). *Boll. Ist. Sieroter. Milan.* **48**, 411.

Amante, L., Ancona, A., and Forni, L. (1972). *J. Immunol. Methods* **1**, 289.

Basten, A., Miller, J. F. A. P., Sprent, J., and Pye, J. (1972). *J. Exp. Med.* **135**, 610.

Cebra, J. J., and Goldstein, G. (1965). *J. Immunol.* **95**, 230.

Coons, A. H., and Kaplan, M. H. (1950). *J. Exp. Med.* **91**, 1.

Coons, A. H., Creech, H. J., and Jones, R. N. (1941). *Proc. Soc. Exp. Biol. Med.* **47**, 200.

Coons, A. H., Leduc, E. H., and Connolly, J. M. (1955). *J. Exp. Med.* **102**, 49.

Courtain, C. C. (1958). *Nature (London)* **182**, 1305.

Courtain, C. C. (1961). *J. Histochem. Cytochem.* **9**, 484.

Forni, L., and Pernis, B. (1975). *In* "Membrane Receptors of Lymphocytes" (M. Seligmann, J. L. Preud'Homme, and F. M. Kourilsky, eds.), p. 193. North-Holland Publ., Amsterdam.

Frye, L. D., and Edidin, M. (1970). *J. Cell Sci.* **7**, 319.

Goldstein, G., Silizys, I. S., and Chase, M. W. (1961). *J. Exp. Med.* **114**, 89.

Knapp, W., Bolhuis, R. L. H., Radl, J., and Hijmans, W. (1973). *J. Immunol.* **111**, 1295.

Loor, F., Forni, L., and Pernis, B. (1972). *Eur. J. Immunol.* **2**, 203.

Mellors, R. C., Arias-Stella, J., Siegel, M., and Pressman, D. (1955). *Am. J. Pathol.* **31**, 687.

Mellors, R. C., Heimer, R., Corcos, J., and Korngold, L. (1959). *J. Exp. Med.* **110**, 875.

Möller, G. (1961). *J. Exp. Med.* **114**, 415.

Nisonoff, A. (1964). *Methods Med. Res.* **10**, 132.

Pernis, B. (1967). *Cold Spring Harbor Symp. Quant. Biol.* **32,** 333.

Pernis, B., Forni, L., and Amante, L. (1970). *J. Exp. Med.* **132,** 1001.

Riggs, J. L., Loh, P. C., and Eveland, W. C. (1960). *Proc. Soc. Exp. Biol. Med.* **105,** 655.

Rowe, D. S., Hug, K., Forni, L., and Pernis, B. (1973). *J. Exp. Med.* **138,** 965.

Taylor, R. B., Duffus, P. H., Raff, M. C., and de Petris, S. (1971). *Nature New Biol.* **233,** 225.

Trasher, S. G., Bigazzi, P. E., Yoshida, T., and Cohen, S. (1975). *J. Immunol.* **114,** 762.

Winchester, R. J., Fu, S. M., Hoffman, T., and Kunkel, H. G. (1975). *J. Immunol.* **114,** 1210.

Wofsy, L., Barker, P. C., Thompson, K., Goodman, J., Kimura, J., and Henry, C. (1974). *J. Exp. Med.* **140,** 523.

10

Radiolabeling and Immunoprecipitation of Cell-Surface Macromolecules

J. Richard L. Pink and Andreas Ziegler

I. INTRODUCTION

If suitable specific antisera are available, cell-surface components can be purified, on a small scale, from lysates of radioactively labeled leukocytes (or other cell types) by a simple three-step procedure.

In the first step, cellular macromolecules are labeled either biosynthetically or by chemical or enzyme-catalyzed incorporation of external isotope. Procedures commonly used for labeling proteins are lactoperoxidase-catalyzed iodination (Section II,A) and biosynthetic incorporation of radioactive amino acids in short-term culture (Section II,B). Glycoproteins and carbohydrates may be labeled by borohydride reduction techniques (Section II,C) or by biosynthetic incorporation of labeled sugars (basically as described for amino acid incorporation).

In the second step, the labeled cells are lysed in a medium usually containing a nonionic detergent, in which membrane components are soluble (Section III). The molecules of interest are purified by passing the lysate over an immunoadsorbent column or, more conveniently, by adding a

IMMUNOLOGICAL METHODS

specific antiserum to the lysate; in the second case, the immune complexes formed are isolated by adding either a second antiserum directed against the immunoglobulins of the first serum (indirect immune precipitation) or a suspension of staphylococci bearing the immunoglobulin-binding protein A (Section III).

It is desirable to remove material that might adhere nonspecifically to an immunoadsorbent column or to an immune precipitate before the specific purification step is carried out. In addition, labeled cell-surface immunoglobulin should be removed from leukocyte lysates [unless it is the object of the researcher's curiosity (see Chapter 2)] or it will appear in any precipitate made with an alloantiserum plus an anti-immunoglobulin reagent or protein A-bearing staphylococci. Therefore, labeled cell-surface immunoglobulin and nonspecifically adsorbable material are usually removed in a preliminary precipitation or absorption step before the specific purification step is performed.

Finally, the purified, radioactive material is characterized, for example, by electrophoresis in sodium dodecyl sulfate-containing polyacrylamide gels (SDS–PAGE) (see Chapter 4).

II. LABELING PROCEDURES

A. Lactoperoxidase-Catalyzed Cell-Surface Iodination

This method, originally applied to the study of erythrocyte surface proteins (Phillips and Morrison, 1970, 1971), has been widely used to characterize lymphocyte cell-surface immunoglobulins (Vitetta *et al.* 1971), major histocompatibility antigens (Silver and Hood, 1974), and various other cell-surface markers (e.g., see Marchalonis *et al.*, 1971; Vitetta *et al.*, 1975). Cell-surface iodination has been reviewed by Morrison and Schonbaum (1976) and Hubbard and Cohn (1976).

In the reaction (whose exact mechanism is unknown), iodide ions are probably oxidized, in the presence of lactoperoxidase and hydrogen peroxide, to give an enzyme-bound reactive intermediate which can convert available protein tyrosine residues into (mainly) the monoiodinated derivatives. Histidine may also be iodinated, but to a much lesser extent than tyrosine (Morrison *et al.*, 1970; Hubbard and Cohn, 1976). The hydrogen peroxide may be added directly to the mixture (Marchalonis *et al.*, 1971) or generated *in situ* using the enzyme glucose oxidase in the presence of glucose (Hubbard and Cohn, 1972).

The method is technically easy to perform, and the results are more convenient to analyze (by γ-counting or autoradiography) than those from experiments in which tritium is used as the label. Furthermore, certain cell types (e.g., erythrocytes and sperm) can incorporate only very small amounts of label biosynthetically; in these cases, iodination is the method of choice for marking membrane proteins.

If viability of the starting cell preparation is good, cell-surface components are preferentially labeled so that the fraction of iodine label in a particular surface component is normally larger than the corresponding fraction in a biosynthetically labeled preparation (for example, 0.05–0.2% of the label in a lysate of iodinated chicken leukocytes is detected in the major histocompatibility antigen peak after SDS–PAGE, whereas the corresponding fraction in a [^{3}H]leucine/[^{3}H]lysine-labeled lysate is 0.02–0.1%) (Ziegler and Pink, 1976). However, this advantage may be offset by the fact that part of certain cell-surface molecules may be inaccessible to the iodination reaction (Walsh and Crumpton, 1977; Schwartz et al., 1978).

Normally, in the procedure described below, about 10–20% of the added radioactivity becomes cell bound in such a way that it cannot be removed by washing. However, a large part of this label becomes dialyzable after the cells are lysed and probably consists of iodinated lipids. After lysis and dialysis, about 1–5% of the input counts are recoverable, essentially all of which can be precipitated by trichloroacetic acid. Thus, for an input of 1 mCi, one might expect to recover 4×10^7 cpm of ^{125}I in the dialyzed lysate. The percentage of these counts in a particular surface component depends on the number and availability of its tyrosine residues at the cell surface; for major histocompatibility antigens, the percentage recovered after purification is about 0.05–0.2% (i.e., about 4×10^4 cpm). This figure corresponds to the iodination of about 0.01–0.1 tyrosine per molecule, assuming the presence of about 10^5 molecules of histocompatibility antigen at the cell surface (Sanderson and Welsh, 1974) and 100% yield during purification.

The procedure given is a modified version of that described by Hubbard and Cohn (1972) for iodination of erythrocytes. Since different batches of lactoperoxidase may have different activities, it is advisable in preliminary experiments to test the effects of different concentrations of the enzyme on iodine uptake.

Procedure

To $1–5 \times 10^7$ viable cells in 1 ml of Dulbecco's phosphate-buffered saline (PBS), pH 7.4, containing 20 mM glucose, add 20 μl of lactoperoxidase (Calbiochem, La Jolla, California, or Sigma, St. Louis, Missouri; stored at $-70°$C in 100-μl aliquots of a 1 mg/ml solution in PBS) and 20 μl of glucose oxidase (Calbiochem or Sigma; stored at $-70°$C in aliquots of 1 U/100 μl.

In a hood equipped for radioactive isotope work, add to the cells 0.5–1 mCi of carrier-free $Na^{125}I$ (freshly diluted with distilled water to give 1 mCi in a volume of 10–20 μl). Incubate the cells in a stoppered tube for 30 min at 20°C.

Stop the reaction by adding 5 ml of precooled PBS containing 10^{-3} M phenylmethanesulfonyl fluoride (PMSF) and wash the cells four times in this solution (5 ml each wash). Aliquots of successive supernatants may be counted to follow the removal of non-cell-bound label.

B. Biosynthetic Labeling of Cell-Surface Proteins

Biosynthetic incorporation of radioactive amino acids into protein has been used to study, for example, cell-surface immunoglobulin (Melchers and Andersson, 1973) and histocompatibility antigens (Brown *et al.*, 1974; Jones, 1977). Leucine and lysine, which are abundant in most proteins and whose tritiated derivatives have high specific activities, are often used, but the remaining essential amino acids are also readily incorporated into protein in short-term leukocyte cultures. Labeling with "nonessential" amino acids is more difficult; for some (alanine, cysteine, and proline), satisfactory incorporation can be achieved, but for others (glycine, serine, aspartate, and glutamate) this is not so (Vitetta *et al.*, 1976). The efficiency of incorporation of label by different cell types into different proteins is very variable. For lymphocytes, in the procedure given below, about 5 to 10% of the [³H]leucine/[³H]lysine label is incorporated into protein in a 6- to 8-hr incubation; of this fraction, about 0.1% can be recovered in major histocompatibility antigens. At first, the amount of label incorporated rises linearly with time, but after about 12 hr the uptake is not significantly increased by further incubation.

Other isotopes can also be used to label protein biosynthetically. [³⁵S]Methionine has the advantages that simple autoradiographic procedures can be used to analyze the purified products [autoradiography of ³H-labeled compounds is less convenient (Laskey and Mills, 1975)] and that the amino acid is available at high specific activity. However, these advantages must be weighed against the fact that most proteins contain relatively few methionine residues. A method for incorporating ¹⁴C label into all 20 amino acids in a single culture, developed to provide material for amino acid sequence studies, has been published by Ballou *et al.* (1976), who used ¹⁴C-labeled amino acids and [¹⁴C]pyruvate to label histocompatibility antigens to activities sufficient for partial amino acid sequence determination.

The procedure given below is that of Ziegler and Pink (1975) for labeling chicken peripheral blood leukocytes with [³H]leucine and [³H]lysine.

Procedure

Viable cells (5×10^7) are incubated in a 10-cm-diameter plastic petri dish in a 5% CO_2/95% air incubator at 37°C in 10 ml of modified Eagle's medium (MEM) lacking leucine and lysine. The medium is supplemented with 10% fetal calf serum (dialyzed overnight against PBS), 2 mM glutamine, and [^{3}H]leucine and [^{3}H]lysine (specific activities, about 20–50 Ci/mmole; 100 μCi of each/ml of culture fluid). If it is desired to label with leucine only, MEM lacking leucine (commercially available) may be used. For labeling with other amino acids, singly or in various combinations, the medium is made up as shown in the tabulation below (the medium given is for labeling with leucine and lycine). The components of the medium are commercially available (for the sources of nonradioactive components see Chapter 27, Section III).

Component	Amount
Earle's balanced salt solution ($10\times$)	1.0 ml
"Essential" amino acids less leucine and lysine ($20\times$)	0.5 ml
"Nonessential" amino acids ($20\times$)	0.5 ml
Vitamins (MEM) ($100\times$)	0.1 ml
[^{3}H]Leucine	1 mCi (ca. 1 ml)
[^{3}H]Lysine	1 mCi (ca. 1 ml)
Fetal calf serum	1 ml
Glutamine (200 mM)	0.1 ml
10% $NaHCO_3$	0.2 ml
Distilled H_2O	To 9.5 ml
5×10^7 cells in PBS	0.5 ml

The amino acid solutions ($20\times$) are made up as given in the following tabulation from 50 mM stock solutions of each amino acid in water, with the omission of the amino acid(s) to be used for labeling.

Essential		Nonessential	
Arginine	(0.2 ml)	Alanine	(0.1 ml)
Histidine	(0.1 ml)	Aspartic acid	(0.1 ml)
Isoleucine	(0.4 ml)	Asparagine	(0.1 ml)
Leucine	(0.4 ml)	Cysteine	(0.1 ml)
Lysine	(0.4 ml)	Glutamic acid	(0.1 ml)
Methionine	(0.1 ml)	Glycine	(0.1 ml)
Phenylalanine	(0.2 ml)	Proline	(0.1 ml)
Threonine	(0.4 ml)	Serine	(0.1 ml)
Tryptophan	(0.04 ml)		
Tyrosine	(0.2 ml)		
Valine	(0.4 ml)		

The cells are incubated for 6–8 hr at 37°C in a 5% CO_2/95% air incubator and then collected, pooled with an equal volume of PBS used to rinse the petri dish, and washed four times with cold PBS containing 10^{-3} M PMSF.

C. Borohydride Reduction Techniques for Labeling Cell-Surface Carbohydrates

Tritiated borohydride has been used to label cell-surface glycoproteins in several ways. Using these methods, the label is introduced either into aldehyde groups or into Schiff bases formed by the reaction of pyridoxal phosphate and the ϵ-amino group of lysines in proteins (Rifkin et al., 1972). The aldehydes are produced by the action of periodate ions on sialic acid residues (Van Lenten and Ashwell, 1971; Blumenfeld et al., 1972) or by the galactose oxidase-catalyzed oxidation of galactose or N-acetyl-galactosamine residues (Gahmberg and Hakomori, 1973). The aldehydes or Schiff bases are then reduced and labeled by the addition of tritiated sodium borohydride.

The efficiency of these reactions is unfortunately very low. An excess of borohydride is needed to incorporate significant amounts of label into the cells (typically less than 0.1% of input radioactivity is taken up by the cells). Thus, to incorporate 10,000 dpm into a protein carrying 0.1% of the sialic acid or galactose available at the cell surface, it is necessary to use at least 10 mCi of NaB^3H_4 in the labeling procedure. Even in the presence of excess borohydride, the fraction of sialic acid or galactose residues that becomes reduced is not more than 10% and is usually less than 1%. However, the method is suitable for labeling carbohydrates and glycoproteins of cells (e.g., red cells and sperm), which do not readily incorporate radioactive sugars.

The procedures given for the periodate oxidation and borohydride reduction steps are from L. Rovis (unpublished data) as modified by Ziegler and Pink (1976); the method given for the galactose oxidase treatment is from Gahmberg et al. (1976), who also describe a very similar periodate oxidation technique together with a milder borohydride reduction step.

Procedure

Suspend 3×10^7 viable cells in 1 ml of PBS and add 1 ml of $NaIO_4$ (4 mM in PBS) or incubate the cells in a solution of galactose oxidase (5 U in 1 ml); keep the cells in suspension (e.g., on a rotary shaker) for 10 min (5 min for red cells) at room temperature for periodate oxidation or for 1 hr at 37°C for galactose oxidase treatment. The efficiency of galactose labeling can be increased severalfold by treating the cells with neuraminidase (12.5 U, 30 min at 37°C) before adding galactose oxidase.

Wash the cells three times with PBS. Resuspend them in 4 ml of PBS and, in a hood suitable for radioactive isotope work, add NaB^3H_4 (about 6 Ci/mmole) to give a final concentration of 1 mM and an activity of 10 to 25 mCi/3 $\times$ 10^7 cells. A suitable procedure is to add 50-μl aliquots of the radioactive NaB^3H_4 dissolved in an appropriate volume of PBS immediately before starting the reaction. Alternatively, aliquots of NaB^3H_4 (e.g., 5 mCi in 0.1 ml) may be stored for several months at $-70°C$ in 0.01 N NaOH if they are frozen immediately after the isotope has been dissolved (Gahmberg et al., 1976); in this case, 10-μl (0.5-mCi) aliquots are used to label 2 $\times$ 10^7 cells (Gahmberg et al., 1976; Gahmberg and Andersson, 1977).

Shake the cells for 15 min at room temperature and then wash the cells four times in cold PBS containing 10^{-3} M PMSF.

III. LYSIS OF LABELED CELLS

The labeled cells are lysed in a nonionic detergent such as Nonidet P-40 (NP-40) (Schwartz and Nathenson, 1971) or Triton X-100 (Simons et al., 1973), which is chemically similar to NP-40. The concentration of detergent should be sufficient to lyse cellular, but not nuclear, membranes (the concentration usually employed for lysing mammalian lymphocytes is 0.5%, but if a new cell type is to be investigated it is wise to make a preliminary check of the yield of intact nuclei after lysis in detergent of various concentrations).

Procedure

After labeling and washing as described in the preceding sections, the cells are suspended at a concentration of 1–3 $\times$ 10^7/ml in PBS containing 1 mM PMSF. One-third volume of NP-40 [2% (v/v) in PBS containing 1 mM PMSF] is added so that the final NP-40 concentration is 0.5%, and the solution is rapidly mixed. The tube is left (without further shaking) at room temperature or at 4°C for 5–10 min, and nuclei are then centrifuged out (1000 g, 10 min).

The supernatant may then be dialyzed against cold PBS containing 1 mM PMSF (two changes of 1–2 liters each). This step is not essential; its purpose is to remove low molecular weight material which may non-specifically bind to immune precipitates made from lysates of iodinated or borohydride-labeled cells (see next section). Handling of the dialysis tubing (which is permeable to the large amounts of isotope it contains) is avoided by first slipping the end of a 15- to 25-cm length of prewet 7-mm dialysis tubing over the tapering end of a Pasteur pipette from which the narrow part has been broken off as shown in Scheme 1.

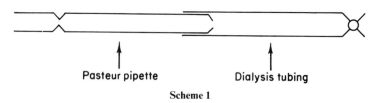

Pasteur pipette   Dialysis tubing

Scheme 1

The pipette is then secured to a holder above the dialysis vessel so that its point is just above the surface of the liquid, while most of the dialysis tubing is submerged. The lysate may now be transferred directly into the dialysis tubing with an intact Pasteur pipette. For removal of the lysate, the tubing is cut and held upright with forceps in a test tube while the lysate is withdrawn.

After dialysis, the lysate is centrifuged again (2000 g, 15 min) to remove any material that may have precipitated, and trichloroacetic acid-precipitable radioactivity in an aliquot of the supernatant is determined. The labeled lysate may be stored at $-70°C$, but the best results are obtained by working as rapidly as possible with material that has not been frozen and thawed.

IV. SPECIFIC PURIFICATION OF LABELED CELL-SURFACE COMPONENTS

Specific antiserum may be added directly to the lysate (Brown *et al.*, 1974). Alternatively, the lysate may be passed over an immunoadsorbent column or treated with insolubilized (e.g., Sepharose-coupled) specific antiserum (Ballou *et al.*, 1976). The latter procedures have the disadvantage that more antiserum is used in preparing the immunoadsorbent than in preparing a simple precipitate, but the advantage that the eluate from the column or insolubilized antiserum contains very little protein. Furthermore, immunoadsorption from the lysate can be accomplished very rapidly, so that the risk of proteolysis during purification is lessened. However, in our experience, the yield of antigen obtained from an immunoadsorbent is not as good as the yield from a specific immunoprecipitation; the need to concentrate material eluted from a column is also a major disadvantage of the method.

Immune complexes formed by the direct addition of antiserum to the lysate may be precipitated by the addition of a second anti-immunoglobulin serum or of protein A-bearing staphylococci (Kessler, 1975, 1976; Cullen and Schwartz, 1976). The use of staphylococci to precipitate immune complexes is described in Chapter 2 and has much to recommend it, particularly rapidity of the procedure, the reduction of nonspecific precipitation of material that binds to Ig–anti-Ig immune complexes, and the elimination of the need to titrate the anti-Ig serum used to form the complexes. However, it should be borne in mind that protein A does not bind to immunoglobulins of all classes or all species (Kronvall and Williams, 1969; Kronvall et al., 1970).

All experiments in which specific antisera are used to precipitate cell-surface components should include a control in which normal (preferably preimmune) sera are substituted for the specific sera and, if possible, a second control in which the specific sera are used to precipitate material from lysates of cells not carrying the desired antigen. In most experiments involving precipitation from leukocyte lysates (see Section I), labeled cell-surface immunoglobulin is removed in a preliminary precipitation step (e.g., Silver and Hood, 1974). If the removal is not complete, this immunoglobulin will be detected in control as well as in specific precipitates. Furthermore, both control and specific precipitates may contain material that is nonspecifically absorbed to any immune complexes. The major nonspecifically bound components are, typically, a protein band with an apparent molecular weight of 45,000, which has been identified as actin (Jones, 1977), plus low molecular weight material, presumably present because dialysis was incomplete. If necessary, these contaminants can be separated from membrane glycoproteins by passing the lysate over a lentil lectin affinity column (Cullen et al., 1976) before the immune precipitation step.

Procedure

Labeled immunoglobulin (Ig) may be removed from the dialyzed lysate as follows. Normal serum from the same species as the labeled cells, containing immunoglobulin acting as a carrier for the precipitation of labeled Ig, is added to the lysate. The amount added (typically 25 μl/10^7 cell equivalents) should equal or exceed the amount of specific antiserum to be added later (see below). Antiserum directed against this immunoglobulin is then added in an amount just sufficient to completely precipitate it. [This amount is determined in a preliminary titration, in which 25 μl of normal serum is mixed with aliquots (e.g., 100, 200, . . . , 1000 μl) of anti-Ig in a total volume of 1 ml (serum + PBS), and the amount of anti-Ig that gives (after overnight formation of a precipitate) a supernatant from which no further Ig can be precipitated by a second addition of 100 μl of anti-Ig is measured.] The precipitate is allowed to form (4–16 hr at 4°C) and is then removed from the lysate by centrifugation (2000 g, 15 min). After removal of labeled Ig, add either specific antiserum or control serum to aliquots of the lysate and incubate for 1–2 hr at 37°C. The amounts to be added are typically 20 μl/10^7 cell equivalents; for serum containing 50 μg/ml of antibody directed against an antigen present in amounts of 5×10^5 molecules/cell, this is a ratio of about two antibody-binding sites per antigen molecule. It is useful to test varying amounts (e.g., 5, 20, and 50 μl/10^7 cells) of serum in preliminary experiments to determine the amount that gives the highest ratio of counts in specific precipitates versus counts in control precipitates. Finally, add the appropriate amount of anti-Ig serum and incubate for 4–16 hr at 4°C.

After the precipitates have formed, they are washed four to six times with 2–4 ml of cold PBS containing 0.1% NP-40 (1000 g, 10 min each wash). They are dissolved in 50 to 100 μl of sample buffer before analysis by SDS-PAGE (see Chapter 4, Section II,B) or in 9.5 M urea containing 5% β-mercaptoethanol, 2% NP-40, and 2% Ampholines (O'Farrell, 1975) before analysis by isoelectric focusing (see Chapter 5). The precipitates can be kept at −70°C until analysis.

REFERENCES

Ballou, B., McKean, D. J., Freedlender, E. F., and Smithies, O. (1976). *Proc. Natl. Acad. Sci. U.S.A.* **73**, 4487.

Blumenfeld, O. O., Gallop, P. M., and Liao, T. H. (1972). *Biochem. Biophys. Res. Commun.* **48**, 242.

Brown, J. L., Kato, K., Silver, J., and Nathenson, S. G. (1974). *Biochemistry* **13**, 3174.

Cullen, S. E., and Schwartz, B. D. (1976). *J. Immunol.* **117**, 136.

Cullen, S. E., Freed, J. H., and Nathenson, S. G. (1976). *Transplant. Rev.* **30**, 236.

Gahmberg, C. G., and Andersson, L. C. (1977). *J. Biol. Chem.* **252**, 5888.

Gahmberg, C. G., and Hakomori, S. (1973). *J. Biol. Chem.* **248**, 4311.

Gahmberg, C. G., Häyry, P., and Andersson, L. C. (1976). *J. Cell Biol.* **68**, 642.

Hubbard, A. L., and Cohn, Z. A. (1972). *J. Cell Biol.* **55**, 390.

Hubbard, A. L., and Cohn, Z. A. (1976). *In* "Biochemical Analysis of Membranes" (A. H. Maddy, ed.), p. 427. Chapman and Hall, London.

Jones, P. P. (1977). *J. Exp. Med.* **146**, 1261.

Kessler, S. W. (1975). *J. Immunol.* **115**, 1617.

Kessler, S. W. (1976). *J. Immunol.* **117**, 1482.

Kronvall, G., and Williams, R. C. (1969). *J. Immunol.* **103**, 828.

Kronvall, G., Seal, U. S., Finstad, J., and Williams, R. C. (1970). *J. Immunol.* **104**, 140.

Laskey, R. A., and Mills, A. D. (1975). *Eur. J. Biochem.* **56**, 335.

Marchalonis, J. J., Cone, R. E., and Santer, V. (1971). *Biochem. J.* **124**, 921.

Melchers, F., and Andersson, J. (1973). *Transplant. Rev.* **14**, 76.

Morrison, M., and Schonbaum, G. R. (1976). *Annu. Rev. Biochem.* **45**, 861.

Morrison, M., Bayse, G., and Danner, D. J. (1970). *In* "Biochemistry of the Phagocytic Process" (J. Schultz, ed.), p. 51. North-Holland Publ., Amsterdam.

O'Farrell, P. H. (1975). *J. Biol. Chem.* **250**, 4007.

Phillips, D. R., and Morrison, M. (1970). *Biochem. Biophys. Res. Commun.* **40,** 284.

Phillips, D. R., and Morrison, M. (1971). *Biochemistry* **10,** 1766.

Rifkin, D. B., Compans, R. W., and Reich, E. (1972). *J. Biol. Chem.* **247,** 6432.

Sanderson, A. R., and Welsh, K. I. (1974). *Transplantation* **17,** 281.

Schwartz, B. D., and Nathenson, S. G. (1971). *J. Immunol.* **107,** 1363.

Schwartz, B. D., Vitetta, E. S., and Cullen, S. E. (1978). *J. Immunol.* **120,** 671.

Silver, J., and Hood, L. (1974). *Nature (London)* **249,** 764.

Simons, K., Helenius, A., and Garoff, H. (1973). *J. Mol. Biol.* **80,** 119.

Van Lenten, L., and Ashwell, G. (1971). *J. Biol. Chem.* **246,** 1889.

Vitetta, E. S., Baur, S., and Uhr, J. W. (1971). *J. Exp. Med.* **134,** 242.

Vitetta, E. S., Uhr, J. W., and Boyse, E. A. (1975). *J. Immunol.* **114,** 252.

Vitetta, E. S., Capra, J. D., Klapper, D. G., Klein, J., and Uhr, J. W. (1976). *Proc. Natl. Acad. Sci. U.S.A.* **73,** 905.

Walsh, F. S., and Crumpton, M. J. (1977). *Nature (London)* **269,** 307.

Ziegler, A., and Pink, J. R. L. (1975). *Transplantation* **20,** 523.

Ziegler, A., and Pink, J. R. L. (1976). *J. Biol. Chem.* **251,** 5391.

11

Haptenation of Viable Biological Carriers

Helmut M. Pohlit, Werner Haas, and Harald von Boehmer

I. INTRODUCTION

This chapter deals with the problem of attaching defined molecules to complex carriers such as proteins, bacteriophages, or cells without interfering with the functional integrity of the carriers.

If the hapten–carrier complex is to be used as a tool for the analysis of immunological specificity, it must be made certain that the observed biological effects are due to the attached hapten and not to side effects of the procedure.

An example is the observation that diazo coupling of haptens to bacteriophage severely reduces infectivity, even at hapten-to-phage ratios at which other haptens would hardly affect viability (Becker *et al.*, 1970). Most likely, this inactivation is due to side reactions and not to the mere presence

IMMUNOLOGICAL METHODS

of the hapten. Other methods may be less harmful, but side effects may still exist.

This chapter describes a method for haptenation of bacteriophage and lymphocytes. Because of its complexity, the use of hapten-coupled lymphocytes to study cytotoxic T cells is discussed in more detail.

A. Commonly Employed Coupling Reactions

The hapten most frequently used in studies on cytotoxic T cells is trinitrophenyl (TNP) sulfonate (Shearer, 1974), about whose coupling reactions very little is known except that, with loss of the sulfonium group, it eventually attaches to primary amines and sulfhydro groups.[1] Other haptens such as NIP were attached to lymphocytes through their acid azides (Koren *et al.*, 1975), and FITC (Starzinski-Powitz *et al.*, 1976) through its isothiocyanate group. In another situation, the haptens TNP and NIP were attached to the amino end of a tripeptide "spacer" whose carboxyl end was coupled to the cell via the acid azide (Rehn *et al.*, 1976). Again, in all of these cases, attachment to primary amines was being observed. Which other reactions occur is not known. In our experience, coupling reactions via diazonium salt have not led to successful hapten-specific lymphocytes. Since for almost every one of the above haptens the coupling reaction is different, the artifacts that might appear as hapten-specific effects must be considered [see, for instance, peroxidase-induced CML determinants (Schmidt-Verhulst and Shearer, 1976)].

B. Coupling via Activated Esters

We have chosen the method of coupling via *N*-hydroxysuccinimide-activated carboxyl (ONS) esters for the reasons listed below.

1. Activated esters are prepared easily. The preparation and isolation of azides (as an example for another mode of activation of the carboxyl group) are clearly more complicated. All ONS esters prepared so far have been found to be soluble in DMF at concentrations of at least 30 mg/ml. These are usually our stock solutions. On the other hand, DMF is infinitely water miscible, thus presenting no problem in the transfer of the activated ester from the organic into the aqueous phase during coupling.

2. Activated esters are very stable in dry solvent. Whether purified or not, stock solutions of esters kept at $-20°C$ have been found to be very stable. This is the basis for reproducible coupling results. If necessary, the

---

[1] There are two reviews on haptenation of carriers and modification of proteins that may serve as sources of general information on related problems: Jacoby and Wilcheck (1974) and Atassi (1977).

activated ester may be transferred without loss of activity into another dry solvent after crystallization or precipitation or after vacuum evaporation of the previous solvent.

3. The hapten-activated esters can be, but often need not be, purified. There is no single solvent system from which all activated esters (which are all solids) may be (re)crystallized. However, warm/cold isopropanol and ethylacetate/petrol ether have been used frequently as recrystallization systems.

On the other hand, we have found that it is not always necessary to purify the activated esters for the present application. Much easier and more important is the purification of the hapten *before* esterification. Excess NHS is not toxic to cells (Dannenberg, 1971) or bacteriophages (H. M. Pohlit, unpublished data) and unreacted DCC can be easily deactivated quantitatively by treatment with HCl in the organic solvent. The urea derivatives (insoluble in DMF, DMSO, THF, and Dioxane) may be filtered.

The preparation of activated esters in pure form may be important when exact quantitation is required or when it is feared that reaction products other than the desired activated forms are present.

4. ONS esters are water compatible. Although ONS esters are generally not water soluble, the ONS moiety transfers a good deal of water compatibility to them, which helps in quickly and reproducibly dispersing the hapten esters, dissolved in DMF, into the coupling reaction mixture. Usually no precipitate occurs. This and the nontoxicity of any of the other chemicals involved are the most decisive factors for the selection of ONS esters over other forms of carbonyl activation.

5. Most haptens may be considered to couple identically. It is difficult to extract from the literature a clear-cut reaction scheme of the ONS-activated esters (Cuatrecasas and Hollenberg, 1976; Wünsch, 1974; Cuatrecasas and Parikh, 1972; Merz and Determann, 1969). This difficulty is caused by the fact that some of the observed effects are due to the synthesis and others are due to the reactions of the activated ester. The situation is further complicated by the different solvent systems to which observations refer (aqueous and nonaqueous conditions). Nevertheless, it seems justifiable to assume that the primary reaction product of DCC with the carboxyl group represents a highly activated state. It may react with many nucleophiles (e.g., also with aliphatic alcohols). *N*-Hydroxysuccinimide, a nucleophile, has, among others, the advantage of retaining some degree of activation of this carbonyl carbon after reacting with the carboxyl group. This lowered degree of activation makes the ONS ester both more stable and more selective with respect to nucleophiles. The differential activation is demonstrated by the inability of an ONS ester to react with aromatic amines, whereas it reacts well with aliphatic amines. On the other hand, a

DCC-activated carboxyl reacts very well with both aliphatic and aromatic amines (Wünsch, 1974).

The ONS-activated esters do not react with aliphatic and phenolic OH groups. There are reports that they react with thiols and are "hydrolyzed" by imidazole (histidine) in an aqueous medium (Cuatrecasas and Parikh, 1972). They react with α- and ϵ-amino acid groups in both organic and aqueous media; this is the preferred reaction over hydrolysis by OH$^-$ ions (in water).

The state of activation of the carboxyl group is determined first by the alcoholic ligand and may be influenced by substitutions at the α-carbon. Thus, whenever inductive or resonance effects may be considered absent or minor, it may be expected that all corresponding ONS-activated esters react identically.

The coupling sites on a cell (or protein) are therefore primary amines with a nucleophilicity of at least that of amino acid α-amines. Thiol side chains may also be coupling sites.

6. Although many haptens may be coupled via the activated ONS ester, there are some restrictions. Many haptens bear a carboxyl group that may be converted immediately to the activated ester. Those with no carboxyl but some other reactive group may be attached to an appropriate bridging molecule bearing both an acceptor group for the hapten and a carboxyl group which is subsequently esterified. Thus, p-sulfodiazobenzene was coupled to p-hydroxyphenylacetic acid, and the product was then esterified; TNP was coupled to ϵ-amino caproic acid followed by esterification of its carboxyl end.

Obviously the variety of haptens that can be coupled by this method is large. However, there are some limitations. Esterification may not succeed in the presence of alcoholic OH groups. Difficulties have also been reported for the imidazole side chain of histidine, for the guanidino side chain of arginine, and for amide in glutamine (Wünsch, 1974; Sakaibara and Inukai, 1965). Of course, the presence of unprotected amino groups would be expected to be detrimental. In general, the nature of the difficulties has not been investigated; instead, a suitable protection of the side chain was employed to circumvent the difficulties. One should, however, clearly distinguish between interference with the formation of the ester and interference with its stability after formation. Either segment of the problem may have its own remedies. For instance, the presence of DCC is avoided in the transesterification method using the ONS ester of trifluoroacetic acid (Sakaibara and Inukai, 1964, 1965; Fujino et al., 1972). Still another method is the oxidation–reduction condensation using triphenylphosphine and 2,2'-dipyridyldisulfide (Mukaiyama et al., 1970a,b).

Esterification (similar in this respect to other activation procedures) at the carboxyl end of a long chain (~10 amino acids) is often very slow (Wünsch, 1974).

Haptens presented on intermediate molecules ("spacers" or "bridges") may have antigenic properties different from those coupled "directly" (Rehn *et al.*, 1976). This may be due to an increased freedom of interaction of the antigen with the combining site of the specific receptor or antibody, as possibly in the case of TNP versus TNP/CAP, both of which presumably attach to identical amino groups and therefore differ only by an additional 6-carbon chain spacer (Becker and Mäkelä, 1975). It also may be due to differences in sites of coupling, as in the case of diazonium salt coupling versus the above-mentioned *p*-hydroxyphenylacetic acid coupling. Finally, it may be due to a changed "specificity," possibly due to "immuno-dominant" portions of the spacer. Which of these conditions prevails is, of course, very important for assessing the specificity of antigenic recognition.

II. PREPARATION OF ONS ESTERS

1. Solvents

Solvents are dried over a molecular sieve.

2. Stock Solutions

NHS (Fluka) and DCC (Fluka, Buchs, Switzerland) are kept in 1 *M* stock solutions in DMF, DMSO, dioxane, or THF (whichever solvent is either necessary for dissolving the carboxylic acid derivative to be esterified or more practical in other respects). All solvents are Merck products. These stock solutions are kept at 4°C. In the course of time some crystallization in the DCC stocks occurs; however, this may be disregarded unless it indicates a substantial loss of solute.

3. Esterification Procedure

Hapten–carboxylic acids are dissolved in a suitable solvent at a concentration of about 0.1 *M*. NHS and DCC stock solutions are added so that both reactants are present at a molar excess of about 10%. The reaction mixture is left for 1 day at room temperature. The progress of the reaction may be judged by the rate at which DCC is converted to its urea derivative, which has a low solubility and therefore crystallizes almost quantitatively. This should occur within a few minutes to 1–2 hr after the start. Should this be delayed considerably and the reaction judged to be slow, possibly harmful side reactions may begin to compete (Gross and Bilk, 1968).

4. Isolation of the ONS Esters for Purification

The precipitated urea derivative is removed from the reaction mixture by filtration, the solvent is evaporated under vacuum, and the remainder is taken up in an appropriate solvent system for recrystallization (e.g., hot/cold isopropyl alcohol). In many cases, it has been found unnecessary for haptenation of cells, and particularly of protein carriers, to purify and isolate the ONS ester, thus avoiding tedious and sometimes low recovery procedures. Crystals are dried in a dry atmosphere at 50°C.

5. Processing of ONS Esters for Coupling to Carriers without Purification and Isolation of the Ester

First, 1 N HCL is added to the esterification mixture (0.5 ml of 1 N HCl for each milliliter of 1 M DCC used) to inactivate any unreacted DCC. After several hours, the precipitated urea derivative is removed by filtration. This solution may be used directly for coupling, provided the coupling buffer has the capacity to bind the additional acid; if it does not, the solvent should be evaporated (lyophilization) and the solids redissolved in the appropriate solvent to remove both HCl and H_2O and, usually, to eliminate more of the (insoluble) DCC–urea derivative. The standard concentration of hapten–ONS ester in these stocks is 0.1 M.

6. Haptens Synthesized and Tested in CML

The haptens that have been prepared in ONS-activated form by the above procedure and used in protein, bacteriophage, and lymphocyte haptenation are listed in Table I. Their formulas are presented in Scheme 1.

The free acids of S/P and PC/P were prepared by the diazotization of sulfanilic acid and the p-amino phenyl ester of phosphorylcholine, respec-

TABLE I

Haptens

Abbreviation	Name (semisystematic)
NIP	3-Iodo-4-hydroxy-5-nitrophenylacetic acid
TNP/CAP	Trinitrobenzene/ε-aminocaproic acid
S/P	p-Sulfanilic acid (PS) derivative
PC/P	Phosphorylcholine (PC) derivative
P	p-Hydroxyphenylacetic acid
A	Acetic acid

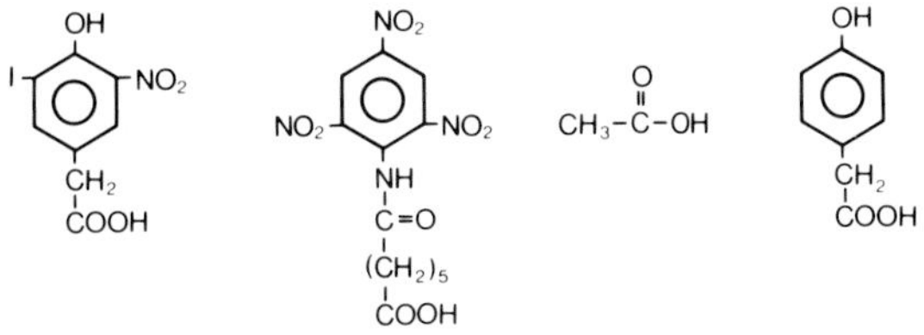

NIP   TNP/CAP   A   P

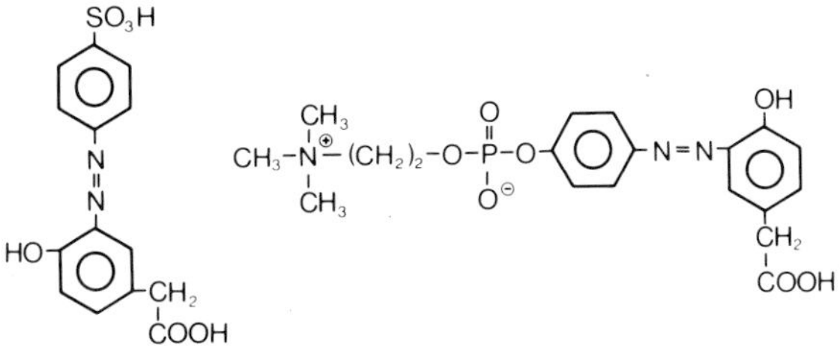

S/P   PC/P

Scheme 1. Structural formulas of haptens.

tively, and coupling these at a concentration of ca. 0.05 M to a 10% excess of p-hydroxyphenylacetic acid (P) in 0.1 M bicarbonate–H_2O at pH 8–9. After repeatedly precipitating at low pH and redissolving at pH 8, the desired product was purified by thick-layer chromatography on silica gel. Chromatography conditions: isopropyl alcohol:H_2O = 7:3 or isopropyl alcohol:NH_4OH:H_2O = 7:2:1; running time, ca. 3 hr. The desired product forms a bright red band, followed by a violet band (most likely a bis-diazo analogue of the desired product). The product was eluted with distilled water and recrystallized at pH 3–4. Analytic TLC runs were developed with Pauly's reagent showing clearly the presence (or absence) of P acid, which runs ahead of the product band. According to such analysis, the presence of P acid from the products could be excluded at levels below 0.2%. Another indicator of purity is the ratio of optical density at 490 nm to that at 330 nm: 0.780 ± 0.005. NIP was prepared according to Brownstone *et al.* (1966). TNP/CAP was prepared by adding a 10% excess of TNP sulfonic acid dissolved in DMF to a 1.0 M solution of ϵ-amino caproic acid in 1 M NaOH–0.2 M bicarbonate–H_2O in an ice bath. The product was precipitated repeatedly at low pH and dried in a vacuum over KOH.

Elemental analyses of all hapten free acids show deviations from the expected values within the experimental error limits (0.5%). Only the A-

and P-ONS esters were purified (hot/cold isopropyl alcohol). Elemental analyses were, by the above criterion, acceptable.

The optical absorption coefficients are shown in Table II.

7. Standard Procedure for Testing the Coupling Efficiency of ONS Esters

Given a method for determining the concentration of hapten in a protein solution (e.g., via optical density or a radioactive label), the following procedure has proved to be simple and reliable.

Ten microliters of the 0.1 M haptens–ONS ester solution (or dilutions of this in DMF) is quickly dispersed into 1 ml of 9 parts 1% BSA in PBS and 1 part 1 M bicarbonate. (Both solutions are kept as stock solutions.) If the hapten absorbs light only in the 280-nm range, polylysine, MW greater than 10,000, is used instead of BSA. The pH of the coupling reaction mixture should be between 8 and 9. After about 30 min an aliquot is removed to determine the "input" hapten concentrations (if it has not been determined independently). The remainder is dialyzed for 24 hr (or possibly longer) against PBS (volume factor, 100–1000). If performed properly, no appreciable volume changes occur in the dialyzing sample. Thus, the determination of hapten concentration after dialysis yields the coupling efficiency. Experience shows that unless some specific reason accounts for lower values, coupling efficiencies lie between 30 and 80%.

Mock coupling (omitting the protein) invariably shows an apparent coupling efficiency of below 0.5%. However, "coupling" is sometimes caused by noncovalent adsorption of the hapten in its acid form (as shown directly by adding hapten acid to the test solution, as above in the case of the hapten–ONS ester, and determining the retention of hapten with the protein). This effect is quite reproducible and depends mainly on the degree of hydrophobicity of the hapten. Thus, noncovalent adsorption is practically absent in S/P; however, it is about 20% (for a 20-hr dialysis period) for P acid and even more for the propionic acid analogue.

TABLE II

Optical Absorption Coeffcients

Hapten abbreviation	$\epsilon\ (M^{-1})$	Wavelength (nm)	Conditions
TNP/CAP	15×10^3	345	PBS
NIP	4.9×10^3	430	PBS
PC/P } S/P }	11.5×10^3	490	0.1 N NaOH
P	1.5×10^3	275	PBS

III. HAPTENATION OF CARRIERS

A. Conditions for Haptenation of Cells

Cells are washed several times in PBS to remove any free protein and other material that might compete with the hapten coupling to cells. Finally, the cells are suspended at 10^7 lymphocytes/ml (or 10% if red blood cells are used) + 2% stock borate buffer (final pH, 8.2). Hapten–ONS esters are added and appropriately diluted (usually in DMF) at a volume ratio of 1 to 20 parts of cell suspension. After 20 min (sufficient for completion of the reaction), washing medium is added and the cells are washed carefully. Usually there is no significant decrease in cell viability, and the overall recovery is 70–100%.

Since DMF dissolves certain plastics, care must be taken in the choice of pipettes and tubes. The activated esters are stable in plastics resistant to this solvent, but glass is still preferable.

B. Testing for the Presence of Haptens on Cells

1. Agglutination

If the hapten density on the cells is sufficiently high (hapten ester final concentration, $\sim 10^{-4}$ M) a qualitative test of successful hapten coupling may be done via agglutination: Two drops of about 10 μl of haptenated cell suspension are placed on a microscope slide. To the first drop, 3 μl of a specific anti-hapten antiserum is added; to the second drop, a control antiserum (normal serum) is added. Both sera are appropriately absorbed with lymphocytes. The microscope slide is slowly rocked back and forth for about 15 sec to allow the cells to move freely. If the haptenation was successful, large aggregates of cells are visible under the microscope in the first drop. However, depending on the strength of the antiserum, low hapten densities may not be detectable this way even though it is sufficient for stimulation and CML.

2. Lysis

Lysis of cells via hapten antibodies plus complement may be observed at a much lower hapten density. Lysis may be judged by the dye exclusion test (trypan blue) or by release of radioactive ^{51}Cr. The latter seems to proceed with difficulty with haptens on normal (unstimulated) spleen cells, whereas haptenated tumor cells or lymphoblasts usually release ^{51}Cr quite easily.

3. Determination of Hapten-Associated Radioactivity

The methods are obvious. It should be borne in mind that all incorporated hapten is determined by this procedure, that is, including the hapten that diffused or was transported into the interior of the cell, and which is therefore presumably not relevant in the present context. The portion of haptens incorporated may be considerable.

C. Haptenation of Bacteriophage

The haptenation of bacteriophage can be described using the following example: hapten S/P on f2 and Qβ. These bacteriophages do not lose infectivity at DMF concentrations as high as 25%. Phage was purified in CsCl gradients, as were the haptenated phages after haptenation. The purified phage preparations were eventually dialyzed extensively against PBS. The haptenation ratio was determined from the absorbance at 490 nm in 0.1 N NaOH (ϵ = 11.5 × 10^3 M^{-1}) and the absorbance at 260 nm (A = 48 at 10^{15} particles/ml). The normal infectivity of these phages is about 15% or lower.

The haptenation procedure is as follows: add 0.5 ml of phage–PBS to 50 μl of 1 M bicarbonate, cool in ice; add 50 μl of S/P–ONS ester dilution in DMF. If the final S/P concentration is 10 or 5 mM, some precipitation may occur, indicating "overcoupling." Figure 1 shows the relevant results. At a low hapten–ONS concentration, the uptake of hapten of phage is almost proportional to the concentration, the coupling yield falling from 43 to 9%. Saturation occurs at about 360 haptens per phage. It is interesting to note that this is just twice the number of phage shell subunits (180 units at 13,700 MW; 6 Lys and 2 Cys per unit).

IV. CML CULTURE CONDITIONS[2]

A. Materials

Medium: RPMI 1640, 10 mM Hepes, 5 × 10^{-5} M 2-mercaptoethanol, glutamine, penicillin + streptomycin (5000 U/ml) and 10% FCS.

Washing medium: RPMI 1640, 10 mM Hepes, and 10% FCS.

PBS: 0.05 M phosphate and 0.9% NaCl.

Stock borate buffer: 13.35 gm of $Na_2B_4O_7 \cdot 10 H_2O$ (0.035 mole) and 4.6 gm of NaCl (0.08 mole) in 1 liter of distilled water; pH, 9.1–9.2.

PBS–borate buffer: 1 part stock borate buffer + 50 parts PBS; pH, approximately 8.

---

[2] See Nabholz *et al.* (1974) for additional information.

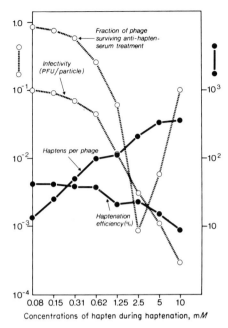

Concentrations of hapten during haptenation, m*M*

Fig. 1. f2 bacteriophages at 10^{15} particles/ml were haptenated with the hapten S/P at various initial concentrations of the hapten (abscissa). The infectivity in plaque-forming units (PFU) per phage particle, the number of hapten molecules per phage particle, the chemical coupling efficiency (amount of hapten on phage per amount of hapten present during haptenation), and the degree by which the haptenated phage may be inactivated by excess anti-S/P antiserum were determined. The nonmonotonous behavior of this plot toward higher haptenation ratios is, as yet, unexplained.

Stimulator cells: Spleen cells [RBS removal by NH$_4$Cl lysis in Gay's solution; dead cell removal by passage through glass wool in low ionic strength buffer (von Boehmer and Shortman, 1973)]; wash twice in PBS; suspend in PBS–borate for haptenation; after careful washing, the cells are irradiated (2000 rad) and washed again; final concentration in culture, 1.5 × 10⁶ cells/ml.

Responder cells: Spleen cells, washed once in BSS; final concentration, 3 to 4 × 10⁶/ml.

Target cells: Tumor cells or 2- to 3-day LPS (50 µg/ml)-stimulated spleen cells (2 × 10⁶ cells/ml); cultured cells are pelleted and 100 µl of sodium [⁵¹Cr]chromate (500–1000 mCi/mg, 10 mCi/ml) is added for 10⁷ cells; incubate at 37°C for 1 hr; cells are purified through a Ficoll gradient (*d* = 1.077) and washed twice in PBS; resuspend the cells in PBS–borate buffer for haptenation.

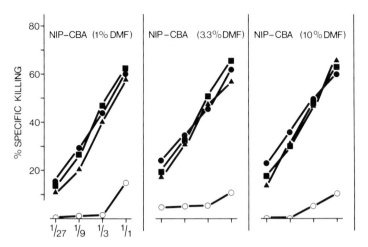

Fig. 2. Normal CBA spleen cells were stimulated *in vitro* with syngeneic spleen cells haptenated with NIP–ONS (50 μM) at a final DMF concentration of 1% (●), 3.3% (■), or 10% (▲) or with allogeneic DBA cells (○). Cytotoxic activity in the cultures was tested after 5 days on 2-day LPS-stimulated blast cells coupled with NIP–ONS under conditions identical to those of the stimulator cells. None of the responder populations killed uncoupled or DMF-treated (10%) target cells (not shown).

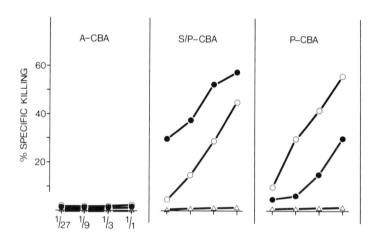

Fig. 3. Spleen cells from CBA mice immunized with 2×10^7 spleen cells coupled with S/P (150 μM) (●), P (1.5 mM) (○), or A (1.5 mM) (△) were restimulated *in vitro* with spleen cells coupled with S/P (50 μM) (●), P (1.5 mM) (○) or A (1.5 mM) (△). Cytotoxic activity was tested 5 days later on 2-day LPS blasts coupled with hapten under conditions identical to those of the stimulator cells.

B. Cytotoxicity Assay

1. Harvesting of Cytotoxic Cells

Usually harvesting is performed 5–6 days after starting the culture; cytotoxic cells are sedimented for 10 min at 1000 rpm and resuspended in ⅓ vol of washing medium.

2. Assay

Place 0.1 ml of target cells (2×10^5 cells/ml) plus 0.1-ml responder cell dilutions (at least three, in steps of 1:3) in washing medium in round-bottom Microtest plates. Spin the plates for 10 min at 100 rpm. Incubate at 37°C in a CO_2 atmosphere for 3–4 hr; spin for 10 min at 1000 rpm and then

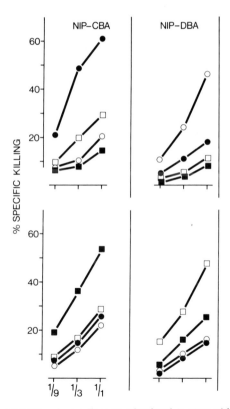

Fig. 4. Normal (CBA × DBA)F_1 spleen cells were stimulated *in vitro* with CBA (●, ■) or DBA (○, □) cells coupled with NIP-ONS (50 μM) (●, ○) or TNP/CAP (50 μM) (■, □). Cytotoxic activity was tested after 5 days on NIP- or TNP/CAP-coupled 2-day LPS blasts, as indicated.

separate 100 μl of the supernatant. The percentage specific killing is the counts per minute per 100 μl of supernatant divided by the total activity incorporated into the target cells; both values are decreased by the ^{51}Cr released spontaneously in the absence of responder cells.

V. OBSERVATIONS ON CML RESPONSES TO HAPTENATED LYMPHOCYTES

1. There is no effect of DMF detectable on hapten-coupled stimulator or target cells (see Fig. 2).
2. There is no effect detectable due to the "chemistry" of haptenation of lymphocytes. Figure 3 shows that cells coupled with acetyl-ONS do not stimulate and that they are not lysed by any syngeneic responder population.
3. The specificity of CML responses to hapten-conjugated cells is not clear. Figure 3 shows a certain degree of hapten specificity of the CML responses to the haptens S/P and P, as would be expected from the structural relationship between these two haptens. Figure 4, however, shows unexplained cross-reactions in CML responses to cells coupled with NIP and TNP/CAP. This figure also demonstrates the incomplete but definite restriction of killing to H-2 homology between target and stimulator cells.

ACKNOWLEDGMENT

H. M. P. gratefully acknowledges Dr. D. Gillesen of Hoffmann–La Roche for his expertise, advice, and frequent helpful critical discussions of many technical problems.

REFERENCES

Atassi, M. Z., ed. (1977). "Immunochemistry of Proteins," Vol I. Plenum, New York.
Becker, M., and Mäkelä, O. (1975). *Immunochemistry* **12**, 329.
Becker, M. J., Conway-Jacobs, A., Wilchek, M., Haimovich, J., and Sela, M. (1970). *Immunochemistry* **7**, 741.
Brownstone, A., Mitchison, N. A., and Pitt-Rivers, R. (1966). *Immunology* **10**, 465.
Cuatrecasas, P., and Hollenberg, M. (1976). *Adv. Protein Chem.* **30**, 295.
Cuatrecasas, P., and Parikh, J. (1972). *Biochemistry* **11**, 2291.
Dannenberg, H. (1971). *Z. Krebsforsch.* **76**, 216.
Fujino, M., Hatanaka, C., and Mitsuno, Y. (1972). *Chem. Abstr.* **76**, 127429.
Gross, H., and Bilk, L. (1968). *Tetrahedron* **24**, 6935.
Jacoby, W. B., and Wilchek, M., eds. (1974). "Methods in Enzymology," Vol. 34., Academic Press, New York.

Koren, H. S., Wunderlich, J. R., and Inman, J. K. (1975). *Transplant. Proc.* **7,** Suppl. 1, 169.

Merz, D., and Determann, H. (1969). *Justus Liebigs Ann.* **728,** 215.

Mukaiyama, T., Matsueda, R., and Suzuki, M. (1970a). *Tetrahedron Lett.* **22,** 1901.

Mukaiyama, T., Goto, K., Matsueda, R., and Ueki, M. (1970b). *Tetrahedron Lett.* No. 60, P5293.

Nabholz, M., Vives, J., Young, H. M., Meo, T., Miggiano, V., Rijnbeek, A., and Shreffler, D. C. (1974). *Eur. J. Immunol.* **4,** 378.

Rehn, T. G., Inman, J. K., and Shearer, G. M. (1976). *J. Exp. Med.* **144,** 1134.

Sakaibara, S., and Inukai, N. (1964). *Bull. Chem. Soc. Jpn.* **37,** 1231.

Sakaibara, S., and Inukai, N. (1965). *Bull. Chem. Soc. Jpn.* **38,** 1979.

Schmitt-Verhulst, A., and Shearer, G. M. (1976). *J. Immunol.* **116,** 947.

Shearer, G. M. (1974). *Eur. J. Immunol.* **4,** 257.

Starzinski-Powitz, A., Pfizenmaier, K., Röllinghoff, M., and Wagner, H. (1976). *Eur. J. Immunol.* **6,** 799.

von Boehmer, H., and Shortman, K. (1973). *J. Immunol. Methods* **2,** 293.

Wünsch, E. (1974). *In* "Methoden der organischen Chemie" (E. Müller, ed.), 4th ed. Vol. XV, p. 149 ff. Thieme, Stuttgart.

12

Production and Assay of Murine Anti-Allotype Antisera

Judith Johnson

The immunoglobulin molecule consists of four polypeptide chains: two identical heavy chains and two identical light chains. In the mouse, six different heavy chains have been found, each of which defines a class of immunoglobulin molecules with unique biological properties. Each of these immunoglobulin classes is found in all mouse strains, but there are structural differences between the heavy chains of a given class from mouse strain to mouse strain, which result from the expression of different allelic genes. When mice of one strain are immunized with immunoglobulin molecules from a second strain, they will produce antibodies that recognize these allotypic differences (Herzenberg *et al.*, 1968). The purpose of this chapter is to detail procedures for the production and assay of murine anti-allotypic sera (Fig. 1). Mice bearing the allotype of interest are hyperimmunized with heat-killed *Proteus mirabilis*. The sera from these mice are mixed with the bacteria, and insoluble immune complexes

IMMUNOLOGICAL METHODS
Copyright © 1979 by Academic Press, Inc.
All rights of reproduction in any form reserved.
ISBN 0-12-442750-2

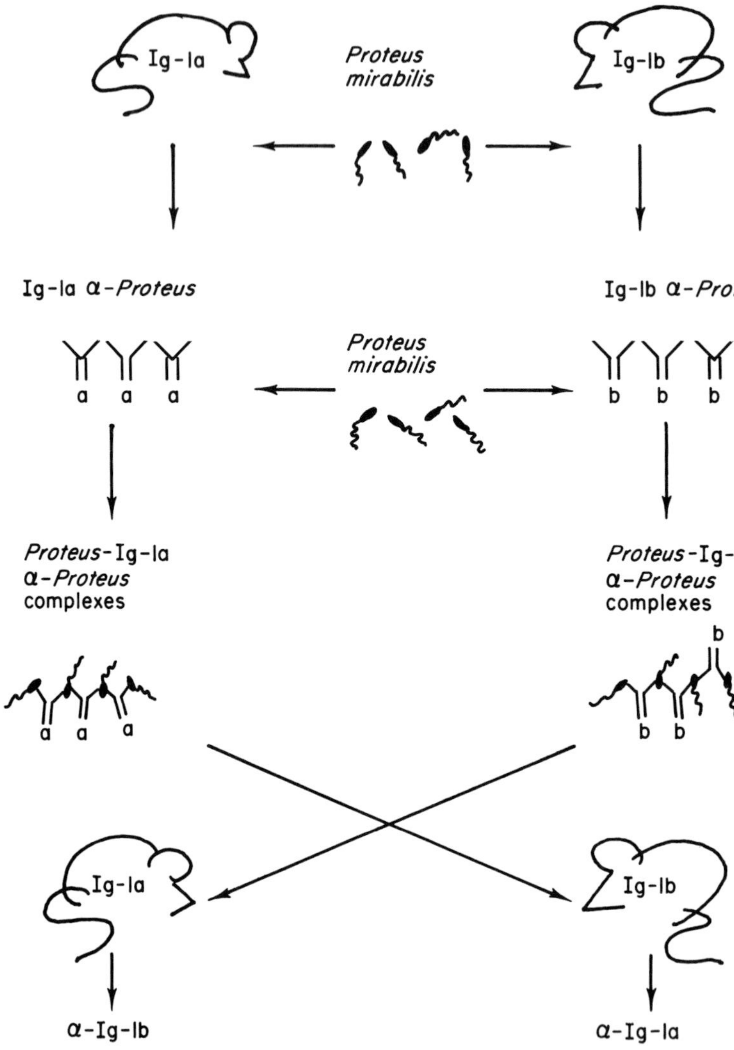

Fig. 1. Production of murine anti-allotype sera.

containing the allotype are formed. The immune complexes are injected into a mouse strain bearing a different allotype; these mice will produce antibody directed to the heavy-chain allotype markers present in the immune complexes. The procedures detailed here will lead to the production of antibodies directed primarily against allotypes of the IgG_{2a} class of heavy chains, which are coded by the *Ig-1* locus (Herzenberg *et al.*, 1968; Herzenberg and Herzenberg, 1973).

I. PRODUCTION OF ANTI-ALLOTYPE SERUM

A. Preparation of Anti-*Proteus* Antisera

1. Materials

Proteus mirabilis (No. 9921, American Type Culture Collection, Rockland, Maryland)
Enriched nutrient agar slants
Enriched nutrient broth
1% $BaCl_2$
1% H_2SO_4, reagent grade
Saline, 0.85% NaCl
Photoelectric colorimeter
37°C water bath or incubator
Ten 10 × 75-mm glass tubes
Ten 120 × 10-mm optically standardized glass tubes

2. Procedure

a. *Proteus mirabilis* cultures are maintained on slants of enriched nutrient agar such as dextrose phosphate. To prepare for use as antigen, 500-ml flasks of broth are inoculated and allowed to grow for 48 hr at 37°C. These cultures are heat-killed and harvested by centrifugation at 6000 rpm for 30 min. They are washed three times in saline, autoclaved, and stored at 4°C. To determine the number of organisms per milliliter, McFarland standards are used (Table I). This is a series of tubes containing various amounts of $BaSO_4$ precipitate, the turbidity of which corresponds to the turbidity of known concentrations of bacteria (Table I; see also Campbell *et al.*, 1970).

TABLE I

Preparation of McFarland Standards

Tube number	1% $BaCl_2$ (ml)	1% H_2SO_4 (ml)	Bacteria × 10^6/ml
1	0.1	9.9	300
2	0.2	9.8	600
3	0.3	9.7	900
4	0.4	9.6	1200
5	0.5	9.5	1500
6	0.6	9.4	1800
7	0.7	9.3	2100
8	0.8	9.2	2400
9	0.9	9.1	2700
10	1.0	9.0	3000

TABLE II

The *Ig-1* Locus

Type/strain	Allele	Specificities											
BALB/c	*a*	1	2	—	—	—	6	7	8	—	10	—	12
C57BL/6J	*b*	—	—	—	4	—	—	7	—	—	—	—	—
DBA/2J	*c*	—	2	3	—	—	—	7	—	—	—	—	—
AKR/J	*d*	1	2	—	—	5	—	7	—	—	—	—	12
A/J	*e*	1	2	—	—	5	6	7	8	—	—	—	12
CE/J	*f*	1	2	—	—	—	—	—	8	—	—	11	—
RIII/J	*g*	—	2	3	—	—	—	—	—	—	—	—	—
SEA/Gn	*h*	1	2	—	—	—	6	7	—	—	10	—	12

The standards are prepared in optically standardized tubes and are stoppered and sealed by dipping in melted paraffin. The concentration of an unknown *Proteus* suspension can be determined by comparing the absorbance (e.g., as measured in a photoelectric colorimeter) of various dilutions of the unknown to a standard curve prepared from the absorbance of the standards.

b. Mice carrying the appropriate *Ig-1* allele (see Table II) are immunized with three to four intraperitoneal injections of 10^9 *Proteus* organisms in saline, spaced 7–10 days apart.

c. After the last injection, the mice are bled and the sera are pooled and tested for anti-*Proteus* activity by bacterial agglutination. Serial twofold dilutions of the antisera are prepared in saline as follows. Ten 10×75-mm tubes are numbered 1 through 10 and 0.5 ml of saline is added to tubes 2–10. To the first tube, 0.95 ml of saline and 0.05 ml of serum are added. The tube is mixed and 0.5 ml is transferred to tube 2. This is mixed and 0.5 ml is transferred to tube 3, and so on. Finally, 0.5 ml of *Proteus* in saline (5×10^8/ml) is added to each tube, and the tubes are mixed and centrifuged at 1000 rpm for 10 min. Agglutination is defined as the presence of a large flocculant precipitate when the tube is gently tapped. The highest dilution in which agglutination has occurred is taken as the titer of the antiserum.

B. Production of Immune Complexes

1. Materials

Anti-*Proteus* antisera
Proteus mirabilis, heat-killed
Saline (0.15 *M* NaCl)
Complete Freund's adjuvant

2. Procedure

a. Anti-*Proteus* sera are diluted in saline to within tenfold of their titer (e.g., if a serum has a titer of 320 it is diluted 1:32).

b. Packed, washed *Proteus* organisms, 10^{10}, are mixed with each milliliter of diluted antiserum and incubated for 30 min at room temperature.

c. These complexes are washed three times in 10 vol of saline (2500 rpm, 10 min) and the pellets are resuspended in 1 ml of saline plus 1 ml of adjuvant per milliliter of diluted antiserum.

C. Production of Anti-Allotype Sera

The selection of mouse strains for the production of anti-allotype sera depends on the presence of H-2-linked immune response genes and non-H-2-linked genes as well as on the allotype allele of the strain (Lieberman and Humphrey, 1971; Dorf *et al.*, 1974). For example, BALB/c mice produce high titers of anti-Ig-1b, whereas C3H mice do not, and LP/J mice produce high titers of anti-Ig-1a antiserum, whereas C57BL/6 mice are low producers. The mice receive 0.1 ml of the immune complexes intraperitoneally every week for 4 weeks. The mice are bled 7 to 10 days after the last injection and tested individually for anti-allotype antibody. The sera from mice producing similar titers of anti-allotype are pooled and these mice are boosted every 4 weeks and bled weekly.

II. QUANTITATION OF ANTI-ALLOTYPE SERUM

Although anti-allotype activity can often be detected by precipitation in gel, not all mice produce precipitating antibody, and passive hemagglutination is more sensitive and more easily quantitated. The use of formalin-treated red cells covalently coupled with purified allotype-bearing immunoglobulin makes it possible to keep indicator cells for at least 6 months. In addition, the use of the microtiter system makes the titration of large numbers of individual serum samples a rapid procedure.

A. Production of Formalinized Sheep Red Blood Cells (FSRBC)

1. Materials

Sheep red blood cells (SRBC)
Phosphate-buffered saline (PBS), pH 7.2, 0.15 M
Neutralized formalin, 3% (formaldehyde is diluted to 3% in saline and the pH is adjusted to 7.0)

37°C water bath or incubator with rocking platform
Thimerosal (ethylmercurithiosalicylate)

2. Procedure

a. SRBC are washed three times in PBS and diluted to 8%. The cells are mixed with an equal volume of 3% neutralized formalin in Erlenmeyer flasks and gently agitated at 37°C for 18–20 hr. The flasks are filled only one-third full and care is taken to avoid foaming.

b. FSRBC are washed five times in PBS and stored as a 10% suspension in phosphate buffer containing 0.01% thimerosal.

B. Preparation of Coupled FSRBC

1. Preparation of Bis-Diazotized Benzidine (BDB) (Campbell et al., 1970)

a. Materials

Benzidine (**Note:** Benzidine is a carcinogen and precautions must be taken to avoid contact with the skin)
$NaNO_2$ (Sodium nitrite)
6 *N* HCl
Acetone–dry ice bath, water–ice bath
Starch iodine paper
0.11 *M* phosphate buffer, pH 7.4

b. Procedure

i. While stirring continuously, add 25 ml of distilled water to 0.23 gm of benzidine, followed by the dropwise addition of 1.5 ml of 6 *N* HCl. Continue stirring for another 5 min. Add another 25 ml of distilled water to the mixture and another dropwise addition of 1.5 ml of 6 *N* HCl. Continue stirring until the benzidine is dissolved completely.

ii. Cool the solution to 0°C in an acetone–dry ice bath. When ice crystals appear, the solution may be kept in an ice–water bath.

iii. Add 2.5 ml of distilled water to 0.25 gm of $NaNO_2$ and pipette 1.5 ml into the benzidine solution with constant stirring. Test for excess nitrite with starch iodine paper and continue to stir the mixture until the test for free nitrite is negative (i.e., the paper does not turn purple).

iv. This stock solution of BDB is standardized by pipetting a 0.5-ml aliquot into a test tube and adding 7 ml of phosphate buffer. The color should change from lemon yellow to a deep reddish brown and turbidity should develop within 90 sec of adding the buffer. If more than 95 sec is required for this change, a few crystals of benzidine should be added. If the reaction occurs in less than 85 sec, a small amount of $NaNO_2$ should be added. In either case, the test should be repeated.

v. The standardized BDB is fractioned into 0.5-ml amounts while keeping the vials in an acetone–dry ice bath. The vials are stored at $-70°C$.

2. Preparation of Isolated γ-Globulins

a. Materials
Sephadex G-200 beads (Pharmacia, Uppsala, Sweden)
$(NH_4)_2SO_4$, ammonium sulfate, saturated solution, pH 7
0.1 M Tris–HCl buffer containing 1.0 M NaCl, pH 8.0 (G-200 buffer)
Chromatography column, 1.0 × 75 cm
Fraction collector with ultraviolet monitor
Spectrophotometer
Polyethylene glycol 20,000

b. Procedure
Immunoglobulin bearing the allotype of interest is isolated from pooled serum or from ascites fluid of myeloma-bearing mice if a myeloma is available. The globulin is isolated by salt fractionation followed by gel filtration.

i. Serum or ascites fluid is diluted with an equal volume of saline and then precipitated by the dropwise addition of an equal volume of saturated ammonium sulfate. This is carried out at 4°C with continuous stirring. The serum is allowed to stir for 2–8 hr at 4°C and the precipitate is collected by centrifugation at 6000 rpm for 20 min. The precipitate is redissolved in saline to the original diluted volume and the precipitation procedure is repeated twice more. The third precipitate is dissolved in a minium volume of saline and placed on a Sephadex G-200 column.

ii. Sephadex G-200 beads are expanded and hydrated in G-200 buffer according to directions. The slurry is deaerated and the column is packed under a constant hydrostatic pressure of 6–8 cm.

iii. The column is washed overnight, the sample is layered on top of the column bed, and the column is run under a pressure of 6–8 cm. Fractions of 5 ml are collected and the absorbance at 280 nm is monitored. Fractions under the second peak are pooled, concentrated, and used as the 7 S IgG preparation. The immunoglobulin preparation is concentrated (e.g., by covering the dialysis bag with polyethylene glycol flakes at 4°C) and analyzed by immunoelectrophoresis and development with rabbit anti-mouse serum. The protein concentration is determined by the Lowry assay.

3. Coupling of FSRBC

The ratio of reagents for FSRBC coupling should be empirically determined. Amounts of protein ranging from 0.01 to 0.5 mg are mixed with 100 μl of 50% FSRBC and incubated in a 37°C water bath. The BDB is thawed and diluted 1:15 with phosphate buffer, and 10–50 μl is added to the cells. The cells are gently agitated for 20 min and then washed five times in 10 vol of phosphate buffer. The coupled cells are stored at 4°C as a 0.1% suspension in phosphate buffer containing 0.01% thimerosal.

C. Titration

1. Materials

Allotype-coupled FSRBC (0.1%)
1% normal rabbit serum in phosphate buffer, 0.11 M, pH 7.4
V-bottom microtiter plates, flexible plastic (Cooke Engineering, Alexandria, Virginia)
Microtiter droppers, 25 μl
Microtiter diluters, 25 μl

2. Procedure

Mice injected with immune complexes are bled individually and tested for the presence of hemagglutinating activity directed to the allotype of interest. Hemagglutination titrations are carried out in V-bottom microtiter plates, using 25-μl diluters. Allotype-coupled FSRBC (25 μl) are added to each well and the plates are mixed and incubated at room temperature. The titer of the serum is reported as the reciprocal of the highest dilution resulting in positive hemagglutination. The immune sera should show no reaction with uncoupled FSRBC. If anti-SRBC agglutinating activity does exist, it can be removed by absorbing the sera with SRBC. However, this activity can generally also be avoided by using the antisera at a starting dilution of 1:20. Titers of anti-allotype sera in this assay will range from 1:125 to 1:10,240.

D. Controls

To ascertain the specificity of the anti-allotype assay, the following controls should be performed.

1. The allotype-coupled FSRBC should not agglutinate in the presence of NRS diluent alone.
2. Serum containing the allotype of interest should be capable of inhibiting the agglutination between antiserum and allotype-coupled cells.

For example, if 25 μl of anti-Ig-1b serum is mixed with 1 μl of Ig-1b normal mouse serum, the subsequently added Ig-1b–FSRBC will no longer be agglutinated by the anti-Ig-1b serum. The addition of serum from mice bearing a non-cross-reacting allotype (e.g., Ig-1a), however, will not inhibit this agglutination. That this activity is in fact due to the immunoglobulin allotypes can be further tested by the use of allotype congenic mice in the inhibition assay. CWB (Ig-1b) and C3H.SW (Ig-1a), and CB.20 (Ig-1b) and BALB/c (Ig-1a) are pairs of mice that differ from each other only in the chromosomal region bearing the immunoglobulin allotype loci. CWB and CB.20 sera will inhibit the anti-Ig-1b assay but not the Ig-1a assay.

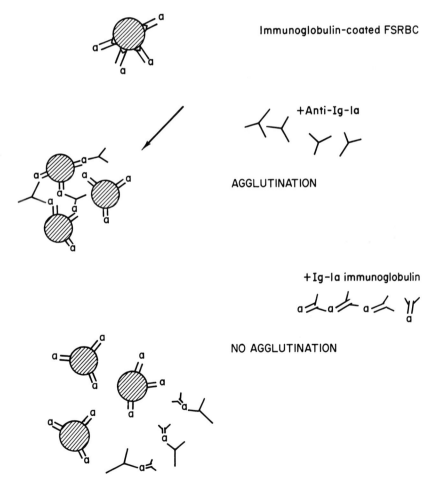

Immunoglobulin-coated FSRBC

+Anti-Ig-Ia

AGGLUTINATION

+Ig-Ia immunoglobulin

NO AGGLUTINATION

Fig. 2. Assay for anti-allotype and allotype.

III. APPLICATIONS

The anti-allotype hemagglutination assay can be modified for use as a quantitative assay for allotype-bearing immunoglobulin. This involves the use of a standard batch of allotype-coupled cells and an anti-allotype serum. Known amounts of a purified allotype-bearing immunoglobulin are added to titration plate wells containing various anti-allotype dilutions and allotype indicator cells. Each concentration of allotype-bearing immunoglobulin is tested for its ability to inhibit the agglutination between allotype-coupled cells and anti-allotype serum (Fig. 2). A standard curve can be prepared relating the micrograms of allotype-bearing immunoglobulin to the reciprocal of the percentage inhibition observed in the standard antisera–indicator cell system. Using this standard curve it is possible to quantitate the amount of allotype present in an unknown sample by determining the percentage inhibition that the unknown can cause.

The quantitation and detection of immunoglobulin allotypes enable the regulation of allelic exclusion and the relationship between allotypes and specific antibodies to be studied. In addition, the allotype can be used as a marker to determine the source of antibody-producing cells in adoptive transfer studies or in chimeric animals.

REFERENCES

Campbell, D. H., Garvey, J. S., Cremer, N. E., and Sussdorf, D. H., eds. (1970). "Methods in Immunology." Benjamin, Reading, Massachusetts.
Dorf, M. E., Dunham, E. K., Johnson, J. P., and Benacerraf, B. (1974). *J. Immunol.* **112,** 1329.
Herzenberg, L. A., and Herzenberg, L. A. (1973). "Handbook of Experimental Immunology." Blackwell, Oxford.
Herzenberg, L. A., McDevitt, H. O., and Herzenberg, L. A. (1968). *Annu. Rev. Genet.* **2,** 209.
Lieberman, R., and Humphrey, W., Jr. (1971). *Proc. Natl. Acad. Sci. U.S.A.* **68,** 2510.

13

Preparation of Mouse Antisera against Histocompatibility Antigens

C. Garrison Fathman

I. OBJECTIVE

From the original description by Gorer (1937) of blood group antigen II, the development of the genetics of the mouse major histocompatibility complex (MHC) has been rapid and exciting (for a review, see Shreffler and David, 1975). The use of anti-alloantisera raised against cell-surface antigens that are products of genes of the MHC has been an invaluable tool in this rapid development. The purpose of this chapter is to present a detailed procedure on the preparation and characterization of such antisera directed against products of the *H-2* loci of the mouse MHC.

IMMUNOLOGICAL METHODS
Copyright © 1979 by Academic Press, Inc.
All rights of reproduction in any form reserved.
ISBN 0-12-442750-2

II. PRINCIPLE OF THE METHOD

It is possible to produce anti-H-2 antibodies by a variety of procedures including skin grafting, inoculation of lymphoid tissue, and/or tumor transplantation. I shall attempt to present methods currently used at the Basel Institute for production of such antisera and will refer the readers to the literature if other procedures are preferred. Assay of such antibody is accomplished by a variety of procedures, which are outlined below. The current methods of serological H-2 typing make use of a battery of oligospecific alloantisera raised in preselected strains of mice (reviewed in Klein, 1975).

III. MATERIALS AND PROCEDURE

A. Mice

Anti-allogeneic antisera are by definition raised in genetically disparate individuals of the same species. I shall outline procedures for the production of anti-alloantisera using conventional inbred mouse strains available at most commercial dealers and using the criteria listed by Klein (1975). Jackson Laboratories in Bar Harbor, Maine, is the source of the animals most commonly used for such antisera production.

B. Skin Grafting

For the skin grafting technique that is used at the Basel Institute, the following materials are used: a scalpel with a No. 10 blade, a pair of forceps with teeth, a pair of small curved-blade scissors, a box of dissecting pins, a cork dissecting board, a box of rubber bands, Vaseline-impregnated sterile gauze, plaster casting material (plaster of Paris strips, 2 cm wide), a 100-W light bulb in a goose-neck lamp, a 10-cm sterile petri dish, 50 ml of sterile PBS, and a bottle of 4% chloral hydrate (0.1 ml/10 gm body weight).

C. Production of Anti-H-2 Antisera

Mice are immunized by skin grafting according to the method of Billingham outlined below and then, 3 weeks after grafting, are given several (Billingham and Silvers, 1961) biweekly intraperitoneal injections of 2×10^7 live lymphoid cells.

1. Preparation of Donor Skin

a. Donor mice carrying the H-2 alloantigen(s) against which antiserum is desired are sacrificed by cervical dislocation.

b. The tail is cleaned by wiping it with a gauze pad soaked in 90% ethanol.

c. An incision through the full thickness of skin is made along the entire ventral surface of the tail using a No. 10 scalpel blade.

d. Circumferential cuts around the tail through the full thickness of skin are made at the distal and proximal ends of this incision (0.5 cm from each end).

e. The skin is seized at the proximal end dorsal side (near the body) by a pair of forceps with teeth and is simply peeled away from the tail.

f. This section of skin is then placed epidermal side down in a 10-cm glass petri dish containing PBS.

g. The tail skin is then simply cut into multiple rectangular sections about 5 × 5 mm using a dissecting needle to control the piece of skin and cutting with a No. 10 scalpel blade.

2. Preparation of Recipient

a. Mice to be grafted (differing in *H-2* type from the donor animals) are anesthetized using 0.1 ml of 4% chloral hydrate ip per 10 gm body weight.

b. The anesthetized animal is then fixed to a dissecting board by looping rubber bands around each of the legs and stretching the rubber bands and pinning them so that the mouse is reasonably firmly attached with its stomach down and back up.

c. A graft bed is then prepared by simply seizing the skin of the back below the shoulders in the dorsal midline with a pair of forceps with teeth, lifting it up, and excising a circular piece of skin (using scissors with a curved blade) that will leave a circular graft bed large enough to accept the donor skin.

d. Place the graft (one of the rectangular sections of tail skin from above) in the graft bed, being careful to keep the epidermal side up and the graft smoothed over the bed.

e. Place several thicknesses of Vaseline-impregnated gauze over the grafted skin, being careful not to shift the position of the graft.

f. Then place a loose-fitting plaster cast around the entire thorax of the mouse by wetting the plaster of Paris strips and gently placing them around the mouse.

g. The mouse is then removed from the dissecting board and placed in an open cage on dry sawdust about 20 cm below the lighted 100-W light bulb.

This light keeps the animal warm while the anesthesia wears off. Transfer the animal into its regular quarters once the anesthesia wears off.

h. Six days following grafting, the case is removed by cutting along one side using scissors. (The animal need not be anesthesized.)

i. Each graft is assessed individually for technical success at this point before immunological rejection has become evident. The graft should be well seated in the bed and attached to the underlying tissue.

j. Rejection will then occur in standard fashion and should be complete by 21 days.

Three weeks following the skin grafting, the animal is immunized ip with 2×10^7 live lymphoid cells (a mixture of spleen, lymph node, and thymus cells) in suspension in medium that does not contain fetal calf serum. A similar immunization is repeated every 2 weeks for a total of four immunizations following the skin graft. The animals are bled from the tail 1 week after each immunization and the successive bleeds are pooled, fractioned, and stored frozen at $-20°C$ until use.

D. Techniques for Assaying Hemagglutinating Anti-H-2 Antibodies[1]

1. Reagents and Equipment

ACD (acid citrate dextrose): 27.2 gm of Na_3-citrate $\cdot 2H_2O$, 1.7 gm of H_3-citrate $\cdot 1\ H_2O$, 2.2 gm of $NaH_2PO_4 \cdot 1\ H_2O$, and 25.0 gm of dextrose. Add distilled water to bring the volume to 1000 ml; filter and store at 4°C in sterile bottles.

PBS (phosphate-buffered saline), pH 6.8.

PVP (polyvinylpyrrolidone), 1.0% in PBS with 0.1% BSA (bovine serum albumin). The PVP is supplied as a 45% aqueous solution. It is made up in PBS to 1% solution, fractioned, and autoclaved. It can be stored at room temperature. Just before using, BSA is added to make the 1% PVP contain 0.1% BSA. After the BSA is added, the PVP will keep in the cold for a few days, but I prefer to make fresh reagents daily. The PVP is available from General Aniline and Film Corporation (140 West 51st Street, New York, New York 10020); specify polyvinylpyrrolidone (PVP), Type K-60, 45% aqueous solution, Lot No. 29. The PVP varies from lot to lot, and lots other than 29 may not work at 1%.

---

[1] Modified from Stimpfling (1961) by Beverly Deak, Stanford University, Stanford, California.

Disposable test tubes, 10 × 75 mm.
Hamilton syringe with automatic dispenser, pipettes, and serial diluter.
Alloantiserum (anti-H-2 serum).

2. Collection of Cells

a. For titering antiserum, the red blood cells are collected in a graduated centrifuge tube containing a large excess of ACD, washed twice in PBS, and resuspended in PBS to a 2% suspension.

b. For typing, the red blood cells are more conveniently collected by bleeding 75 μl from the retro-orbital plexus into 2.0 ml of ACD. The cells are then washed twice with 2-ml aliquots of PBS and resuspended in 2 ml of PBS. This gives a 2% suspension.

3. Titering Antiserum

The test is set up in duplicate with a normal mouse serum (NMS) control. For example, let us assume serial dilutions from $\frac{1}{10}$ to $\frac{1}{5120}$ (10 tubes across). Dispense 0.18 ml of PVP solution into the first tube and 0.1 ml in the remaining tubes. Add 20 μl of alloantiserum to the first tube and serially dilute across the row by transferring 0.1 ml, discarding the final 0.1 ml. Repeat for each row. For each *set* (two rows of antiserum dilution and one row of NMS dilution) add 0.05 ml of 2% RBC suspension to each tube. Shake the rack, incubate at room temperature for 2 hr, and read.

4. Typing Red Cells

Again the test is set up in duplicate with an NMS control, but this time only the dilution of antiserum that gives optimal agglutination is used. For each tube, 0.1 ml of serum dilution is added (either antiserum or NMS). Then, 0.05 ml of a 2% suspension of test cells is added to each set, and the rack is shaken, incubated at room temperature for 2 hr, and read.

5. Controls

In addition to NMS for a serum control, it is advisable in titering and typing to use known positive and known negative cell controls.

6. Reading

To read, tubes are "stroked" smoothly across the length of an Rh-typing box 8 or 10 times and scored for red cell agglutination on a scale of 1 to 4. I consider clarity of the suspending medium as well as clump size in scoring. Generally, a good positive will be in clear suspension. Always use an NMS control.

E. Antibody-Mediated Cytotoxicity[2]

1. Reagents

a. Tris-Buffered NH₄Cl

Tris: 20.6 mg of Tris per liter (Schwarz–Mann, Orangeburg, New York). Fill a 1-liter volumetric flask one-half to three-quarters full and adjust the pH to 7.2–7.4 with concentrated HCl (starting pH, about 11.0) and adjust the volume to 1 liter.

NH_4Cl: 8.3 gm of NH_4Cl per liter in distilled H_2O (Allied Chemicals, Morristown, New Jersey).

To prepare the buffer, mix 9 parts of Tris stock solution with 1 part of NH_4Cl stock solution and store at 4°C. It is good for several weeks and is used at 37°C.

b. Medium

1% gelatin: 1 gm of gelatin (Nutritional Biochemical Corp., Cleveland, Ohio) is heated in 100 ml of distilled H_2O, with stirring to just below boiling. Filter hot through S and S fluted filter paper No. 588 (S and S, Keene, New Hampshire). Store frozen in 5- or 10-ml aliquots.

To prepare the gelating medium, mix 100 ml of medium TC-199 with 10 ml of 1% gelatin. (Melt in either 55° or 37°C water bath before adding.)

c. Trypan Blue (Allied Chemicals No. 0508)

Use stock solution of 1% in distilled H_2O. Dilute the stock solution 1:5 in saline for daily use.

d. Complement

Rabbit or guinea pig serum selected for low spontaneous lytic activity is used as the source of complement.

2. Cell Preparation

a. Remove the spleens of the appropriate animals and place them in a petri dish on ice.

b. Perfuse each spleen (5-ml syringe, 22-gauge needle) with Tris-buffered NH_4Cl (at 37°C); use approximately 3.0 ml. *Note:* For a mouse spleen, the yield by this method is 2 to 4 × 10⁷ cells.

c. Incubate the cells in Tris-buffered NH_4Cl for 5 min at 37°C (15-ml conical tubes, Falcon Plastics).

d. Fill the tubes with medium and gel and spin at 1400 rpm for 6–8 min.

e. Decant the supernatant and resuspend the cells to 2.0 ml with medium and gel for counting.

[2] Modified from Gorer and O'Gorman (1956) and Sachs *et al.* (1971).

f. Determine cell count and viability with trypan blue. (Continue only if viability is 90% at this stage.)

g. Adjust the cells to 5×10^6/ml for cytotoxicity test.

3. Two-Stage Cytotoxicity Procedure

This is performed in microtiter plates (Cooke Engineering, Alexandria, Virginia) and may be done with either 25- or 50-μl equipment.

a. Add 25 μl of medium and gel to all wells. Include wells for medium, serum, and complement controls for each titer.

b. Add 25 μl of the anti-H-2 antiserum to be tested (decomplemented, 56°C for 30 min) to the serum control well.

c. Add 25 μl of the antiserum to be tested to one well (generally well No. 4).

d. Dilute the serum out using 25-μl serial dilutions to the end of the plate.

e. Add 25 μl of target cells to each well and mix on a Micromixer (Cooke Engineering) for 10 sec at speed 3.

f. Add the coverplate and incubate for 15 min at 37°C.

g. Remove from the incubator and add 150 μl of medium and gel to all wells.

h. Spin at 1000 rpm for 5 min using microtiter plate holders (Cooke Engineering).

i. Remove the supernatant by suction or by flicking.

j. Add 25 μl of complement, diluted for use, to all titered wells plus complement control.

k. Mix all wells with the plate covered by self-adhering tape (Cooke Engineering or NIH stock). This requires vigorous mixing for 30 sec at full speed on a Micromixer.

l. Incubate for 30 min at 37°C.

m. Spin down at 10°C at 1500 rpm (450 g for 5 min).

n. *Read:* Remove the supernatant from five wells. Add 10 μl of trypan blue to each well, mix, and remove 5 μl for counting. Eppendorf pipettes (Brinkmann Instruments, Westbury, New York) are convenient for this purpose. Counting is done an F500 white slide (Roboz Surgical, Washington, D.C.) using a Kimble No. 1 cover glass (12-mm circle).

F. Chromium Release Assay for Antibody-Mediated Cytotoxicity[3]

1. Reagents

Use the following: [51]Cr (Amersham/Searle Corp.) at 300 μCi/ml in a cell concentration of 10^8/ml and medium TC-199 with 0.1% gelatin (see above).

---

[3] Modified from Wigzell (1965), Sanderson (1969), and Kaliss (1969).

2. Cell Preparation

This is the same as Section III,E,2.

3. Cytotoxicity Assay

a. Label the cells with ^{51}Cr at 300 μCi/ml at a cell concentration of 10^8/ml for 40 min at 37°C in medium 199. Shake the cells every 10 min.

b. Wash three times (450 g) in medium 199 containing 0.1% gelatin and resuspend in the same medium following the final wash at 5×10^6/ml.

c. Perform the cytotoxicity assay in Cooke microtiter plates (round bottom) by adding 25 μl of the cell suspension to 25 μl of antisera diluted serially as in the previous method. Be sure to leave wells for medium and complement controls.

d. Incubate the cells and antisera for 15 min at 37°C and wash once by filling the wells with cold TC-199 containing 0.1% gelatin; flick off the supernatant (remember it is radioactive).

e. Add 25 μl of complement at the appropriate dilution to each well including complement control well but excluding medium control, which gets 25 μl of TC-199 with 0.1% gelatin.

f. Incubate at 37°C for 30 min.

g. Spin down the cells (450 g) and collect the supernatant from each well.

h. Assay the ^{51}Cr counts (standard γ-counting) per supernatant and as a control the counts contained in 25 μl of labeled cells.

i. Percentage lysis is then calculated using the following formula:

$$(\% \text{ lysis})_N = 100 + [(\text{supernatant}_N/\text{total}_N - \text{supernatant}_M/\text{total}_M)/(\text{supernatant}_Z/\text{total}_Z - \text{supernatant}_M/\text{total}_M)]$$

where N, experimental well; M, medium control; Z, potent anti-H-2 control; total, radioactivity (cpm) of 25 μl of labeled cells. For convenience, the entire supernatant is not assayed, only an aliquot (i.e., 10 μl), and the counts per minute are then adjusted to the total volume of the supernatant.

IV. CONTROLS

As pointed out in Section III, it is necessary to have controls in each type of assay for anti-H-2 antisera. In every instance, a medium control is included. This will account for unexpected lysis due to some problem with the medium. In addition, the complement control is included to test the possibility of inappropriate lysis due to complement alone (or in combination with the medium) and, finally, a potent anti-H-2 serum of known specificity and titer is included to check specificity of the reaction and to ascertain that the expected complement activity is present. In addition to these internal controls, the cells used for specific targets in the assay will be controlled by the known anti-H-2 antiserum used as serum control; however, the specificity of the unknown antiserum must be controlled by using inappropriate targets. Usually these are of two types:

1. Cells from the antiserum-producing strain are used to test for autoantibodies (i.e., antibodies that will react with self).
2. Cells from an inappropriate (i.e, non-*H-2*-matched) strain are used to test for nonspecific antibodies that might be directed toward non-H-2 antigens. This control is best accomplished using cells from *H-2* congenic strains that are similar in background to the strain against which the antiserum is directed, but carry the *H-2* type of the strain producing the antibody.

When such inappropriate antibodies (i.e., directed at cell-surface antigens other than the specific H-2 antigen against which it was purportedly raised) are detected, they can generally be removed by absorption and, in fact, specific absorption is quite often used to increase the specificity of anti-H-2 antisera. Furthermore, specific absorption [i.e., absorption with cells from strains bearing the H-2 antigen(s) against which the antiserum is directed] is a critical test of specificity. For a detailed analysis of such absorptions, see Klein (1975, pp. 81–93). For a detailed methodology of absorptions, see Sachs and Cone (1975).

V. CRITICAL APPRAISAL

The ultimate goal of serological analysis should be the definition of a certain *H-2* haplotype. Each of the methods described in this chapter has certain advantages and certain limitations to reaching this goal. The advantage of skin grafting for the primary immunization is the potency of an allogeneic skin graft as an immunogen; the disadvantage is the laboriousness of the procedure. The ultimate plateau titer of anti-H-2 antibodies raised by skin grafting is no different from that seen using multiple ip injections but is simply reached faster. If simple repeated ip immunization is used, it is widely held that female recipients are better antibody producers than males. The various techniques used for assay of anti-H-2 activity all have certain disadvantages. I have outlined the three most widely used techniques, but there are many more techniques and modifications of these techniques that can be used [see Klein (1975) and Chapter 17 for a more complete listing of the techniques and references].

H-2 antibodies were originally discovered as anti-erythrocyte antibodies. The various technical difficulties encountered in early techniques of hemagglutination have largely been circumvented by the use of a colloid as diluent in the procedure reported here. The problems inherent in hemagglutination techniques are largely due to the fragility of mouse RBC.

The problems with cytotoxicity are somewhat more varied than those observed in hemagglutination, but these techniques have become standard in many laboratories due either to their simplicity and speed or to quantitation and objectivity in the case of ^{51}Cr release. The biggest problem in both types of cytotoxicity studies is the complement that is used. Most laboratories use rabbit or guinea pig serum as a source of complement. The activity varies from animal to animal and from batch to batch. Each pool first must be tested for spontaneous cytotoxicity (usually due to anti-mouse antibodies) and then frozen at $-70°C$ in small aliquots. These aliquots are thawed just prior to use and the excess serum is then discarded after use.

Each test has proponents that claim quantitation and reproducibility. It is better for an investigator to attempt several separate assays and choose the one that provides him with reproducibility and the sensitivity he desires.

REFERENCES

Billingham, R. E., and Silvers, W. K., eds. (1961). "Transplantation of Tissue and Cells." Wistar Inst. Press, Philadelphia, Pennsylvania.

Gorer, P. A. (1937). *Br. J. Exp. Pathol.* **18**, 31.

Gorer, P. A., and O'Gorman, P. (1956). *Transplant. Bull.* **3**, 142.

Kalis, P. (1969). *Transplantation* **8**, 526.

Klein, J. (1975). "Biology of the Mouse Histocompatibility-2 Complex," pp. 67–127. Springer-Verlag, Berlin and New York.

Sachs, D. H., and Cone, J. (1975). *J. Immunol.* **114**, 165.

Sachs, D. H., Winn, H. J., and Russell, P. S. (1971). *J. Immunol.* **107**, 481.

Sanderson, A. R. (1969). *Br. J. Exp. Pathol.* **45**, 398.

Shreffler, D. C., and David, C. S. (1975). *Adv. Immunol.* **20**, 125.

Stimpfling, J. H. (1961). *Transplant. Bull.* **27**, 109.

Wigzell, H. (1965). *Transplantation* **3**, 423.

14

Technique of HLA Typing by Complement-Dependent Lympholysis

John W. Stocker and Domenico Bernoco

I. INTRODUCTION

Detection of the HLA antigens carried on the cell surface of a variety of human cells may be performed by several techniques. In this chapter the complement-dependent lympholysis technique will be described. This test has gained widespread acceptance as a reproducible, convenient means of histocompatibility typing in man since its introduction by Terasaki and McClelland (1964). The test to be described uses the incubation conditions and reagent quantities of the NIH standard procedure (Brand *et al.*, 1970; Terasaki *et al.*. 1978).

IMMUNOLOGICAL METHODS
Copyright © 1979 by Academic Press, Inc.
All rights of reproduction in any form reserved.
ISBN 0-12-442750-2

II. PRINCIPLES OF THE TEST

Human blood lymphocytes are separated from heparinized peripheral blood following (a) elimination of the adherent cell population by a nylon-wool column and (b) lymphocyte purification by density gradient centrifugation (Bøyum, 1968).

The separated lymphocytes are incubated in the wells of plastic trays with typing alloantisera containing anti-HLA antibodies of defined specificity. In each test, a battery of different antisera including monospecific and oligospecific reagents is used. These sera are obtained from multiparous women and from planned immunization, and their specificity has been previously determined by comparing their reaction pattern with that of defined antisera and by analyzing the pattern of segregation within families. The miniaturization of the system, requiring only 1 μl of antiserum for each test, has permitted extensive international exchange of antisera.

Complement is added to the cell–antisera mixture and incubation is continued. After incubation with complement, eosin solution is added to allow identification of viable cells that exclude the dye. The preparation is then fixed by adding formaldehyde solution.

The test is read by inspecting each well under a phase-contrast microscope. The proportion of viable (unstained) lymphocytes is estimated and recorded for each individual well.

The HLA phenotype of the individual is established by comparing the pattern of positive cytotoxicity reactions with the specificities of the antisera in the positive wells.

A flow diagram of the steps in the test is given in Table I.

TABLE I

Flow Diagram for the Lymphocyte Cytotoxicity Test

Step	Procedure	Conditions
1	Typing trays set up	Stored at $-80°$C
2	8–10 ml of peripheral blood	Heparinized
3	Adherent cell removal on nylon column	37°C, 30 min
4	Lymphocyte-rich suspension prepared by density gradient	
5	Lymphocytes incubated with antisera	Room temperature, 30 min
6	Complement added, incubated	Room temperature, 60 min
7	Eosin added	5 min
8	Formaldehyde added	
9	Test result read	Inverted phase-contrast microscope

III. DETAILS OF THE TEST

A. Materials Required

Microtest plates, Cat. No. 3034 (Falcon Plastics, Division of BioQuest, 5500 West 83rd Street, Los Angeles, California 90045)

Hamilton syringes (needle point style 3)

50 lambda 705 N
100 lambda 710 N
250 lambda 725 N
500 lambda 750 N

Hamilton repeating dispenser PB 600-1 (Hamilton Co., P.O. Box 307, Whittier, California 90608)

Cornwall 5-ml syringe plus repeating dispenser (Beckton–Dickinson Co., Waltham, Massachusetts 02150)

Mineral oil: Olio di Vaselina, Code No. 200 466 (Carlo Erba, Divisione Chimica Industriale, Milano, Italy)

McCoy's 5 A medium, Cat. No. 166 (Grand Island Biological Co., 3175 Stanley Road, P.O. Box 68, Grand Island, New York 14072)

Eosin Y, pure for histology and blood staining, No. 45380 (Serva, Feinbiochemica, Heidelberg, Germany)

Formaldehyde solution, 37% acid free, Cat. No. 3999 (E. Merck A. G., Darmstadt, Germany)

Microscope cover glasses, 45 × 65 mm (Gerhard Menzel, Glas-bearbeitungswerk K. G., D-3300 Braunschweig, Saarbrückner-strasse 248, Germany)

TC Hank's solution, 10×, Cat. No. 5774-72 (Difco Laboratories, Detroit, Michigan)

TC bicarbonate solution, 10%, Cat. No. 5788-60 (Difco Laboratories, Detroit, Michigan)

Ficoll 400 (Pharmacia, Uppsala, Sweden)

Urovison, 58% (Schering AG, Berlin/Bergkamen)

7X Detergent (Linbro Chemicals Scientifique Co., P.O. Box 6187, 143 Leederhill Drive, Hamden, Connecticut 06517)

Complement source: Normal rabbit serum, a pooled bleed from approximately 100 rabbits, is stored at −80°C in small aliquots or is lyophilized, stored at −20°C, and reconstituted immediately before use

B. Test Procedure

1. Setting Up Typing Trays

Mineral oil, approximately 2 μl, is added to each well of the Microtest plate by means of a repeating dispenser. Typing trays are conveniently set up in batches in multiples of 48 trays. They contain mineral oil to prevent evaporation of the small volume of reagents used in the test and are stored at $-80°C$ until immediately before use.

One microliter of each typing serum is dispensed into every well using a 50-μl Hamilton syringe. The position of a particular serum is uniform in each tray. Negative control wells containing McCoy's medium and positive controls with human anti-lymphocyte serum (ALS) prepared in rabbits are also included. High-titer ALS must be diluted before dispensing to avoid contamination by anti-lymphocyte antibodies of adjacent wells during cell and complement addition.

2. Cell Separation Technique

a. Removal of Adherent Cells. To a 20-ml disposable syringe 1.5 gm of washed nylon wool is added. The wool is washed by soaking in $7\times$ detergent solution for 24 hr followed by rinsing under running tap water for 48 hr and then soaking in distilled water for a further 48 hr with frequent changes of distilled water. The washed wool is dried at $37°C$. Heparinized blood, 8 ml, is added to the nylon-wool column and distributed through the wool by means of the plunger. The column is then incubated for 30 min at $37°C$.

Nonadherent cells are washed through the column by rinsing with Hank's solution at room temperature. Twenty milliliters of Hank's solution is used for each column.

b. Density Gradient Separation of Lymphocytes. The Urovison–Ficoll solution is made by dissolving 18.47 gm of Ficoll in 238.8 ml of distilled water. Urovison, 50 ml, is added and the mixture is stirred for 60 min at room temperature in the dark. The density of the solution is adjusted to 1.077 by adding distilled water or Ficoll. The solution is Millipore-filtered and stored in aliquots at $4°C$. For the separation procedure, 3.5 ml of Urovison–Ficoll is added to centrifuge tubes and 10–12 ml of the cell suspension obtained after adherent cell separation is layered over the gradient. The Urovison–Ficoll should be at room temperature at the time of cell overlay. The tubes are then centrifuged at $1000\,g$ at $20°C$ for 20 min.

After centrifugation, the lymphocyte-rich layer can be seen at the interface between the medium and the Urovison–Ficoll and is transferred to a fresh tube. The cells are then washed twice in Hank's solution, resuspended in McCoy's medium, and counted, and the cell concentration is adjusted to approximately 2×10^6/ml. An approximate estimation of cell concentration may be performed without counting the cells by transferring 1 μl of the cell suspension to a chamber containing mineral oil and inspecting from beneath with an inverted phase-contrast microscope. The proportion of granulocytes and erythocytes contaminating the lymphocyte suspension can be determined with the high-power objective.

3. The Cytotoxicity Test

To each well of the typing trays is added 1 μl of lymphocyte suspension using the dispensing syringe. The cell–antiserum mixture is held at room temperature for 30 min, after which complement is added. The complement is thawed rapidly, immediately before use, and held on ice. Complement, 5 μl, is transferred to each well and incubation at room temperature is continued for a further 1–1.5 hr, the duration of this incubation depending on the strength of the complement batch. This is determined by comparing the reaction of a lymphocyte sample in a typing tray using a known complement batch and the new batch. The incubation time in the new complement is adjusted to produce identical reactions with the standard.

After complement incubation, 5% eosin Y solution in distilled water is added. This solution is filtered after preparation and stored at room temperature. Four microliters of eosin is added to each well. Five minutes later, the reaction is terminated and the cells are fixed by adding 10 μl of formaldehyde solution. This is prepared by adjusting the pH of the stock 37% solution by shaking with sodium bicarbonate powder until the pH is 7.2. A layer of mineral oil, added to prevent contact with air, helps stabilize the pH of the solution. The formaldehyde is filtered immediately prior to use. A cover glass is placed over each tray and the trays are allowed to stand for several hours before being read.

4. Reading the Cytotoxicity Test

The trays are read using an inverted phase-contrast microscope and scored according to the shown in the following tabulation.

Score	Observation	Interpretation
1	0–19% Dead cells	Negative reaction
2	20–29% Dead cells	Negative reaction; high background
4	30–49% Dead cells	Weakly positive reaction
6	50–79% Dead cells	Positive reaction
8	80–100% Dead cells	Strongly positive reaction
0	Not readable	Invalid test

The proportion of positive cells (i.e., stained with the dye) is estimated without counting individual cells. With practice, a high degree of reproducibility can be achieved within the observations of a single observer and between observers.

5. Interpretation of the Results

HLA specificities are assigned to the cells according to the antigens recognized by the typing sera. Antigens at loci *HLA-A*, *-B*, and *-C* are ascribed discrepant reactions and loci where only a single antigenic determinant is detected are noted. The latter situation arises when the individual is homozygous for the locus controlling expression of an HLA antigen or, if heterozygous, when the second specificity cannot be detected using the available sera. This can only be resolved by typing other family members of the cell donor.

IV. FAMILY STUDIES

Progress in detecting and characterizing new HLA specificities, as well as in some cases the typing of an individual (e.g., *HLA* homozygote), depends on family studies. When several members of the family are available, it may be possible to determine the *HLA* genotype of the individual family members. An example of a family study in which this type of analysis was performed is depicted in Table II and Fig. 1. The HLA typing of the children revealed only one HLA specificity at each of the *A* and *B* loci for children C-2, C-9, and C-10. That these children were homozygous at each locus was revealed by typing the parents and siblings, where the pattern of segregation could be reconstructed (Table II; Fig. 1).

V. SOME COMMENTS ON THE CYTOTOXICITY TEST

A. Typing Sera

While the available typing sera allow the use of monospecific reagents for detection of some of the defined specificities, the need to rely on chance alloimmunization through pregnancy results in a low probability of generating such sera in the individual case. Planned immunization suffers the drawbacks of exposure of recipients to the risk of infection and of the uncertainty of production of antisera of narrow specificity. In all typing sera, anti-HLA antibodies of a wide range of avidities would be expected to be present and hence to have different cross-reactivities. Ideally, homogenous, monoclonal antibodies should be produced, an approach that may in the future be rendered possible by *in vitro* techniques involving cell

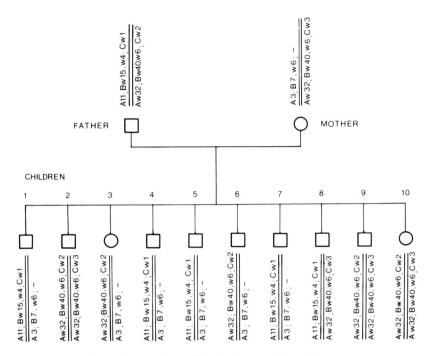

Fig. 1. Segregation of HLA haplotypes within a family.

fusion between anti-HLA antibody-forming cells and tumor cell lines. This method has been described for anti-sheep erythrocyte antibody-forming cells by Köhler and Milstein (1975).

Another approach to the production of typing sera has been the raising of xenogeneic anti-HLA sera by immunizing animals with purified HLA antigens (Ferrone *et al.*, 1973). The disadvantages of this method include several of the above, as well as the presence in the sera of a number of species of heterophil antibodies reacting with human lymphocytes.

B. Complement

1. Heterophil Antibodies

Rabbit complement is especially effective in the lymphocytotoxicity test and it has been suggested that anti-human lymphocyte heterophil antibodies normally present in rabbit serum may act synergistically with anti-HLA

TABLE II

HLA Haplotype Analysis of a Family

| Family member | HLA specificities | | | | | | | | | | | | | | | | | | | | | | | | | | | | | | | | | | | | Chromosomes[a] |
| | A Locus | | | | | | | | | | | | | B Locus | | | | | | | | | | | | | | | | | C Locus | | | | | |
	1	2	3	w23	w24	w25	w26	11	28	29	w30	w31	w32	5	7	8	12	13	14	18	27	w15	w16	w17	w21	w22	w35	w40	w4	w6	w1	w2	w3	w4	w5	
Father	−	−	−	−	−	−	−	+	−	−	−	−	+	−	−	−	−	−	−	−	−	+	−	−	−	−	−	+	+	+	+	+	−	−	−	a/b
Mother	−	−	+	−	−	−	−	−	−	−	−	−	+	−	+	−	−	−	−	−	−	−	−	−	−	−	−	−	−	+	−	−	+	−	−	c/d
Child																																				
1	−	−	+	−	−	−	−	+	−	−	−	−	−	−	+	−	−	−	−	−	−	+	−	−	−	−	−	−	+	+	+	−	−	−	−	a/c
2	−	−	−	−	−	−	−	−	−	−	−	−	+	−	−	−	−	−	−	−	−	−	−	−	−	−	−	+	−	+	−	+	+	−	−	b/d
3	−	−	+	−	−	−	−	−	−	−	−	−	+	−	+	−	−	−	−	−	−	−	−	−	−	−	−	+	−	+	−	+	−	−	−	b/c
4	−	−	+	−	−	−	−	+	−	−	−	−	−	−	+	−	−	−	−	−	−	+	−	−	−	−	−	−	+	+	+	−	−	−	−	a/c
5	−	−	+	−	−	−	−	+	−	−	−	−	−	−	+	−	−	−	−	−	−	+	−	−	−	−	−	−	+	+	+	−	−	−	−	a/c
6	−	−	+	−	−	−	−	−	−	−	−	−	+	−	+	−	−	−	−	−	−	−	−	−	−	−	−	+	−	+	−	+	−	−	−	b/c
7	−	−	+	−	−	−	−	+	−	−	−	−	−	−	+	−	−	−	−	−	−	+	−	−	−	−	−	−	+	+	+	−	−	−	−	a/c
8	−	−	−	−	−	−	−	+	−	−	−	−	+	−	−	−	−	−	−	−	−	+	−	−	−	−	−	+	+	+	+	−	+	−	−	a/d
9	−	−	−	−	−	−	−	−	−	−	−	−	+	−	−	−	−	−	−	−	−	−	−	−	−	−	−	+	−	+	−	+	+	−	−	b/d
10	−	−	−	−	−	−	−	−	−	−	−	−	+	−	−	−	−	−	−	−	−	−	−	−	−	−	−	+	−	+	−	+	+	−	−	b/d

[a] Chromosomes: Father—(a) *A11; Bw15,w4; Cw1*; (b) *Aw32; Bw40,w6; Cw2*. Mother—(c) *A3; B7,w6; —*; (d) *Aw32; Bw40,w6; Cw3*.

alloantibodies in the typing sera to cause the cytotoxicity reaction (Ferrone *et al.*, 1974).

2. Pathway of Complement Activation

Depending on the nature of the alloantiserum and precise conditions of incubation with complement during the cytotoxicity reaction, the classical or alternative pathways of complement activation may be initiated (Ferrone *et al.*, 1974; Bernoco *et al.*, 1976). Thus, incubation of the reagents under the conditions of the NIH test may produce unexpected reactions (positive or negative) when sera are used that have been selected for activity at higher temperatures [e.g., according to the method of Kissmeyer-Nielsen and Kjerbe (1967)].

C. Other Techniques for Detection of HLA-A, -B, and -C Antigens

There is a wide range of alternative methods for the detection of these antigens. The choice of a method other than the standard NIH technique may be dictated by a particular experimental protocol (e.g., the need to observe movement of HLA antigens at the cell surface, or the more ready detection of a particular antigen on cells other than lymphocytes). For detailed descriptions of these techniques and discussions of their advantages and limitations, the reader is referred to the NIH publication "Manual of Tissue Typing Techniques" (Ray *et al.*, 1974).

VI. TECHNIQUE FOR DETECTING B-CELL ANTIGENS OF THE HLA SYSTEM

A new family of antigens, controlled by the HLA system, has been described (van Rood *et al.*, 1975a). These antigens are expressed predominantly on B lymphocytes and may be homologues of the mouse Ia antigens. Several techniques have been proposed for their serological detection. B lymphocytes comprise a minority population in normal blood and may be as low as 5–10% of peripheral blood lymphocytes. This necessitates a modification of the lymphocyte cytotoxicity test described above, because a 5–10% decrease in viability caused by a cytotoxic reaction with an anti-B-cell antigen alloantiserum would be indistinguishable from the "background" of the test. A further problem is that many antisera with activity against these B-cell antigens contain anti-HLA (A, B, and C) antibodies.

One proposed modification (Bernoco *et al.*, 1976) depends on the observation that antisera to β_2-microglobulin are able to block lympholysis due to HLA. In this technique, the HLA-A, -B, and -C antigens are "blanketed" by treating the cells with avian anti-human β_2-microglobulin or $F(ab')_2$ fragments of rabbit anti-human β_2-microglobulin. Each preparation is incapable of fixing complement and causing lympholysis during incubation at 20°C, but they allow a subsequent cytotoxicity reaction between non-HLA (A, B, and C) antibodies. The test is conveniently performed on suspensions of peripheral blood lymphocytes enriched for B cells (van Rood *et al.*, 1975b).

A different approach uses two-color fluorescence, with a fluorescein-labeled anti-immunoglobulin allowing detection of B cells and the uptake of ethidium bromide being used as a marker for dead cells. This test has the advantages of avoiding the need for lengthy B-cell enrichment procedures prior to the cytotoxicity test and of allowing positive identification of individual killed cells as B cells (van Rood *et al.*, 1976).

REFERENCES

Bernoco, D., Bernoco, M., Ceppellini, R., Poulik, M. D., van Leeuwen, A., and van Rood, J. J. (1976). *Tissue Antigens* **8**, 253.
Boyum, A. (1968). *Scand. J. Clin. Lab. Invest.* **21**, Suppl., 97.
Brand, D. L., Ray, J. G., Hare, D. B., Kayhoe, D. E., and McClelland, J. D. (1970). *In* "Histocompatibility Testing" (P. I. Terasaki, ed.), p. 357. Munksgaard, Copenhagen.
Ferrone, S., Pellegrino, M. A., Götze, D., Mittal, K. K., Terasaki, P. I., and Reisfeld, R. A. (1973). *Ser. Immunobiol. Stand.* **18**, 218.
Ferrone, S., Cooper, N. R., Pellegrino, M. A., and Reisfeld, R. A. (1974). *Transplant Proc.* **6**, 13.
Kissmeyer-Nielsen, F., and Kjerbe, K. E. (1967). *In* "Histocompatibility Testing" (E. S. Curtoni, P. L. Mattiuz, and R. M. Tosi, eds.), p. 381. Munksgaard, Copenhagen.
Köhler, G., and Milstein, C. (1975). *Nature (London)* **256**, 495.
Ray, J. G., Hare, D. B., Pederson, P. D., and Kayhoe, D. A., eds. (1974). "Manual of Tissue Typing Techniques," NIAID Transplant. Immunol. Branch DHEW. Publ. No. (NIH) 75-545. USDHEW, Washington, D.C.
Terasaki, P. I., and McClelland, J. D. (1964). *Nature (London)* **204**, 998.
Terasaki, P. I., Bernoco, D., Park, M. S., Ozturk, G., and Iwaki, Y. (1978). *Am. J. Clin. Pathol.* **69**, 103.
van Rood, J. J., van Leeuwen, A., Parlevliet, J., Termijtelen, A., and Keuning, J. J. (1975a). *In* "Histocompatibility Testing" (F. Kissmeyer-Nielsen, ed.), p. 629. Munksgaard, Copenhagen.
van Rood, J. J., van Leeuwen, A., Keuning, J. J., and Blussé van Oud Albas, A. (1975b). *Tissue Antigens* **5**, 73.
van Rood, J. J., van Leeuwen, A., and Ploem, J. S. (1976). *Nature (London)* **262**, 795.

15

The MLR Test in the Mouse

Tommaso Meo

I. THE CONVENTIONAL PRIMARY MLR

A. Principles

The immunobiology of histocompatibility has found a fundamental *in vitro* tool in the study of the interactions that take place in cultures of allogeneic lymphocytes, collectively called the mixed lymphocyte reaction (MLR). This designation broadly refers to a number of metabolic events occurring in such cultures, most manifestly expressed by an increment of

IMMUNOLOGICAL METHODS

macromolecular synthesis and cell proliferation. More restrictive requirements for the definition of the reaction are genetic and immunologic: The
mixed cell populations are obtained from donors not deliberately
presensitized to one another and carry allotypic codominant stimulatory
determinants encoded by a limited number of polymorphic genes.

The phenomenon depends on two major properties of the mixed
lymphocyte populations: (1) the expression of cell-surface stimulatory
determinants and (2) the capacity to recognize them. These two
characteristics were first distinguished empirically by the so-called
unidirectional MLR test, in which one of the two allogeneic populations is
prevented from undergoing activation and can only provide a source of
stimulation for the other. This can be achieved by two approaches:
genetically by the use of lymphocytes from a heterozygote F_1 animal
(stimulator) cultivated with cells from an inbred parental strain (responder),
or biochemically by inhibiting DNA synthesis in one of the two cell
populations (stimulator) with X irradiation or mitomycin C treatment. The
structures responsible for the recognition and stimulation properties of
lymphocytes are not known with certainty; however, they appear to be
attributes of distinct cell populations. While it is generally admitted that the
responding cells belong exclusively to restricted subpopulations of the T-cell
pool and that B cells possess only strong stimulatory determinants, the
possibility that T cells also carry some stimulatory determinants is not
excluded by all of the available evidence.

Other cells contribute to the total reaction, although their role is
considered to be accessory and perhaps immunologically nonspecific.
Nonactivated phagocytic adherent cells, ubiquitous in the lymphoid system,
and probably also B cells, produce a soluble mediator(s) necessary for the
activation of T cells by allogeneic stimulators. It is not clear whether in all
types of cultures the requirement for these cells can be met by the addition
of 2-mercaptoethanol. In addition, it should be considered that, although
the recognition of the allogeneic determinants appears to be a property of
only one subclass of T cells, other cells are undoubtedly activated by the
subsequent production of numerous factors that can be elaborated independently of DNA synthesis.

The genetic analysis of inbred and congeneic mouse strains has allowed
the isolation of two short chromosomal segments within which reside the
genes (or group of genes) responsible for the MLR stimulatory capacity of
lymphocytes. These genes and their products are usually referred to with the
uncommitted terms of "MLR loci" and "MLR determinants," respectively.
The murine major histocompatibility complex, H-2 (on chromosome 17),
encodes the group of determinants, which appear to be the most important
both in terms of their stimulating capacity and because a functional

homologue thereof has been found to be associated with the major histocompatibility complex in many species, spanning orders as diverse as amphibia, birds, and mammals. In the mouse genome, another genetically independent system exists with no defined counterpart in other species. This was designated the *Mls* locus (on chromosome 1) and appears to be less polymorphic (or less complex) than the H-2-associated *MLR* loci.

This introduction represents a brief outline of the basic information relevant to the design and interpretation of an MLR experiment. Comprehensive information is available in the following references: Bach *et al.* (1972), Sorensen (1972), Meo *et al.* (1973), Festenstein (1974), Klein (1975), and Snell *et al.* (1976); these references are the source of most uncited data reported here.

B. Methods

A variety of methods are used in different laboratories. The criteria used for establishing the conditions to be described are inevitably empirical. Instructions are based on personal experience and are not generalized to include all published variations. Although this description illustrates an assay with mouse cells, the methods have been successfully used as well for the rat and the guinea pig MLR.

C. Media

RPMI 1640 has become the most popular medium for cultivating mouse lymphocytes. It is supplemented with antibiotics, glutamine, and serum, which are stored in concentrated stock solutions and added to achieve the final concentrations listed in Table I.

Note also that when the medium is purchased as a solution containing glutamine, this amino acid should be replenished, unless the medium is kept frozen. The choice of the serum is one of the most important variables in the assay. Positive MLR can be detected in serum-free medium, but the system has not been adequately tested. We routinely supplement the medium with human serum: It has proved to be less mitogenic than the more popular fetal calf serum. To prepare human serum, donors are bled and the blood is aseptically collected directly into conical, 50-ml, sterile tubes and allowed to clot for not more than 2–3 hr at room temperature (sera obtained after prolonged clotting accumulate inhibitory substances). The clots are freed from the walls of the tubes and the tubes are centrifuged for 1 hr at 2000 g. The supernatant sera are aspirated aseptically with a "propipette" bulb, collected separately, and assayed for sterility; they are then pooled, heat-inactivated (56°C for 30 min), fractioned, and stored at

TABLE I

Tissue Culture Medium for Mouse MLR

Stock ingredient	Concentration	Storage temperature (°C)	Final concentration
Heat-inactivated human serum	Undiluted	−20	2.5%
Penicillin	10^4 U ml^{-1}	−20	100 U ml^{-1}
Streptomycin	10 mg ml^{-1}	−20	100 μg ml^{-1}
L-Glutamine	$2 \times 10^{-1} M$	−20	$2 \times 10^{-3} M$
2-Mercaptoethanol	Undiluted	4	$3 \times 10^{-5} M$
Hepes	$2 M$	4	$25 \times 10^{-3} M$

−20°C. Since it is difficult to control the variations in the quality of the serum from different individuals, it is recommended to pool serum from various donors in order to minimize these differences. When the experimental design requires the use of iso- or allogeneic serum, it is possible to use mouse serum-supplemented medium. Serum should be obtained and maintained in the cold after a clotting period of 20–30 min and added at a final concentration that generally is kept at a maximum of about 2%. Commercial preparations of mouse serum cannot be recommended for supplementing culture media. Cell washes can be done with the same culture medium or any common balanced salt solution, for example, Ca^{2+}- and Mg^{2+}-free Dulbecco's PBS. The pH of the culture medium, 7.2–7.4, is stabilized by 25 mM Hepes.

D. Mice

The major advantage of working with mice is the availability of inbred and genetically well-defined strains. Most of the common strains have been typed for the MLR determinants associated with the *H-2* or the *Mls* loci. A list of these strains typed for both systems is given in Table II. Since MLR responsiveness in mice declines with age, we use animals 6 weeks to 6 months old.

E. Preparation of Cell Suspensions

Mice are sacrificed immediately before dissection. When lymph nodes are to be collected, animals should be killed by less traumatic means than cervical dislocation to prevent undue internal hemorrhages, which can complicate the isolation of the cervical nodes. The dead mice are dipped in

70% aqueous ethanol and transferred, in an aseptic environment, onto an anatomical board covered with a sheet of aluminum foil that is sterilized by flaming and replaced after each operation. To collect lymph nodes, proceed as follows (use sterilized instruments).

The abdominal skin is lifted with forceps, incised, and cut with straight dissecting scissors along the midline in a transverse plane around the body. The animal is turned on its left side and the upper part of the skin is pulled gently toward the head on only the right side of the animal in order to uncover the right axillary region. One or two nodes will protrude and remain adherent to the muscular plane but detached from the skin. They are removed with forceps, freed from connective tissue, placed into a sterile plastic dish (Falcon No. 3002) containing 5 ml of medium, and kept on ice. The skin is lowered and the animal is turned on the other side to operate in an identical fashion on the left axillary region. Then the skin is lifted gently upward to expose the ventral surface of the cervical region. Here, four nodes, readily identified in close proximity to the salivary glands, are removed.

To isolate the inguinal nodes, the lower part of the abdominal skin is dissected (without opening the peritoneum) along the vertical midline. Under each of the two lower quadrants of the abdominal skin, one or two nodes embedded in the adipose tissue will be easily recognized. To isolate the mesenteric nodes, the peritoneum is cut and removed from the entire abdominal area. The intestines are gently lifted and dislodged from the central and lower parts over the left upper quadrant. In this way, the mesentery will be easily exposed. At least three large nodes should be

TABLE II

List of Common Inbred Mouse Strains Typed for both *H-2*- and *Mls*-Associated MLR Determinants

Mls alleles	*H-2* haplotypes					
	a	*b*	*d*	*k*	*q*	*s*
a			DBA/2	AKR BRVR/DK	DBA/1	
b	B10.A	C57BL/6 C57BL/10 C57L	BALB/c B10.D2	B10.K B10.BR CBA/H CBA/HLacSto CBA/HT6T6		
c	A/J			C3H/HeJ C3H/HeLac		SJL
d				CBA/J		

identified and removed without bleeding. At this stage the spleen can also be removed if desired, from the left flank of the animal, and placed in a separate dish.

When all the organs are collected from one mouse strain, all lymph nodes and spleens are aseptically transferred separately to plastic tubes (Falcon No. 2001; inside diameter, 15 mm), minced with scissors in the presence of 3 ml of medium, and gently squeezed against the wall with a loose-fitting Teflon pestle (diameter, 13 mm) until all the cells are extruded from the capsulae. To rapidly remove clumps and tissue debris, we filter the cell suspensions through sterile No. 100 nylon mesh or through nylon wool. Plastic syringes (10-ml) are filled halfway with loosely packed nylon wool that has been washed with $7\times$ detergent and extensively rinsed in tap or deionized water and finally in triple-distilled water; the syringes are then autoclaved with the plungers in place. The nylon wool is moistened with 2 ml of medium, and the cell suspensions are transferred into the syringe with a Pasteur pipette and forced through, with the plunger, into a new plastic tube (Falcon 3033, 15 ml, or Falcon 2070, 50 ml). The syringe is washed with 5 ml of medium, and the cells are resuspended by drawing them up repeatedly with a 5-ml pipette and then centrifuged at 150 g for 20 min at 4°C. The supernatant is aspirated to remove the fat layer (when abundant, it is recommended that the tube be changed), and the cells are resuspended by tapping the bottom of the tube first gently and then vigorously to break the pellet. Medium is added (10 ml to Falcon 3033 tubes and 20 ml to Falcon 2070 tubes) and the cells are mixed by pipetting; centrifugation is then repeated.

Total cell counts and cell viability are assessed simultaneously. An aliquot of cell suspension is diluted with an equal volume of 0.5% eosin Y in PBS. The viable and dead cells (showing dye uptake) are enumerated under phase-contrast microscopy and the original suspension is adjusted at a final concentration of 10^7 viable cells ml^{-1}, after a final centrifugation. The yield of lymph node lymphocyte fluctuates within a wide range. However, for planning an experiment, it is safe to expect an average minimum yield of $3-4 \times 10^7$ viable lymphocytes per animal and an average viability of 75–90%. Dilute an aliquot of cell suspension to 5×10^6 ml^{-1} to obtain the final preparation of responding cells required in the experiment.

F. Preparation of Stimulator Cells for the Unidirectional MLR Test

1. Mitomycin C Treatment

An aliquot of cells corresponding to at least 1.5 times the total number of stimulators required by the experimental design is transferred to a separate tube (Falcon No. 3033) at 10^7 ml^{-1} (or up to two to four times this concentration). Mitomycin C is added from a stock solution (500 μg ml^{-1} of PBS) at a ratio of 0.05 ml (that is, 25 μg) per milliliter of cell suspension. The tube is incubated at 37°C for 30 min and occasionally agitated. Following incubation, add cold medium and centrifuge as before. The cells are washed at least three times after the first centrifugation with a large excess of cold wash medium (kept on ice), counted as before, and then resuspended at 10^7 ml^{-1} of viable cells.

2. X Irradiation

If an X-ray source is available, stimulator cells can be more efficiently prepared. We routinely suspend the required amount of cells at 10^7 ml^{-1} in capped plastic flasks (Falcon 3012) (up to 8 ml) and lay the flasks on their larger sides under the tube of a Phillips RT305 X-ray machine. A total of 3300 R is delivered at 250 kV, 10 mA, through 4.0 mm of aluminum and 1.1 mm of copper, at a rate of 90–100 R per minute, at 30 cm from the source. Following treatment, the cells are resuspended and kept at the same concentration in flasks, on ice, until distribution in the final cultures.

G. MLR Combinations

Cultures are set up in Falcon 3040 tissue culture plates, which contain a matrix of 96 flat-bottom wells. Using a serological plastic pipette (Falcon No. 7521), aliquots of 0.1 ml of responding lymph node cells (i.e., 0.5 × 10^6) and 0.1 ml of stimulating lymph node cells (i.e., 10^6) are dispensed into each well of the microplates so that triplicate or quadruplicate cultures are plated for each combination. Responding and stimulating splenocytes are used at half the amount, respectively. Each donor should be tested for the capacity to respond and to stimulate a control strain unrelated to those under investigation. Other control cultures include autologous or syngeneic combinations, which provide a measure of background activation, cultures of each responding cell preparation with a nonspecific soluble T-cell mitogen (i.e., concanavalin A at a final concentration of 2 μg ml^{-1}), and finally pairwide allogeneic combinations of all the stimulator cells prepared for the experiment in order to assess the efficacy of mitomycin C or the X-ray treatment. Depending on the number of strains included in the experiment, it may be preferable to premix responder–stimulator combinations at double concentrations, in separate tubes, and distribute them together in volumes of 0.2 ml per well. This additional step has the advantage of eliminating one source of experimental variation among the replicas. The plates are covered with loose-fitting plastic lids that allow gas exchange along the edges (Falcon 3041) and placed in a humidified 5% CO_2/95% air incubator at 37°C.

H. Quantitation of the Response

The stimulation of quiescent lymphocytes entails a sequence of metabolic activations connected with their entering the mitotic cycle and possibly acquiring differentiated functions. Cell growth is commonly monitored by measuring the synthesis of any of the three major classes of macromolecules, DNA's, RNA's, and proteins, that are physiologically interrelated in dividing cells.

We routinely determine DNA synthesis by labeling the cultures with tritiated thymidine 18–24 hr prior to termination of the culture period. A dilution of stock [^{3}H]methyl thymidine (specific activity, 1.9 Ci mmole^{-1}) is made with culture medium at 40 μCi ml^{-1}. The solution is equilibrated at 37°C and distributed in aliquots of 50 μl per well (2 μCi per well) with plastic, autoclavable dropping pipettes of the type generally employed for agglutination tests (Cooke M17 microtiter pipettes).

The kinetics of DNA synthesis varies with cell types and the degree of stimulation: An earlier proliferative response is generally correlated with greater stimulation. It is recommended that the experiments, especially with unknown combinations, be assayed at different time intervals. We routinely pulse the lymph node MLR cultures after 4 and 6 days of incubation. The cultures are terminated by transferring the plates to a refrigerator at 4°C. Harvesting can be conveniently delayed for as long as a week. The cells are harvested by collecting them from the culture well with a semiautomatic sample precipitator (Hartzman *et al.*, 1971; Miggiano *et al.*, 1975).

Several collectors are available commercially; we recommend the types available from Otto Hiller Scientific Equipment (Box 1294, Madison, Wisconsin 53701). The cultures are aspirated onto glass-fiber filters (934 AH grade, Reeve Angel, 9 Bridewell Place, Clifton, New Jersey) and the supernatant is removed with distilled water.

The filters are dried on a hot plate and the portion of filter for each well is transferred into counting vials for liquid scintillation spectrometry. Using minivials and Plexiglas adaptors, the usual volume (10 ml) of the toluene-based scintillation fluid can be reduced to 2.5 ml with negligible loss in counting efficiency.

I. Evaluation and Presentation of the Data

The incorporation of the label in each culture is expressed as counts per minute (cpm) and every combination can be represented by the mean or the median value of its replicate determinations. The presence of a response is evaluated by estimating the average incorporation in the experimental allogeneic mixtures (E) versus the average of the unstimulated control cultures (*C*). The difference between the two groups can be statistically analyzed using Student's *t* test on log converted data to stabilize the variances.

The degree of stimulation is generally presented either as the Δ value, that is, the difference between the average cpm of stimulated and unstimulated cultures ($D = E - C$), or as their ratio or stimulation index (SI = E/C). The latter is a dimensionless number and is thus generally preferred for comparing different sets of data. However, its weakness is due to the fact that it is greatly influenced by the magnitude of the background control values. Presentation of raw data is a better solution; alternatively, any pairwise combination of Δ's, ratios, and control and experimental values will convey the same information. These values can be easily interconverted considering that

$$C = \frac{D}{SI - 1} \quad \text{and} \quad E = \frac{D}{1 - (1/SI)}$$

II. *IN VITRO* SECONDARY MLR

New techniques have allowed long-term culture of lymphocytes. It is thus possible to prime a population of alloreactive lymphocytes *in vitro* and rechallenge them in secondary MLR cultures (Alter *et al.*, 1976; Fathman *et al.*, 1977). These primed responder cells are greatly enriched for responsiveness to the primary stimulating cell. This technique has proved to be extremely useful in defining MLR in quantitative rather than qualitative terms. In addition, it has been possible to obtain cultures of primed cells exhibiting limited specificities and functions compared to primary MLR cultures. It should be possible to identify the many interactions and metabolic events that take place in primary MLR using such secondary MLR cultures.

A. Principle

Using cells that have been primed in MLR cultures as a source of responder cells (called primed responder cells, PRC), it is possible to rechallenge them with a variety of different stimulator cell types to further define the reactivity and specificity of alloreactive lymphocytes. Using this method, it might be possible to examine further the nature of MLR-stimulating determinants and T-cell receptors for such determinants.

B. Materials and Methods

The techniques used in the primary culture are identical to those outlined above with the exception that fetal calf serum (FCS) is used (10% final volume) instead of human serum in the MLR medium. The FCS selected must be screened for low spontaneous mitogenic activity prior to use. If the FCS contains mitogenic substances, the results obtained will be irreproducible and invalid as far as specificity and kinetics of response are concerned.

C. Primary Culture

Lymph node responder cells (40×10^6) obtained as above are cultured with 80×10^6 irradiated (3300 R) stimulator spleen cells. This primary culture is carried out in plastic flasks (Falcon No. 3024) containing 15 ml of MLR medium (containing 10% heat-inactivated FCS instead of 2.5% human serum). The flasks are incubated upright. After 4 days of culture, 100-μl aliquots can be removed and given a 4-hr pulse of [^{3}H]thymidine, as above, to assay the primary MLR reaction.

After 9 days, proliferation can usually no longer be detected above control levels. Fourteen days following initiation of the culture, the cells are harvested and viability is assayed. We usually assay viability using fluorescein diacetate (FDA). This assay is described elsewhere (Rotman and Papermaster, 1966). Briefly, FDA is added to an aliquot of cells to give a final concentration of 5 μg ml^{-1}. (We routinely keep FDA at 5 mg ml^{-1} in acetone at $-20°C$ stored in a foil-covered bottle. This is diluted 1:100 in saline and 10 μl is added to a 100-μl aliquot of a cell suspension.) Viable cells will fluoresce when observed in a hemocytometer chamber using a standard fluorescence microscope equipped with a vertical illuminator and appropriate excitation and barrier filters. Recovery of viable cells ranges from 10 to 50% of the original input of responder cells. Viable cells are called primed responder cells (PRC).

D. Secondary MLR

PRC are recultured in secondary MLR in 0.2 ml of MLR medium in flat-bottom microtiter plates (Falcon No. 3040) in the presence of 1×10^6 irradiated stimulator cells (either syngeneic or allogeneic to the PRC). The number of PRC per well should be varied depending upon the experiment. We commonly make serial dilutions of PRC and test duplicate cultures of at least three concentrations for each proposed day of harvest. Under similar conditions, 50×10^3 PRC react as well as 1×10^6 unprimed responder cells. Thus, many fewer PRC are required for each culture and statistically significant responses can be obtained with as few as several hundred PRC per well (Watanabe *et al.*, 1977). The secondary cultures can be harvested (as above) after 2, 3, and 4 days of culture. Peak responses are usually observed at day 3 of culture (harvested 72 hr after initiation of culture).

E. Controls

The controls are similar to those described above for primary MLR. It is important not only to include syngeneic controls but to have a positive control on PRC responses. This is achieved by including as one stimulator combination the cells against which the PRC were primed. The results obtained in the absence of dose–response curves may be misleading (Corley, 1977); thus, it is important to include several PRC dilutions and assay more than one point in time for each experiment.

III. CRITICAL COMMENTS

Preparation and handling of cell suspensions should be performed with great care so as to minimize cell damage and the possibility of contamination. It is not generally realized that the role of the stimulator cells is more than the mere presentation of the allogeneic determinants. The MLR requires, at least in the initial period of culture, intact viable cells as stimulators or cells in which only DNA synthesis has been irreversibly blocked. We have shown (unpublished results) that, in the human system, where the peak of DNA synthesis in primary allogeneic cultures occurs after 6–7 days of incubation, treatment of the cultures at various times with cytotoxic anti-HLA antibodies reacting only with stimulator cells causes a strong suppression of the response even after 3 days of incubation. Killing of the stimulator has little effect from the fourth day on. Several treatments were shown to block the MLR-stimulating capacity of lymphocytes without drastically altering the cell surface. Heat and iodoacetic acid (Shellekens and Eijsvoogel, 1970), gluteraldehyde (Hardy *et al.*, 1970), ultraviolet light (Lindahl-Kiessling and Safwenberg, 1971), and lantanum chloride and colchicine (Ranney and Pincus, 1975) all abolish the stimulating properties of allogeneic lymphocytes.

Interpreting the MLR results requires recognizing the fact that, in a given allogeneic combination, stimulation is not only the result of the interactions between the responder and the stimulator cells, but is also strongly influenced by the "general" capacity of each party to respond and stimulate, respectively. This demands that attention be paid to the "specificity" of a poor or high response by taking into account the performance of each partner, responder and stimulator, in other combinations, in the same experiment. When typing an unknown strain, a particular problem is the criteria adopted for establishing a negative (specific) response, especially for the combinations where a very small level of stimulation is detected. In this instance, it is advisable to repeat the experiment and, if possible, to test unpooled cell suspensions from several individual donors for the particular combination under study, as well as to estimate the consistency of the response, using comparisons also between *autologous* and *syngeneic* control cultures. This may allow ranking of an inconsistent level of allogeneic stimulation within the range of responses of syngeneic cultures compared to the autologous cultures and therefore assist in establishing "nonstimulatory" combinations. Due to the great variability of the control counts, occasional syngeneic mixtures with a statistically significant SI (as high as 2) are frequently found. Considering the great interexperimental variability, conclusions based on a single test should be tempered with caution.

Cell division and macromolecular synthesis are magnified events that bear only a remote relationship to the initial process of the allogeneic interactions. Spurious positive MLR can be detected in cultures of heterozygous F_1 responding to the parental inbred strains or of homozygous nude mice responding to allogeneic cells. These reactions were proved to result from "back stimulation" of the responder cells mediated by an abortive allogeneic activation of the irradiated stimulator by the untreated responder.

Bidirectional MLR cultures with spleen cells can be a useful tool, especially when a large number of animals must be tested. For a large-scale application, see, for instance, Meo *et al.* (1976).

ACKNOWLEDGMENT

I thank Dr. C. G. Fathman for his advice and for having kindly provided the material for the secondary MLR cultures.

REFERENCES

Alter, B. J., Grillot-Courvalin, C., Bach, M. L., Sondel, P. M., and Bach, F. H. (1976). *J. Exp. Med.* **143**, 1005.
Bach, F. H., Widmer, M. B., Bach, M. L., and Klein, J. (1972). *J. Exp. Med.* **136**, 1430.
Corley, R. B. (1977). *Eur. J. Immunol.* **7**, 93.

Fathman, C. G., Collavo, D., Davies, S., and Nabholz, M. (1977). *J. Immunol.* **118**, 1232.

Festenstein, H. (1974). *Transplantation* **18**, 555.

Hardy, D. A., Knight, S., and Ling, N. R. (1970). *Immunology* **19**, 329.

Hartzman, R. J., Segall, M., Bach, M. L., and Bach, F. H. (1971). *Transplantation* **11**, 268.

Klein, J. (1975). "Biology of the Mouse Histocompatibility-2 Complex." Springer-Verlag, Berlin and New York.

Lindahl-Kiessling, K., and Safwenberg, J. (1971). *Int. Arch. Allergy Appl. Immunol.* **41**, 670.

Meo, T., Vives, G., Rijnbeck, A. M., Miggiano, V. C., Nabholz, M., and Shreffler, D. C. (1973). *Transplant. Proc.* **5**, 1339.

Meo, T., David, C. S., and Shreffler, D. C. (1976). *In* "The Role of Products of the Histocompatibility Gene Complex in Immune Responses" (D. H. Katz and B. Benacerraf, eds.), p. 167. Academic Press, New York.

Miggiano, V. C., Meo, T., Birgen, I., and Nabholz, M. (1975). *Tissue Antigens* **5**, 173.

Ranney, D. F., and Pincus, J. H. (1975). *Fed. Proc., Fed. Am. Soc. Exp. Biol.* **34**, 1011.

Rotman, B., and Papermaster, B. W. (1966). *Proc. Natl. Acad. Sci. U.S.A.* **55**, 134.

Shellekens, P. T. A., and Eijsvoogel, V. P. (1970). *Clin. Exp. Immunol.* **7**, 229.

Snell, G. D., Dausset, J., and Nathenson, S. (1976). "Histocompatibility." Academic Press, New York.

Sørensen, S. F. (1972). *Acta Pathol. Microbiol. Scand.* **230**, 1.

Watanabe, T., Fathman, C. G., and Coutinho, A. (1977). *Immunol. Rev.* **35**, 3.

16

A Sensitive Method for the Separation of Rosette-Forming Cells

Bruce E. Elliott[1]

[1] Research fellow of the National Cancer Institute of Canada.

I. OBJECTIVE

The technique described here is designed to separate erythrocyte rosette-forming cell (RFC) populations for analytical and functional studies.

II. PRINCIPLE OF THE METHOD

The technique of velocity sedimentation at unit gravity is used to separate rosettes from single cells on the basis of size (Osoba, 1970; Elliott and Haskill, 1973; Elliott *et al.*, 1973). The sedimentation velocity of a rosette is proportional to both the number of erythrocytes bound and the size of the RFC. Rosettes therefore sediment faster than single cells. Furthermore, by this method, it is possible to separate subpopulations of RFC differing with respect to the number of erythrocytes bound.

To determine whether cells defined by certain functions (e.g., precursors of antibody-forming cells or helper T cells) are RFC, two separations are carried out: (1) without prior rosette formation (sham) and (2) with prior rosette formation. The relative functional cell activity is determined by testing cells from each fraction in the appropriate assay. Any cell detected in the functional assay that binds erythrocytes will sediment as a rosette faster than that single cell alone, and the distribution curve of the relative functional activity for that cell population will shift to fractions of faster sedimentation velocity. The function of rosette populations can thus be determined.

In the following detailed descriptions, it is shown that the rosette technique and functional assays are designed to study antigen-specific sheep erythrocyte (SRBC) rosettes formed by T and B cells involved in the anti-SRBC immune response. However, the general separation principle can be applied to a wide number of rosette systems.

III. FORMATION OF ROSETTES

A. Medium

For all living tissue, Eagle's minimal essential medium (MEM) [Grand Island Biological Co. (Gibco), Grand Island, New York] buffered to pH 7.2

with tris(hydroxymethyl)aminomethane (Trizma base, Gibco) was used. The following volumes per liter were added: 2.19 M NaCl, 9.6 ml; 10 × isotonic Trizma base, 10 ml.

Eagle's balanced salt solution (see Section VI,D,3) was made from the following stock solutions (2 liters each): solution I—120 gm of Tris reagent (Sigma), 17.8 gm of $Na_2HPO_4 \cdot 2 H_2O$, phenol red, 0.2 gm; solution II—4.92 gm of $MgSO_4 \cdot 7 H_2O$, 5.8 gm of $CaCl_2 \cdot 2 H_2O$; solution III—140 gm of NaCl, 9.0 gm of KCl. The final solution consisted of equal volumes of solutions I, II, and III. Solutions II and III were mixed separately, before adding to solution I.

B. Sodium Azide

A 1% (w/v) solution of sodium azide (Fisher Scientific Co., Pittsburgh, Pennsylvania) in phosphate-buffered saline (PBS) was used in some of the experiments described.

C. Neuraminidase Treatment

In some experiments, SRBC (8×10^8) were incubated in a solution of neuraminidase (General Biochemicals Division, Chagrin Falls, Ohio) (50 U/ml in phosphate-buffered saline, pH 7.4) for 30 min at 37°C. The cells were washed three times in 10 ml of MEM, and spleen cells were added for rosette formation as described below.

D. Erythrocytes

SBRC obtained from a single donor animal were stored in Alsever's solution at 4°C for at least 1 week. Any clots or fibrinogen coagulates were removed. For each experiment, a sample was removed and washed three times in MEM at 800 g for 10 min. One milliliter of packed pellet contained 2×10^{10} SRBC.

E. Preparation of Cell Suspensions

Spleens were removed from at least three mice per experiment and placed in 10 ml of cold MEM in a plastic petri dish on ice. Each spleen was held at one end with fine curved-tip forceps, and the connective tissue sheath at the other end was cut with scissors. The cells were teased through the opening by rubbing gently on the surface of the spleen with a second pair of fine forceps. In this way, the cells were protected by the connective tissue from any mechanical abrasion from the forceps. Cell clumps were dispersed by firmly pipetting the suspension with a small-bore Pasteur pipette. The petri dish was tilted and the remaining cell aggregates were allowed to settle for 10 min. The single cells in the upper two-thirds of the suspension were removed and washed three times in MEM, and the nucleated cell count was determined in 5% acetic acid. Viability (70–90%) was assessed after mixing a cell sample with an equal volume of 1% eosin Y (in PBS).

F. Rosette Formation

Since many variables, such as the shape and size of the tube, the erythrocyte and nucleated cell concentrations, and the volume of medium, can significantly alter the number and morphology of RFC formed (Wilson, 1971; Charreire *et al.*, 1973), a standard procedure must be used in all experiments.

The following method was used for preparing large numbers of cells for functional studies. Rosettes were made in MEM with no serum present. Nucleated cells (8×10^7) were mixed in 2 ml of MEM with 8×10^8 SRBC. This ratio of SRBC to nucleated cells (10:1) was found to be optimal. In some experiments, SRBC were pretreated with neuraminidase before rosette formation (see Section VI,C,4). The cell suspension was centrifuged at 4°C in a 15-ml plastic centrifuge tube (No. 2057, Falcon Plastics, Division of BioQuest, Oxnard, California) at 100 *g* for 6 min to form a clear pellet at the bottom of the tube. After an incubation at 0°C for 1 hr, the pellet was gently resuspended by pipetting six times with a large-bore Pasteur pipette. In some experiments, 0.1 ml of 1% sodium azide in PBS was added immediately before resuspending the pellet (see Section VI,C,3). This rosette suspension was subjected to cell separation as described below.

IV. CELL FRACTIONATION

A. Theory

The theory of velocity sedimentation at unit gravity has been reviewed extensively elsewhere (Miller, 1973). The general principle is that, when a particle is moving at terminal velocity in a fluid, the sedimentation velocity, *s* (in millimeters per hour), is given by the following equation:

$$s = \frac{2(\rho - \rho^1)gr^2}{9\eta}$$

where ρ is the cell density (in grams per cubic centimeter), ρ^1 is the fluid density, *g* is the acceleration due to gravity (980 cm/sec²), η is the coefficient of viscosity of the fluid, and r is the radius (in micrometers) of a sphere equivalent to the volume of the particle. Under physiological conditions, most mammalian cells have radii between 2.5 and 10 μm and densities between 1.05 and 1.10 gm/cm^3. In an aqueous medium (ρ^1 = 1.01 gm/cm^3), size variations can give rise to as much as a 16-fold variation in terminal velocity, whereas the density varies only 2-fold (Miller, 1973). Therefore, variations in s are primarily due to size.

If the density and size of a cell are known, s values can be directly calculated from this formula. Thus, a typical nucleated cell (ρ = 1.06 gm/cm^3) would sediment in an aqueous medium (ρ^1 = 1.01 gm/cm^3; η = 1.567 cP) with an s value of $r^2/4$. Calculated s values have been found to correlate very well with those obtained experimentally (Miller, 1973).

B. Apparatus

The objective is to form a thin layer of cell suspension on top of a fluid column, to let the cells sediment under the influence of gravity for an appropriate length of time, and to collect fractions containing cells which have moved different distances.

The sedimentation chamber (O. H. Johns Scientific, Toronto) used in the present procedure was 22 cm in diameter, with an angle of 30° in the cone

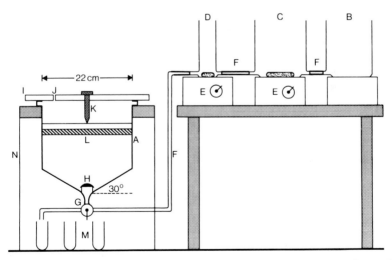

Fig. 1 The velocity sedimentation apparatus used for rosette separation. A, sedimentation chamber; B, dense fluid reservoir; C, light fluid reservoir; D, intermediate vessel; E, magnetic stirrers; F, silicone rubber tubing (Silastic, Dow–Corning); G, three-way valve; H, flow baffle; I, chamber lid; J, vent hole in chamber lid; K, screw; L, cell band shortly after loading completed; M, collecting tubes; N, stand.

(Fig. 1). All tubing interconnections were made with silicone tubing (Silastic, Dow–Corning, Toronto, Ontario, Canada) because of the very low tendency of cells to stick to silicone rubber.

The cells were loaded in 100 ml of sample buffer directly into the sedimentation chamber (Fig. 1,A) and lifted into the starting position (L) by a shallow density gradient (between 1.007 and 1.011 gm/cm³), introduced by gravity from the reservoirs of the gradient maker (B,C). This shallow density gradient was generated by connecting, in series, two large reservoirs containing 1.5% (B) and 0.75% (C) Ficoll (1.2 liters each) as in Fig. 1. The purpose of this gradient is to protect the cells during sedimentation from convection and mechanical jarring; it has no effect on the sedimentation rate of the cells.

To stabilize the cell band, the gradient was "rounded off" just below the cell layer by introducing into the intermediate vessel (D) 50 ml of a 0.35% Ficoll solution. In this way an attenuated step gradient was formed (Fig. 2).

The stainless steel baffle (H) deflects the flow to prevent mixing during filling. In experiments in which a direct comparison between two sedimentations is required, the chamber can be reproducibly filled to the same volume by stopping the flow when the screw tip (K) just touches the rising gradient.

C. Detailed Procedure

The protocol we use in separating rosettes is described in detail below.

1. Set up the apparatus as shown in Fig. 1. We use gradient reservoirs

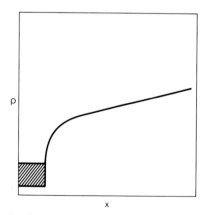

Fig. 2. Density distribution for attenuated step gradient immediately after loading. The part contributed by the cells is shown hatched. (Reproduced with permission from Miller, 1973, Separation of Cells by Velocity Sedimentation, *in* "New Techniques in Biophysics and Cell Biology" edited by R. H. Pain and B. J. Smith. Copyright © 1973 by John Wiley & Sons Ltd.)

TABLE I

Serum and Ficoll Concentrations for Velocity Sedimentation Medium

Vessel	% BSA	% FCS	% Ficoll	Volume (liters)
Dense reservoir (B)[a]	2.0	30	1.5	1.2
Light reservoir (C)[a]	1.0	15	0.75	1.2
Intermediate vessel (D)[a]	0.5	7.5	0.37	0.15
Cell sample buffer[b]	0.25	3.7	0.17	0.1

[a] See Fig. 1.
[b] See Section IV,C.

and an intermediate vessel with internal diameters of 12 and 2.5 cm, respectively. For sterile work, the complete apparatus is autoclaved before use.

2. Prepare solutions of Ficoll in MEM at the concentrations listed in Table I, cool to 4°C, and adjust the pH to 7.2. [Add sodium azide to a final concentration of 0.5%, if required (see Section VI,C,3).]

3. Fill the connecting tubing between D and H with 0.35% Ficoll in MEM, making sure to eliminate all air bubbles.

4. Center carefully the flow baffle (H) inside the cone of the sedimentation chamber.

5. Clamp the lines between vessels B, C, and D. Load 1.2 liters of 1.5% Ficoll into B and 1.2 liters of 0.75% Ficoll into C; fill the intermediate vessel with 0.35% Ficoll to the level of B and C.

6. Gently mix by pipetting the rosette cell suspension (prepared as in Section III, E and F) into 100 ml of cell sample buffer (0.17% Ficoll in MEM) and load it directly into the chamber (A), taking care not to disturb the baffle. [For experiments involving functional analysis, set up a parallel separation of the same number of cells mixed with erthrocytes (without rosette formation) in a second chamber, about 30 min later.]

7. Start the flow into the chamber at an initial rate of 2–3 ml/min. Turn on magnetic stirrers.

8. Remove all clamps and record time (t_1). The gradient will rise rapidly from 0.35 to 0.75% Ficoll and slowly thereafter to 1.5% Ficoll. Once the cells have been lifted off the bottom, the flow rate can be increased. Loading should take place as rapidly as possible, without disturbing the cell band (20–30 min with this chamber size). The time elapsed between loading the cells and starting the gradient should be as short as possible.

9. After a sedimentation time of 1.5 hr, start unloading the chamber through the bottom. Discard the chamber volume. Collect 40-ml fractions in glass conical tubes (Bellco, Vineland, New Jersey) at a rate of about 30

ml/min. Record the time the first fraction started (t_2) and the last fraction finished (t_3). Record the number and volume of the last fraction.

D. Calculation of s Values

The increment of sedimentation velocity per fraction (s) is calculated according to the following formula (Miller, 1973):

$$s = V_F/(KT)$$

where V_F is the fraction volume, T is the mean time of sedimentation, and K is a constant equal to the volume in milliliters per millimeter of the chamber cylinder (38.0 ml/mm for a chamber 22 cm in diameter).

Since the sedimentation of the cells continues during the fraction collection, an average sedimentation time, T, must be calculated as follows:

$$T = \frac{t_3 - t_2}{2} - t_1$$

where t_2 and t_3 are the times the first and last fractions were collected, respectively, and t_1 is the time loading started. This approximation of sedimentation time is sufficient for the rosette separations described, in which the sedimentation time is short and the s value per fraction is large (1.2 mm/hr/fraction). For sedimentations involving longer times, the s value per fraction is less (<0.4 mm/hr/fraction); more accurate s values can be calculated by considering the loading and unloading times during which the cells sediment in the cone (Miller, 1973).

The $s = 0$ point is defined as the middle of the input cell band. Therefore, the corrected volume of the last fraction (corresponding to the top of the gradient) is determined by subtracting one-half the volume of the starting cell band (i.e., 50 ml in the above experiments).

The velocity corresponding to this (corrected) fraction volume is calculated, and increments of s are added for each additional fraction to determine the mean velocity per fraction in millimeters per hour.

E. Preparation of Cells for Counting and Functional Assays

It is important to count rosettes in each fraction without washing, since rosettes may dissociate during centrifugation. Therefore, a portion (0.5 ml) was removed from each fraction, 100 μl was stained with 10 μl of a filtered saturated crystal violet solution in PBS, and a known volume was dropped onto a glass slide and covered with a glass coverslip. Rosettes were scored as single nucleated cells (staining with crystal violet) with at least four SRBC bound. The number of rosettes per fraction was determined.

To the remaining cells in each fraction, 1 ml of FCS and 0.1 ml of a 0.1% SRBC suspension were added; this step increased the recovery of cells during centrifugation. The cells were centrifuged at 250 g, 4°C, for 20 min, the supernatants were removed, and the cells were resuspended in 1 ml of fresh medium. Viable nucleated cells per fraction were counted after staining with 1% eosin Y (as in Section III,F).

After the cell distribution per fraction was determined, equal numbers of fractions were pooled as required, and cells were tested in the appropriate assay. For many *in vitro* assays (e.g., helper cell activity or precursors of antibody-forming cells), the variable number of erythrocytes in each fraction was not important because excess erythrocytes subsequently added for immunization. However, some assays [e.g., tests for cell-mediated cytotoxicity or delayed-type hypersensitivity (Elliott *et al.*, 1975)] required that the erythrocytes be removed. This was achieved by resuspending the cells in a red cell lysing buffer (0.01 M KHCO$_3$, 0.155 M NH$_4$Cl, 0.1 mM EDTA) to yield a cell concentration of no more than 10^7/ml. The cells were incubated at 0°C for 1 min; excess cold MEM was added, and the cells were washed three times before use.

F. Counting the Number of Erythrocytes per RFC

1. Fixation

The number of erythrocytes bound and the morphology of each RFC were determined on fixed and stained preparations. Glutaraldehyde [50% (w/w), Fisher Scientific Co.], a reagent that causes protein cross-linking (Sabatini *et al.*, 1963), was used as a fixative. The stock solution was adjusted to a concentration of 25% with distilled water and stored in the dark at 4°C over activated charcoal (one-fifth volume). For each experiment, a 1:10 dilution of the stock glutaraldehyde was made in phosphate-buffered saline (pH 7.4) at 4°C. Any charcoal remaining was removed by centrifugation.

This fixing solution was added to yield a final concentration of 0.6% glutaraldehyde. The suspension was gently mixed and left for 20 min at 4°C.

Fixation was terminated by diluting the suspension in distilled water. The pellet was carefully dispersed by pipetting, and the cell concentration was adjusted by accurate dilutions with distilled water to approximately 5×10^5 total cells (i.e., nucleated cells plus erythrocytes) per milliliter. After careful mixing, equal volumes were dropped onto clean glass slides with a Pasteur pipette and allowed to dry. The concentration of rosettes in the original suspension was calculated from the number of rosettes per drop and the known dilutions.

2. Staining and Cell Morphology

The dried preparations were washed with methanol in order to adhere the cells to the slide. Each sample was then stained with methyl green pyronine (British Drug Houses Ltd., Toronto) for 15 min. Rosettes were located on the slide by scanning under low magnification. At a magnification of 1000 (under oil immersion), the presence of a lymphocyte in the center of each rosette was confirmed and morphological examinations were carried out. With a micrometer eyepiece, the diameter of each RFC was measured. RFC were categorized on the basis of lymphocyte size: small (less than 7 μm), medium (7–11 μm), and large (greater than 11 μm) (Metcalf and Wiadrowski, 1966). The number of SRBC per RFC was counted. All RFC scored should not be in contact with other nucleated cells and should be morphologically intact.

3. Determination of Rosette Recovery

The recovery of rosettes during the separation was carefully monitored: Two samples (10 μl each) of the unfractionated rosette suspension were transferred to tubes containing 1 ml of cell buffer (0.17% Ficoll in MEM). One was fixed immediately; the other was kept at 4°C during the separation and then fixed. Each preparation was scored, and the number of T and B RFC before and after the separation time was determined. The recovery of B RFC after the separation period was 100%. Good recovery of T RFC only occurred when sodium azide (0.05%) was added after resuspending the rosette pellet (Section VI,C,3). The recovery of rosettes from the gradient (Section V,B) was calculated in comparison with the number of rosettes in the unfractionated suspension after the separation period.

V. RECOVERY, DEPLETION, AND ENRICHMENT

A. Nucleated Cell Distribution

The recovery of nucleated cells from the gradient ranged between 50 and 85%. The mean sedimentation velocity in the present system of small lymphocytes (equal to or less than 7 μm in diameter for mouse cells) was 3.7 mm/hr (Fig. 3A). Because of the short period of sedimentation, most of the nucleated cells in a normal cell population sedimented in a narrow band between 2.5 and 4.5 mm/hr. Medium cells (7–11 μm in diameter) sedimented between 5 and 6 mm/hr. In normal animals, this represented 10–20% of the total nucleated cells. Less than 2% of the cells sedimented faster than 8 mm/hr.

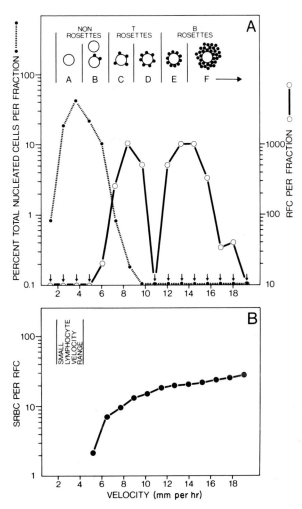

Fig. 3. (A) Separation of rosettes by velocity sedimentation: Normal mouse spleen cells (DBA/2) were subjected to rosette formation with neuraminidase-treated SRBC and separated by velocity sedimentation. The number of nucleated cells per fraction is expressed as the percentage of the total nucleated cells loaded. The number of rosettes per fraction was determined by counting methyl violet-stained cells in suspension without washing. (B) Fixed and stained preparations were made from 0.5-ml samples from each fraction as described in Section IV,F. The number of SRBC per RFC was determined. Each point represents the average SRBC binding ability of at least 15 rosettes.

The cells recovered from the gradient were greater than 98% viable; dead cells and cell debris sedimented at less than 2.5 mm/hr.

B. RFC Distribution

In sham separations without prior rosette formation, the majority of RFC sedimented as single cells between 2.5 and 4.5 mm/hr.

When rosette formation preceded separation, rosettes (consisting of four or more erythrocytes bound to a single nucleated cell) sedimented at greater than 6 mm/hr (Fig. 3A). The sedimentation velocity of each rosette was proportional to the number of SRBC bound (Fig. 3B). The recovery of rosettes from the gradient was between 70 and 100%.

C. Depletion and Enrichment

All cells sedimenting at less than 5 mm/hr were completely depleted of rosettes. The rosette fractions, particularly between 6 and 8 mm/hr, contained some single nucleated cells (Fig. 3A). In the fractions of faster sedimentation velocity (i.e., greater than 8 mm/hr), the proportion of rosettes approached 25 to 50%. This proportion was greatly improved (75–90%) if the faster-sedimenting single cells were removed by a preliminary separation before rosette formation.

VI. APPLICATIONS, SENSITIVITY, AND LIMITATIONS

A. Determination of Functional Activity

Functional activity in each cell fraction (or pools of an equal number of fractions) can be measured in two ways, depending on the experimental design.

1. Activity per Fraction

Activity per fraction can be measured directly by assaying a constant proportion of cells in each fraction. The values obtained in the assay are directly proportional to the total activity in the fraction and can be expressed as the relative activity per fraction. Recovery of functional activity is determined by comparing the total sum of activity detected in all the fractions with that of a sample of unfractioned cells equivalent to the total number of cells loaded onto the sedimentation gradient.

2. Frequency of Activity per Fraction

Alternatively, the frequency of activity per fraction can be measured directly by assaying a constant number of cells in each fraction. The values thus obtained are directly proportional to the frequency of activity per fraction and can be expressed as relative activity per 10^5 cells per fraction. Total activity per fraction is calculated by multiplying this frequency by the cell number per fraction. This calculation of course includes the error of cell counting, and the value of activity per fraction thus obtained is therefore less accurate than that obtained directly (see Section VI,A,1). With this experimental design, the recovery of functional activity can be determined only after calculating the activity per fraction; the same comparison with unfractionated cells can then be made as above (Section VI,A,1).

B. Summary of Results

The above procedures have been used to characterize quantitatively antigen-specific SRBC rosette-forming lymphocytes (0.01–0.05% of normal peripheral mouse lymphocytes) and to determine their function in the immune response. The following results have been obtained.

1. Normal splenic T RFC [which are depleted in mice treated with adult thymectomy (ATx) and anti-lymphocyte serum (ALS), and which are sensitive to anti-Thy 1.2 serum and guinea pig complement treatment] bind fewer erythrocytes than B RFC (which are resistant to ATx and ALS or anti-Thy 1.2 serum and guinea pig complement treatment) (Haskill et al., 1972). T RFC also form less stable rosettes than B RFC (Elliott and Haskill, 1973).

2. Most precursors (i.e., more than 80%) of 19 S hemolytic anti-SRBC antibody-forming cells in normal adult spleen sediment as single cells at less than 5 mm/hr. However, most AFC precursors (more than 80%) form single-layered rosettes (with 10 to 18 SRBC bound) that sediment between 6 and 10 mm/hr. The majority of 19 S AFC (detected by a hemolytic plaque-forming cell assay) form multilayered rosettes, binding greater than 18 SRBC per RFC and sedimenting at greater than 12 mm/hr (Elliott and Haskill, 1973).

For this study, SRBC were not treated with neuraminidase and sodium azide was not added to the medium. Under these conditions, B-cell functions correlate well with RFC populations binding greater than 10 SRBC.

3. The separation of T RFC for functional studies requires the presence of a reversible metabolic inhibitor, sodium azide (0.05% final concentration), in the suspension medium to prevent the dissociation of T rosettes

(Elliott and Haskill, 1973). Furthermore, rosettes are made with neuraminidase-treated SRBC to increase the resolution of separation between T and B rosettes (Fig. 3A). Helper T cells (i.e., T cells that interact with B cells in the production of anti-SRBC AFC) in both normal (Elliott *et al.*, 1973) and immune (Elliott and Haskill, 1975) animals always sediment as *non*-rosette-forming single cells. In contrast, a population of medium lymphocyte effector T cells, active in delayed hypersensitivity (assayed by the transfer of immune cells to SRBC-challenged recipients) and in *in vitro* cytotoxicity (assayed by specific killing and growth inhibition of sheep fibroblasts that express SRBC determinants), forms T-type rosettes with 8 to 10 SRBC bound and which are sensitive to anti-Thy 1.2 and guinea pig complement. Thus, helper T cells in the (19 S) humoral response are distinct from effector T cells involved in cellular immune responses (i.e., delayed hypersensitivity and *in vitro* cytotoxicity).

C. Sensitivity

Several features of the above procedure contribute to its high degree of sensitivity.

1. Time of Sedimentation

In contrast to the longer sedimentation times (3.5–4 hr) required to obtain optimal resolution of small and medium lymphocyte separations (Miller, 1973), the duration of the rosette separation is short (1.5 hr). Therefore, most single cells remain in a relatively narrow band between 2.5 and 5 mm/hr. In contrast, the rosettes move much farther in this time, sedimenting at velocities greater than 6 mm/hr. Thus, good depletion can be obtained.

2. Erythrocyte Volume

An SRBC [32 μm^3 in volume (Altman, 1961)] sediments at a mean velocity of 1.5 mm/hr; a small lymphocyte [172 μm^3 in volume (Metcalf and Wiadrowski, 1966)] sediments at a mean velocity of 3.7 mm/hr. Therefore, any lymphocyte with even one, two, or three erythrocytes bound sediments at a significantly faster velocity than a single cell [i.e., 4.5–6 mm/hr (see Fig. 3 and Elliott *et al.* 1973)]. Thus, by comparing sedimentation profiles of functional activity before and after rosette formation, very weak SRBC binding can be detected. Furthermore, significant differences in sedimentation velocity between rosette populations with different numbers of SRBC bound can be detected (Section VI,B).

3. Sodium Azide

Some RFC [e.g., T RFC (Elliott and Haskill, 1973)] are unstable in that they dissociate within minutes after resuspension from the pellet at 0°C. However, if sodium azide (0.05% final concentration) is added to the tube while resuspending the pellet, and to the sedimentation medium, this dissociation is prevented. This procedure might also be applicable in other systems in which a rapid rate of membrane turnover renders rosettes unstable. The effect of sodium azide is reversed after washing three times in azide-free medium. The functional activity of T and B cells is completely recovered as assessed in the functional assays above (Elliott *et al.*, 1973, 1975; Elliott and Haskill, 1975).

4. Size of Rosette

The resolution of the separation of T and B rosettes is improved when the erythrocytes are pretreated with neuraminidase. This treatment in the present system increases the number of SRBC bound by B RFC but not by T RFC, without altering the total RFC frequency. In this way, greater resolution between T RFC (mean of 4–10 SRBC bound) and B RFC (more than 10 SRBC bound) is obtained (Elliott *et al.*, 1973, 1975; Elliott and Haskill, 1975). This process also yields greater enrichment of B rosettes since these cells sediment at faster velocities and are separated further from the single-cell fraction. However, neuraminidase treatment was not used in the experiments involving separation and comparison of distinct B RFC populations distinguishable by SRBC-binding ability [e.g., PFC precursors and mature PFC (Section VI,B)].

5. Cell Size

If RFC are of heterogeneous size, then some overlap in cell populations might be observed. For example, a small lymphocyte with 18 SRBC bond (750 μm^3) has a mean volume similar to that of a medium lymphocyte with 10 SRBC bound (720 μm^3). Both sediment at 12 mm/hr (Elliott *et al.*, 1975).

Improved resolution can be obtained by sedimenting the cells before rosette formation (for 3.5–4 hr) to obtain a population of small (2.5–4 mm/hr) or medium (4–5 mm/hr) cells, more homogeneous with respect to size. Rosettes can then be made from this selected population and separated by the above procedures (Elliott and Haskill, 1973). However, this PFC population may represent only a select proportion of unfractionated RFC and care must be taken in the interpretation of these results.

D. Reproducibility

The results described above are highly reproducible both qualitatively and quantitatively. However, the following important points are critical.

1. pH

Since erythrocytes are sensitive to pH, each buffer solution must be carefully adjusted using a pH meter.

2. Temperature

Since sedimentation velocity is proportional to temperature (Miller, 1973), all separations should be carried out in a sensitively monitored cold room. Optimal recovery of viable cells is obtained at 4°C.

3. Medium for Rosette Formation and Velocity Sedimentation

The medium should be a buffered isotonic medium. Although a Trizma base buffer was used in the present procedure (see Section III,A), phosphate-buffered saline (PBS) is also suitable. Hepes in the absence of serum is sometimes toxic to cells (see Chapter 21) and therefore should not be used in erythrocyte rosette separations. The same medium should be used for both rosette formation and separation procedures. The medium should contain amino acid nutrients, as, for example, in MEM (see Section III,A) or TC-199 (Difco), to ensure optimal recovery of functional RFC.

Various laboratories have used three main reagents to generate the shallow density gradient required to stabilize the sedimentation of cells: bovine serum albumin, fetal calf serum, and Ficoll. Table I lists these reagents and their required concentrations for use in the sedimentation medium. Bovine serum albumin (BSA) and fetal calf serum (FCS, Gibco) are proteins that act as strong buffers. BSA is obtained in the form of lyophilized material from Cohn fraction V (Pentex), dissolved in Eagle's balanced salt solution (see Section III,A) to a concentration of 20%, filtered, and stored at 4°C. The pH is neutralized with 1 N NaOH, and the required amounts are added to the sedimentation medium as indicated in Table I.

Ficoll (Pharmacia, Uppsala, Sweden) is a high molecular weight (400,000) polysaccharide. Since it has relatively few charged groups compared to protein, it does not act as a pH buffer. This reagent is also relatively inert in that it does not adhere to, or alter the charge of, surface membrane proteins. Ficoll is therefore useful in the separation of cells for membrane studies. It is also much cheaper than BSA or FCS. All BSA, FCS, and Ficoll reagents should be pretested to show that they are nontoxic and do not interfere with the function of the cells being tested.

Since medium with serum has a greater viscosity than medium with Ficoll, the sedimentation velocity of cells in medium with Ficoll is faster (by a factor of about 1.2) than that in medium with serum (see Section IV,C). This factor must be considered when comparing results between laboratories.

4. Streaming and Cell Load Limitations

Streaming is a phenomenon in which, shortly after loading, large numbers of filaments a few millimeters long can be seen hanging down from the cell band (Miller, 1973). When viewed from above, the cell band has a mottled appearance. This phenomenon occurs if the cell concentration in the cell band at the time of loading exceeds a certain number, the streaming limit.

The streaming limit varies with the cells being sedimented and in all systems so far tested is inversely proportional to the average cell volume. For sheep erythrocytes, the streaming limit is 1.5×10^7 cells/ml when an attenuated step gradient is used (Section IV,B). Cells from normal animals must be loaded at cell concentrations of no more than 1.5×10^6 nucleated cells/ml. Cultured cells, or cells from immune animals, have larger volumes; the streaming limit for these cells is therefore less than that for normal cells.

E. The Nature of the Erythrocyte

An obvious advantage of the antigen-specific erythrocyte rosette system is that different specificities can be compared by using erythrocytes from different species. Care must be taken concerning the following points.

1. The isotonicity and storage requirements may vary and should be carefully controlled before use in the rosette assay.
2. The optimal ratio of erythrocytes to nucleated cells, cell concentration, volume, and centrifugation force may be different and should be standardized.
3. Since erythrocytes from different species vary in size, the streaming limits and sedimentation rates of each type of erythrocyte must be carefully tested.

F. Comparison with Density Separation Techniques

The separation of rosettes from a cell mixture by density centrifugation over a Ficoll solution (density, 1.09 gm/ml) has been described elsewhere by Parish and Hayward (1974). The cells are gently layered over the Ficoll solution and centrifuged at 2000 *g* for 15 min. Single cells remain at the interface or in the Ficoll, whereas the rosettes (and free erythrocytes), which are more dense than single nucleated cells, concentrate in the pellet. Excellent recoveries, depletion, and enrichment of rosettes have been reported. In addition, this method requires less time than the velocity sedimentation procedure.

However, the velocity sedimentation method described here has the following unique advantages.

1. Rosette populations can be separated and classified according to the number of erythrocytes bound.
2. Cells with even one or two erythrocytes bound can be detected, since they sediment significantly faster than single cells. This point is particularly important in studying the function of cells that bind erythrocytes at the lower limit of detection by the rosette assay.
3. Shearing forces present at high centrifugation speeds required for Ficoll separations are absent in separation experiments at unit gravity. Cells that form unstable rosettes can be separated in medium with a metabolic inhibitor (sodium azide) present (see Section VI,C,3).
4. Velocity sedimentation may be more sensitive for separating rosettes present in the unfractionated cells at low frequencies (less than 1%), as in the antigen-specific erythrocyte rosette system.

Thus, in experiments where these advantages are important, velocity sedimentation can be a useful technique for separating rosette populations.

VII. CONCLUSION

A sensitive method is described to separate rosettes by sedimentation at unit gravity. Since a rosette sediments at a velocity related to the number of erythrocytes bound, RFC populations can be defined and separated on the basis of this parameter.

The principle of this procedure is applicable to many rosette techniques, including those to detect receptors for complement [EAC rosettes (Nussenzweig, 1974)] or for the Fc component of Ig [EA rosettes (Cohen *et al.*, 1971; Krammer *et al.*, 1975)].

ACKNOWLEDGMENTS

I thank Dr. J. S. Haskill for his helpful advice and encouragement during the development of these techniques and Ms. T. Stakowski for her excellent technical assistance.

REFERENCES

Altman, P. L. (1961). *in* "Blood and Other Fluids," p. 119. Fed. Am. Soc. Exp. Biol., Washington, D.C.

Charreire, J., Dardenne, M., and Bach, J.-F. (1973). *Cell. Immunol.* **9**, 32.

Cohen, D., Gurner, B. W., and Combs, R. R. A. (1971). *J. Exp. Pathol.* **52**, 41.

Elliott, B. E., and Haskill, J. S. (1973). *Eur. J. Immunol.* **3**, 68.

Elliott, B. E., and Haskill, J. S. (1975). *J. Exp. Med.* **141**, 599.

Elliott, B. E., Haskill, J. S., and Axelrad, M. A. (1973). *J. Exp. Med.* **138**, 1133.

Elliott, B. E., Haskill, J. S., and Axelrad, M. A. (1975). *J. Exp. Med.* **141**, 584.

Haskill, J. S., Elliott, B. E., Kerbel, R., Axelrad, M. A., and Eidinger, D. (1972). *J. Exp. Med.* **135**, 1410.

Krammer, P. H., Elliott, B. E., and von Boehmer, H. (1975). *Eur. J. Immunol.* **6**, 138.

Metcalf, D., and Wiadrowski, M. (1966). *Cancer Res.* **26**, 483.

Miller, R. G. (1973). *In* "New Techniques in Biophysics and Cell Biology" (R. H. Pain and B. J. Smith, eds.), p. 87. Wiley, New York.

Nussenzweig, V. (1974). *Adv. Immunol.* **19**, 217.

Osoba, D. (1970). *J. Exp. Med.* **132**, 368.

Parish, C. R., and Hayward, J. A. (1974). *Proc. R. Soc. London, Ser. B.* **187**, 65.

Sabatini, D. D., Bensch, K., and Bernett, R. J. (1963). *J. Cell Biol.* **17**, 19.

Wilson, J. D. (1971). *Immunology* **21**, 233.

17

The Use of Protein A Rosettes to Detect Cell-Surface Antigens

Judith Johnson

I. INTRODUCTION

Methods used to detect cell-surface antigens are techniques with wide applications for many aspects of biological research. The products of the major histocompatibility complex were among the first cell-surface antigens to be described, and these molecules can be used to distinguish cells of one individual from those of all other individuals (Klein, 1975). In addition to these universal surface antigens, many cell populations within a single

IMMUNOLOGICAL METHODS
Copyright © 1979 by Academic Press, Inc.
All rights of reproduction in any form reserved.
ISBN 0-12-442750-2

individual can be defined and distinguished by the presence of unique cell-surface antigens. This approach is being used in an attempt to dissect the nervous system (Schachner *et al.*, 1975) and has been particularly useful in identifying numerous subpopulations of morphologically indistinguishable lymphocytes (Raff, 1971).

To detect a particular cell-surface antigen, one requires an antibody with specificity for the antigen and a method to ascertain the number of cells that bind the antibody in any given population. The preparation of antiserum directed against cell-surface antigens is detailed in Chapter 13. Antigen-bearing cells are generally detected in one of two ways. The serum can be labeled with a fluorochrome so that the cells of interest will be fluorescent when excited by ultraviolet light (see Chapter 9). Alternatively, the cell population can be treated with antiserum together with complement, and the dead cells (i.e., those cells that have bound the antiserum) can be visualized by staining with a vital dye such as trypan blue. The purpose of this chapter is to detail a method for the detection of cell-surface antigens that uses sheep red cells (SRC) to indicate the cells that have bound antibody. This method has the advantage of using unmodified antibody, and it is highly sensitive and allows rapid screening of large numbers of cells. In addition, cells bearing the specific antigens can be readily isolated from the rest of the cells in the population.

II. PRINCIPLE OF THE METHOD

This method involves treating a cell population with antiserum directed to the surface antigen of interest and then labeling the cells that have bound the antiserum with SRC. The antigen-bearing cells are thus easily visualized in the microscope as *rosettes*, or lymphoid cells surrounded by red cells. Cells in the population that lack the antigen do not bind the antiserum and therefore do not bind the indicator SRC. The indicator red cells are produced by coating SRC with protein A (SpA), a 42,000 MW protein that forms part of the cell wall of the bacterium *Staphylococcus aureus*. This protein binds specifically to the Fc portion of immunoglobulins of the IgG class of several species (Sjöquist *et al.*, 1972).

III. MATERIALS

Protein A (Pharmacia, Uppsala, Sweden), diluted to 0.25 mg/ml in saline and stored at $-70°C$

Chromic chloride, $CrCl_3 \cdot 6\ H_2O$

Sheep red cells (SRC)

Hank's balanced salt solution containing 10% heat-inactivated fetal calf serum (HBSS–FCS)

Normal saline, 0.15 M NaCl

Phosphate-buffered saline, pH 7.2, 0.15 M (PBS)

Alsever's solution (pH adjusted to 6.1): 0.103 M glucose, 0.027 M sodium citrate, and 0.072 M sodium chloride

Ficoll–Urovison (density, 1.090) containing 0.1% sodium azide: 50 gm of Ficoll 400 (Pharmacia) and 75 ml of Urovison 58% (Schering, Zürich) made up to 360 ml with distilled H_2O; the density must be checked with a hydrometer

Crystal violet stain: stock solution, 10% in methanol; working solution, 1:20 in PBS

Sodium azide, NaN_3

Red cell lysing buffer: 0.01 M $KHCO_3$, 0.155 M NH_4Cl, and 0.1 mM EDTA; pH adjusted to 7.5

IV. PROCEDURES

A. Preparation of Protein A-Coated SRC

Protein A is coupled to SRC using chromic chloride. Since phosphate ions interfere with the coupling reaction, it is important to use normal saline in the preparation of all reagents.

1. SRC are washed three times in saline and finally adjusted to 50% in saline.

2. Chromic chloride is made up to 1 mg/ml (3.8×10^{-3} M) in saline just prior to use.

3. Equal volumes of SRC, chromic chloride, and protein A are mixed and left at room temperature (without shaking) for 4 min. (It is advisable to initially determine the optimal time of coupling because this parameter may vary with the batch of protein and the source of red cells.)

4. The reaction is stopped by adding 20–50 vol of PBS and the coupled cells are washed three times (in PBS) and then resuspended to a final concentraion of 0.5% in HBSS–FCS. The cells are stored at 4°C and are not washed prior to use. They are stable for 7 to 10 days.

B. Cell Preparations

1. Organs

Single-cell suspensions are prepared in HBSS–FCS by teasing the tissue with needles or pressing the tissue through fine wire mesh. Clumps are removed by allowing the cell suspension to settle on ice for 5 min and removing the supernatant. The cells are washed three times (1000 rpm, 10 min, 4°C) and then counted. If spleen cells are used, the red cells should be lysed. The washed cell pellet is resuspended in lysing buffer (0.5 ml/spleen) and left on ice for 10 min. The suspension is diluted with 10 ml of HBSS–FCS and the cells are washed three times.

2. Peripheral Blood Lymphocytes

A sample of blood (0.2–0.3 ml) is added to 1 ml of Alsever's solution. The cells are washed three times in HBSS–FCS and the red cells are lysed with two rounds of lysing buffer treatment. The lymphocytes are then washed three times and counted.

3. Cultured Cells

Viable cells are isolated from cultured cells by flotation on Ficoll 1.090 containing sodium azide. The cells at the interface are collected, washed three times in HBSS–FCS, and counted. For rosetting, all cell preparations are adjusted to $2–5 \times 10^6$ cells/ml.

C. Antisera

Antisera directed against cell-surface antigens are produced by the procedures described in Chapter 13. The sera are tested for the optimal dilution for rosette formation by titrating the serum against a cell population that is known to bear the antigen of interest. This is done by incubating cells with dilutions of antisera ranging from 1:10 to 1:1000. At the lowest dilutions, the percentage of rosetted cells will be low. This figure will rise with increasing serum dilution and should reach a plateau of 85–95% (for anti-histocompatability sera). At very high serum dilutions, the percentage of rosettes will again fall. The dilution used for standard testing should correspond to the plateau region. Hyperimmune anti-H-2 sera are generally used at a dilution of 1:1000 to 1:250.

D. Rosette Formation

1. Fifty microliters of cell suspension is mixed with a suitable amount of antiserum in round-bottom glass test tubes (12 × 75 mm) and incubated for 30 min at 4°C.

2. The cells are washed twice with 1 ml of HBSS–FCS and the tubes are drained on paper towels.

3. The cell pellets are resuspended and 50 ml of SpA–SRC is added to each tube. The tubes are mixed and centrifuged at 500 rpm for 10 min at 4°C.

4. Without disturbing the pellets, the tubes are incubated at 4°C overnight or at 37°C for 45 min. If the 37°C incubation is used, it is necessary to add sodium azide (2 mM) to the SpA–SRC to prevent capping of the red cells.

E. Reading

The pellet is gently resuspended and a drop of crystal violet is added (this can be done with a sample taken from the tube of rosetted cells). A wet mount is prepared by placing a drop of the cell suspension on a clean glass slide and covering this with a cover slip. Using a magnification of 160–250×, the number of rosetted and nonrosetted lymphocytes (stained cells) is counted. A cell is considered to be rosetted if it is surrounded by four or more red cells. A minimum of 100 cells should be counted and any clumps should be disregarded. Permanent preparations can be made by smearing the rosettes on acid-cleaned microscope slides, allowing them to dry, and fixing them in methanol. The cells can then be stained with any routine blood cell stain.

V. CONTROLS

To be certain that the assay and the SpA–SRC are working properly, it is important to include a control consisting of murine spleen or lymph node cells incubated with an appropriate anti-H-2 serum. The percentage of rosettes in these samples should be greater than 85%. Additional controls should include incubation of the test cells with an inappropriate antiserum and incubation of cells from a population known to lack the antigen in question with the test serum. Under these conditions, no more than 2–3% of the lymphocytes should be rosetted.

VI. CRITICAL ASPECTS

1. Since nonviable cells often do not form rosettes under these conditions, it is necessary that the cell suspensions be of high viability. If necessary, the cell preparations can be depleted of dead cells by passage over Ficoll.

2. The antiserum used must contain antibody of the IgG class because IgM molecules do not have a high affinity for protein A. If the antiserum used is primarily of the IgM class, it is possible to incubate the antibody-coated cells with an anti-immunoglobulin serum of the IgG class prior to

incubation with SpA–SRC. In this case, the cells are washed after each 30-min incubation.

VII. APPLICATIONS

A. Genetic Typing for Murine Histocompatibility Antigens

Murine peripheral blood lymphocytes are incubated with the appropriate anti-H-2 sera and SpA–SRC. This is a rapid assay method which has the advantage that scoring of the test need be only qualitative: Positive animals will have 80–90% rosettes, whereas negative animals will have less than 5% rosettes, a difference that is obvious from a brief scan of a wet mount.

B. Examination of the Surface Antigens of Dividing Cells

The protein A rosette method can be combined with autoradiography to allow the surface antigens of dividing cells to be examined. Dividing cells are labeled with tritiated thymidine *in vitro* (specific activity, 2–5 Ci/mmole) or *in vivo* (specific activity, 50–60 Ci/mmole) and then processed as described above for rosette formation. To prepare autoradiographs, 0.1 ml of fetal calf serum is added to the rosette pellet after incubation and the tubes are centrifuged for 10 min at 1000 rpm. The tubes are drained and the concentrated cell pellet is gently resuspended. This is smeared on an acid-cleaned, gelatin-coated microscope slide (0.1% gelatin in distilled water) and allowed to dry. The slides are fixed in methanol, dried, and then dipped in an appropriate dilution of emulsion (for tritium, Kodak NTB2 or Ilford K5, diluted 1:2 to 1:4 in distilled water) and exposed for an appropriate length of time (7–10 days). The slides are fixed and developed (Kodak K-19) and stained for 5 min with Giemsa stain. The slides are examined for the numbers of rosetted and nonrosetted labeled cells.

C. Isolation of Cells Bearing a Given Surface Antigen

The cells that have formed rosettes can be selectively removed from the cell population by sedimentation at 1 *g* (see Chapter 16) or by flotation on Ficoll–Urovison 1.090 containing 0.1% sodium azide. Rosettes in 2–5 ml of HBSS–FCS are layered onto 5 ml of Ficoll and centrifuged at 2500 rpm for 20 min at room temperature (20°C). The rosetted cells and free red cells will be found in the pellet, whereas the nonrosetted lymphocytes will be at the interface. The rosetted lymphocytes can be recovered by adding 4 parts of freshly prepared 0.83% ammonium chloride, pH 7.2, to 1 part of cells.

Cells are kept for 5 min on ice and then washed in medium. This method has been used to remove B cells from lymph node and spleen populations by treating the population with anti-immunoglobulin serum and rosetting the immunoglobulin-bearing B cells (Ghetie et al., 1975).

REFERENCES

Ghetie, V., Stålenheim, G., and Sjöquist, J. (1975). Scand. J. Immunol. 4, 471.
Klein, J. (1975). "Biology of the Mouse Histocompatibility H-2 Complex." Springer-Verlag, Berlin and New York.
Raff, M. C. (1971). Transplant. Rev. 6, 52.
Schachner, M., Wortham, K. A., Carter, L. D., and Chaffee, J. K. (1975). Dev. Biol. 44, 313.
Sjöquist, J., Meloun, B., and Helm, H. (1972). Eur. J. Biochem. 29, 572.

18

Hapten–Gelatin Gels Used as Adsorbents for Separation of Hapten-Specific B Lymphocytes

Werner Haas

I. PRINCIPLE

The principle of the "gelatin technique" for separation of specific receptor-bearing lymphocytes is shown in Fig. 1. The technique is based, like all other cellular immunoadsorbent techniques, on the binding of cells to insolubilized ligands. The general experience with such techniques has been, with few exceptions, that cells once trapped specifically cannot be eluted by free antigen or by mechanical means without affecting cell viability. The use of gelatin as a matrix allows the recovery of bound cells by melting the adsorbent. Gelatin forms an insoluble network at sufficiently high concentrations below a critical temperature. The melting point depends mainly on the gelatin concentration and is relatively sharp, as is characteristic for network gels that are stabilized by secondary forces such as hydrogen bonds (Veis, 1964). Melting of 5 to 10% gelatin occurs at

IMMUNOLOGICAL METHODS

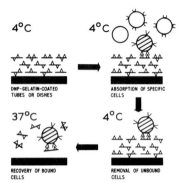

Fig. 1. Principle of the method used for specific cell separation. Lymphoid cells are moved over thin layers of DNP–gelatin, which is insoluble at 4°C. The binding cells are recovered by melting the gel at 37°C; this does not affect the cell viability.

physiological temperatures. Haptens may be coupled to gelatin without affecting its melting characteristics. Gel layers of hapten–gelatin conjugates that are insoluble at low temperature can be prepared readily and used as adsorbents for specific lymphocyte separation. The technique described here was developed in the Walter and Eliza Hall Institute (Haas *et al.*, 1974; Haas, 1975; Haas and Layton, 1975; Nossal and Pike, 1976, 1978). Other techniques based on the same principle have been described by several authors (Edelman and Rutishauser, 1974; Gold *et al.*, 1974; Webb *et al.*, 1975).

II. DESCRIPTION OF THE TECHNIQUE

A. Preparation of the Adsorbent

1. Gelatin

Bovine gelatin may be obtained from empty gelatin capsules, which melt in distilled water at 40° to 60°C. Pure gelatin from other sources is also suitable but has not been used extensively. The gelatin solutions are stored at a concentration of 20 gm/100 ml of distilled water at 4°C after sterilization by filtration of the hot solutions through Millipore filters (0.45-μm pore size). The concentration of gelatin solutions may be calculated from the light extinctions of appropriate dilutions at 215 nm using an extinction coefficient of $E_{1\,cm}^{1\%} = 17.50$.

2. Conjugation of Haptens to Gelatin

The details of two standard procedures are described below.

a. Preparation of DNP–gelatin (according to Eisen, 1964). Twenty milliliters of a 20% (w/v) gelatin solution is mixed with 10 ml of 8% (w/v) K_2CO_3 and 10 ml of a 10 mg/ml solution of sodium 2,4-dinitrobenzene sulfonate (DNBS). The mixture is stirred gently for 16 hr at 37°C and then dialyzed extensively against distilled water and phosphate-buffered saline at 4°C. The molar concentration of DNP is determined by light absorption at 360 nm using an extinction coefficient of 2,4-DNP-lysine of $E_{1\,cm}^{1\,M}$ = 17,400. The conjugation ratio of DNP–gelatin is then determined assuming an average molecular weight of 10^5 for gelatin. The described procedure gave a conjugation ratio of approximately four DNP groups per gelatin molecule. Lower substitutions are obtained by reducing the concentration of DNBS or the reaction time.

b. Preparation of NIP–gelatin (according to Brownstone et al., 1966). Fifty milliliters of gelatin (10%, w/v) is mixed with 140 ml of 0.2 M bicarbonate buffer (pH 9.2) and 100 mg of 4-hydroxy-3-iodo-5-nitrophenylated (NIP) azide in 2 ml of dimethyl formamide (DMF). The mixture is stirred gently at room temperature for 12 hr and then dialyzed extensively against phosphate-buffered saline (PBS, pH 7.3). The conjugation ratio of this preparation is approximately one NIP per molecule of gelatin as determined spectrophotometrically using an extinction coefficient of 5.6×10^3 at 430 nm for NIP.

The conjugation of other haptens to gelatin may be performed according to other techniques described elsewhere in this book (see Chapter 8). Diazo haptens may be used despite the paucity of tyrosine residues in gelatin since high coupling ratios are not desirable in most cases.

For purification of antibody-forming cell precursors, low coupling ratios, such as one hapten per molecule of gelatin, are advantageous because too many low-affinity cells bind to highly hapten-conjugated gelatin (Haas, 1975).

3. Coating of Petri Dishes with Gelatin

Gelatin, hapten–gelatin, or mixtures of gelatin and hapten–gelatin (5%, w/v) are heated to 40° to 60°C and portions of 1 to 2 ml are pipetted into sterile petri dishes (Sterimed, 85-mm diameter, or Falcon 3003 Optilux tissue culture dishes, 100 × 20 mm). The plates are swirled immediately to distribute the solution over the whole base surface and as much solution as possible is aspirated from the edge of the dish so that only a very thin uniform layer remains at the base of the dish. The coated dishes are then stored at 4°C overnight for the gel to "age" (Veis, 1964). The dishes are rocked twice with 5 to 10 ml of cold glycine–HCl buffer (pH 2.2) for 5 min and then washed several times with cold PBS (pH 7.4). The gel-coated dishes may be stored with PBS for up to 2 days at 4°C and rinsed again with glycine–HCl (pH 2.2) and PBS (pH 7.4) just prior to use for cell fractionation. The extensive washing procedures are essential to remove any hapten–gelatin from the dishes that is not firmly incorporated in the gel structure. Traces of solubilized hapten–gelatin would be sufficient to prevent binding of high-affinity receptor-bearing cells.

4. Cross-Linking of Gelatin Gels

For some purposes it may be advantageous to use cross-linked hapten–gelatin layers that no longer melt. Hapten–gelatin-coated dishes are prepared as described and rinsed several times with cold PBS (pH 7.3). The PBS is then poured off and 3 ml of a 2.5% solution of glutaraldehyde in PBS is added to each dish. The gel is cross-linked almost instantaneously (Avrameas and Ternynck, 1969). The glutaraldehyde is kept in the dishes for 10 to 20 min at room temperature and then the dishes are rinsed with glycine–HCl and PBS as described.

B. Preparation of Single-Cell Suspensions

Mice are killed by cervical dislocation and the spleens are removed into cold Eisen's balanced salt solution (EBSS). The spleens are dissociated into small segments with scissors and the cells are extruded from the capsule of the organ by gently pressing the fragments with the flat upper end of the plunger of a glass syringe through a stainless steel sieve into cold EBSS. Large cell aggregates are removed by adding the solution to centrifuge tubes containing 1 ml of 100% FCS and centrifuging for 10 min on ice. Red cells may be removed using Gey's solution; however, this is not essential for the subsequent cell separation. For dead cell removal, the pellet is resuspended in low ionic strength medium (0.3 M glucose in 100 ml of deionized water mixed with 10 ml of PBS) to a maximum concentration of 5×10^7 cells/ml (von Boehmer and Shortman, 1973). The suspension is then immediately filtered through a siliconized glass Pasteur pipette with a small loosely packed cotton wool plug above the constriction. For preparation of large numbers of cells, larger siliconized glass columns may be used, which are packed loosely with a 1- to 2-cm layer of cotton wool on the end. Immediately after the filtration, the cells are recovered from the low ionic strength medium by centrifugation and resuspended in EBSS. Dead cell removal is important to avoid cell clumping and nonspecific binding of viable cells to the adsorbent via "sticky" dead cells or their released "sticky" DNA. The procedure described allows the preparation of single-cell suspensions of 95 to 100% viability with only a few very small cell aggregates.

C. The Separation Procedure

1. The Medium

For separation, the cells are suspended in EBSS or PBS without fetal calf serum (FCS). FCS should be avoided since it tends to increase nonspecific binding of spleen cells to gelatin layers for unknown reasons. Gelatin that is soluble at 4°C may be included at low concentrations (0.1%) to inhibit binding of cells specific for gelatin determinants. Removal of Ca^{2+} and Mg^{2+} by chelating with EDTA (5 mM) reduces cell aggregation, and adding it does not appear to interfere with specific and nonspecific interactions of cells with the adsorbent.

2. The Mechanics of the Separation Procedure

Dishes with the cells to be separated are placed on a shaker–rocker, which moves in two directions. The shaker moves horizontally through 1.5 cm at 80 Hz and is mounted on a rocker that moves vertically through 20° at 20 Hz. Using this procedure, the cells do not accumulate in the center or at the edge of the dish but move continuously over the whole gel layer surface. The movement of the cells should be not too fast, since this would interfere with binding of specific cells, and not too slow, to avoid nonspecific binding.

3. The Number of Cells Separated per Dish

Up to 10^8 spleen cells in a volume of 3 ml of EBSS may be separated per dish. The number of binding cells is proportional to the number of cells separated per dish as long as not more than 10^6 cells bind per dish. With 2×10^6 or more binding cells per dish, the adsorbent surface becomes limiting.

4. The Separation Time

With not more than 10^8 cells per dish the number of binding cells increases with time for up to 60 min and then remains constant (Haas and Layton, 1975). However, the peak number of binding cells is almost reached after 15 min of fractionation. Moreover, with cells fractionated for 15 min optimal antibody-forming cell precursor activity could be demonstrated

(Nossal and Pike, 1976). Separation for more than 15 min may result in preferential release of specific receptor-bearing cells from the adsorbent.

5. *The Recovery of Unbound Cells*

The separation is terminated by pouring off the cell suspension. Each dish must then be washed several times to remove all nonbinding cells. The dishes are swirled gently with 10 ml of EBSS. The washing medium may be poured off each time without affecting the bound cells since a thin layer of medium always remains on top of the gel layer. The effect of washing should be controlled using an inverted microscope, through which bound and unbound cells can be distinguished easily since the unbound cells move in relation to the dish when the medium is gently agitated.

6. *The Recovery of Bound Cells*

After the last wash, 10 ml of EBSS (37°C) is added to each dish. The gel layer melts immediately and the binding cell population is suspended in the medium by gentle pipetting. The cells are then transferred to tubes, centrifuged, resuspended, and pooled with cells recovered from replicate dishes.

D. Treatment of Separated Cells with Collagenase

Hapten–gelatin remains bound to cells recovered from hapten–gelatin layers by melting and cannot be removed from the cells by washing through FCS. However, hapten–gelatin may be removed from the cell surface after treatment with trypsin or collagenase. For most purposes, the use of highly purified collagenase (A grade) is required, which does not affect any cell-surface proteins. Up to 10^7 cells are suspended in 0.9 ml of EBSS (or PBS) and 0.1 ml of collagenase (1 mg/ml) is added. Much lower collagenase concentrations may be sufficient depending on the activity of the colla-genase preparation. The mixture is kept for 10 min at 37°C and the cells are then washed twice through 1-ml underlayers of FCS. Siliconized glass tubes should be used to avoid a substantial loss of cells during the washing procedure. For some purposes it may be advantageous to treat the cells with collagenase at 4°C for 20 min. This procedure also effectively removes all hapten–gelatin from the cells.

III. APPLICATIONS

Hapten-specific B cells enriched by the gelatin technique described here have been used to facilitate studies on antigen-binding cells (Nossal and

Layton, 1976; Goding and Layton, 1976), to study anti-hapten antibody responses *in vitro* (Nossal and Pike, 1976; Pike and Nossal, 1976; Fidler and Pike, 1977), and in attempts to obtain colonies of cells derived from hapten-specific B cells (Metcalf *et al.*, 1975). Several other applications are obvious. However, before using the technique it is important to consider its limitations.

IV. LIMITATIONS

1. It is difficult to prepare large numbers of highly purified cells.
2. The efficiency of the technique to separate from a heterogeneous population of lymphocytes *all* cells bearing receptors for a particular hapten is low since a substantial number of specific cells are found in the nonbinding population. Thus, the technique is not suitable for depletion of specific cells (Haas, 1975).
3. The technique allows hapten-specific antibody-forming cell precursors to be enriched up to a frequency of 30% (Nossal *et al.*, 1977). However, considering the idiotypes of the receptors of the purified cells and their affinities for the hapten, even highly purified populations are still rather heterogeneous.
4. Some studies on antigen–lymphocyte interactions may be limited by the exposure of the cells to hapten–gelatin at melting temperature and/or the treatment with collagenase.

REFERENCES

Avrameas, S., and Ternynck, T. (1969). *Immunochemistry* **6**, 53.
Brownstone, A., Mitchison, N. A., and Pitt Rivers, R. (1966). *Immunology* **10**, 465.
Edelman, G. M., and Rutishauser, U. (1974). *In* "Methods in Enzymology" (Jakoby and Wilchek, eds.), Vol. 24, p. 195. Academic Press, New York.
Eisen, H. N. (1964). *Methods Med. Res.* **10**, 94.
Fidler, J. M., and Pike, B. L. (1977). *Cell. Immunol.* **31**, 163.
Goding, I. W., and Layton, I. E. (1976). *J. Exp. Med.* **144**, 852.
Gold, F., Kleinman, R., and Ben-Efraim, S. (1974). *J. Immunol. Methods* **6**, 31.
Haas, W. (1975). *J. Exp. Med.* **141**, 1015.
Haas, W., and Layton, J. E. (1975). *J. Exp. Med.* **141**, 1004.
Haas, W., Schrader, J. W., and Szenberg, A. (1974). *Eur. J. Immunol.* **4**, 565.
Metcalf, D., Nossal, G. J. V., Warner, N. L., Miller, J. F. A. P., Mandel, T. E., Layton, J. E., and Gutman, G. A. (1975). *J. Exp. Med.* **142**, 1534.
Nossal, G. J. V., and Layton, J. E. (1976). *J. Exp. Med.* **143**, 511.
Nossal, G. J. V., and Pike, B. (1976). *Immunology* **30**, 189.
Nossal, G. J. V., and Pike, B. L. (1978). *J. Immunol.* **120**, 145.

Nossal, G. J. V., Pike, B. L., Stocker, J. W., Layton, J. E., and Goding, J. W. (1977). *Cold Spring Harbor Symp. Quant. Biol.* **41**, 237.

Pike, B., and Nossal, G. J. V. (1976). *J. Exp. Med.* **144**, 568.

Veis, A. (1964). "The Macromolecular Chemistry of Gelatin." Academic Press, New York.

von Boehmer, H., and Shortman, K. (1973). *J. Immunol. Methods* **134**, 66.

Webb, C., Teitelbaum, D., Rauch, H., Maoz, A., Arnon, R., and Fuchs, S. (1975). *J. Immunol.* **114**, 1469.

19

Assay for Plaque-Forming Cells

Ivan Lefkovits and Humberto Cosenza

I. OBJECTIVE

The objective of the plaque assay is to enumerate and study individual antibody-forming cells, specially in situations where only a few such cells are present among millions of cells that do not release antibody.

II. PRINCIPLE OF THE METHOD

The plaque assay was developed by Jerne and Nordin in 1963. Lymphoid cells are mixed with a suspension of red blood cells and immobilized in a gel

IMMUNOLOGICAL METHODS
Copyright © 1979 by Academic Press, Inc.
All rights of reproduction in any form reserved.
ISBN 0-12-442750-2

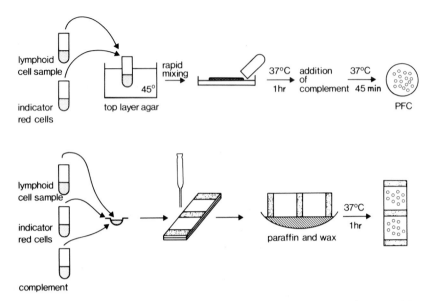

Fig. 1. Flow diagram of the plaque-forming cell assay. The standard method (top) and Cunningham's modification (bottom) are shown.

(usually agar) or in a liquid medium enclosed in a sealed chamber (Fig. 1). The specific antibody synthesized by some of the lymphoid cells is released and diffuses from the central cell; antibody is trapped by antigen in the areas immediately surrounding the plaque-forming cell (PFC). In the presence of complement, plaques will appear as a consequence of lysis of sensitized red cells.

The original two papers of Jerne and Nordin (1963) and Jerne et al. (1963) should be consulted before introducing the plaque technique. For any further modification, especially for the indirect techniques, fluorescent stainings of plaques, and autoradiography, as well as for theoretical questions, the detailed review by Jerne et al. (1974) should be consulted.

III. MATERIAL

For a given modification of the hemolytic plaque assay, only a few of the following items are needed.

Petri dishes, 100 × 15 mm or 85 × 15 mm (most of the types
   are suitable, i.e., Falcon Plastics 1001, Sterilin, or Greiner)
Agar (Bacto agar, Difco No. 0140-01)

Agarose (Indubiose)

Eagle's medium (Difco TC minimal Eagle, dried No. 5675-24)

Glass tubes (volume, 5–10 ml; preferentially so-called Wasserman tubes)

DEAE-dextran (Pharmacia, Uppsala, Sweden)

Alsever's solution

Phosphate-buffered saline, PBS

Balanced salt solution, BSS

Guinea pig complement (dilution 1:10 in Dulbecco PBS)

Microscope slides

Double-face Scotch tape

Paraffin

Wax

Türk's solution (0.01% gentian violet in 3% acetic acid)

Trypan blue (4 parts of 0.2% trypan blue and 1 part of 4.5% NaCl)

Glutaraldehyde

Plaque counter

Dissecting microscope with fluorescent lamp (Bausch and Lomb)

IV. PREPARATION OF CELL SUSPENSIONS

A. Lymphoid Cell Suspensions

The cell concentration of the lymphoid cell suspensions is adjusted so that the aliquot plated would yield about (i) 400 PFC per petri dish, (ii) 150 PFC per microscope slide, or (iii) 100 PFC per Cunningham chamber. If it cannot be predicted how many PFC will be present in the sample, a preliminary test is often necessary. As a rule of thumb, one should use 1% of a spleen per sample and one-twentieth of the content of a 1-ml culture. The lymphoid cells are washed twice by centrifugation (500 g for 10 min at 4°C), resuspended in cold BSS, and kept on ice until they are used for plaquing.

Cell counts may be done two ways: (a) The number of nucleated cells in each cell suspension is determined by diluting a sample in Türk's solution and counting at least 100 stained cells in a hemocytometer. (b) The number of viable cells is determined in another sample by the trypan blue exclusion test. [A drop of cell suspension is mixed with a drop of trypan blue solution. The number of dead (stained) cells is counted after allowing the mixture to stand at room temperature for 1–3 min.]

B. Indicator Cells

As far as uncoated erythrocytes are concerned, fresh red cells are considerably less susceptible to lysis than aged red cells, and one should use at least 1-week-old red blood cells, stored in Alsever's solution, as indicator cells. Prior to plaquing, the red cells are washed three times by centrifugation (2500 g for 10 min at room temperature) before being resuspended in PBS or BSS to 20% (v/v) if using the agar technique or as an 8–10% suspension for use in the Cunningham modification of the plaque technique.

V. PLAQUING PROCEDURES

A. Plating on Petri Dishes

This is the original standard method of Jerne and Nordin (1963).

1. Agar Bottom Layer

During the week preceding the experiment, petri dishes are coated with a 1.4% agar layer. Bacto agar, 2.8% in distilled water, is autoclaved, cooled to 45°C in a water bath, and mixed with an equal volume of Eagle's medium of double concentration, equilibrated previously to 45°C. The agar is then poured in 10- to 15-ml portions into petri dishes (100 × 15 mm). The plates can be stored at 4°C for 2–3 weeks. On the day to be used, the plates are incubated upside down without covers at 37°C for about 1.5 hr, in order to evaporate 1–2 gm of water from the agar.

2. Agar Top Layer

Agar for the top layer should be made fresh on the day it will be used. Bacto agar, 1.4% in distilled water, is autoclaved, cooled to 45°C in a water bath, and mixed with an equal volume of Eagle's medium of double concentration, equilibrated previously to 45°C. Note that the final concentration of the agar top layer is 0.7%. To prepare the top layer more quickly, the agar can also be boiled instead of autoclaved. In this case, the agar suspension should be boiled until foam appears, the flame is then removed, and, when the foam subsides, the boiling is continued. The procedure is repeated until no more foam appears or until only large foam bubbles are formed. The boiling procedure usually takes 5 min.

3. Plaquing

Wasserman tubes (usually a 5-ml volume) containing 0.1 ml of DEAE-dextran solution are placed in a 45°C water bath. Then 2 ml of the agar top layer is dispensed with a prewarmed pipette into each of the tubes containing DEAE-dextran.

In rapid sequence, 0.1 ml of the indicator red cell suspension and 0.01–0.5 ml of the lymphoid cell suspension are added to the agar containing tube kept at 45°C. This mixture is poured rapidly over the bottom layer. Care should be taken to spread the top layer mixture quickly over the whole surface of the petri dish, otherwise the solidified top layer will be faulty. The agar is allowed to solidify evenly by placing the petri dish on a leveled horizontal bench.

The covered plate is incubated for 1 or 2 hr at 37°C. The plate is then flooded with 2 ml of guinea pig complement, diluted 1:10 in phosphate-buffered saline, and returned to the incubator for 0.5 hr. At this time, the plaques are visible as small, round, pale areas against the red cell background. The plates are left at room temperature for 1 to 2 hr and then, after pouring off the complement, can be stored at 4°C. The plaques can be counted with the naked eye, but the use of a low-power dissecting microscope is preferable. The central cell in each plaque can be found by examination under a microscope. The PFC's can be fixed by adding 2 ml of 0.25% (v/v) glutaraldehyde.

B. Plating on Slides

Microscope slides should be coated with a thin layer of 0.1–0.2% agarose and allowed to dry. This procedure ensures the firm attachment of the agar layer, containing the cell suspension, to the slide. A 0.5% solution of agarose in balanced salt solution is distributed as 0.5-ml aliquots into prewarmed tubes kept in a 45°C water bath. Fifty microliters of a 15% (v/v) SRC suspension and lymphoid cells (10–100 μl) are added, and the mixture is spread on a coated slide. The spreading is conveniently performed by sliding the rim of the inverted tube on the surface of the microscope slide. The agarose on the slides is allowed to solidify on a horizontal surface, and then the slides are inverted in special Lucite racks provided with a shallow (21.5 × 4.7 × 0.1 cm) well. The space between the slides and the bottom of the well is filled with guinea pig complement, diluted 1:10 in BSS. The racks are stacked and placed inside plastic boxes containing a base layer of wet paper towels to provide a moist atmosphere. The containers are incubated for 2–3 hr at 37°C. For counting, the slides are dipped in saline, the backs are wiped dry, and the slides are held under strong indirect light. Counting is most satisfactory with 40 to 100 plaques per slide.

C. Cunningham's Plaque Assay

Cunningham (1965) proposed a modification of the hemolytic plaque technique, where lymphoid cells and indicator erythrocytes are incubated without supporting gels as monolayers in chambers. The method is simple, sensitive, and rapid for the enumeration of plaque-forming cells and is also suitable for studies involving micromanipulation or examination under the light microscope of living undistorted cells.

The incubation chambers are prepared by placing three strips of narrow double-face tape on a microscope slide (75 × 25 mm), dividing it into two areas of roughly equal surface. A second slide is pressed onto the first so that the two slides are face to face and separated only by the thin strips of tape. The total volume of the two chambers is about 180–200 μl.

The liquid layer containing the cell suspension is mixed in plastic microtiter plates as follows: (a) 100 μl of balanced salt solution, (b) 50 μl of the lymphoid cell suspension, (c) 20 μl of an 8–10% suspension of SRC, and (d) 20 μl of a 1:2 dilution of GPC (previously absorbed with SRC). The above cell suspension is mixed and placed (by capillary action) into both chambers of a set of slides with a Pasteur pipette. The chambers are sealed by carefully dipping the slide edges into a melted mixture of equal portions of paraffin and wax. The chambers are then placed in a tray and incubated at 37°C for 1–2 hr before scoring the plaques under a dissecting microscope. A total of 100–200 plaques can be scored with ease. Careful handling of the chambers avoids any distortion in plaque morphology. The plaques should be counted within 4 hr after development since after a longer time lapse the plaques tend to become unclear due to movement of cells in the liquid layer.

VI. CALCULATIONS

The plaques are expressed either as PFC per spleen or as PFC per 10^6 nucleated cells. If the samples are taken from cultures, then the number of PFC may be expressed: (a) per culture, (b) per 10^6 input cells, or (c) per 10^6 recovered viable cells.

VII. CRITICAL FACTORS

A. DEAE-Dextran and Complement

The use of unrefined agars like Difco, Bacto, Noble, or Ionagar demands the addition of DEAE-dextran (MW about 2 × 10^6). This polycation overcomes the anticomplementary properties of the agar, probably by binding to the sulfuric ester groups on the galactan strands. Agarose is not anticomplementary and its use obviates the necessity to add DEAE-dextran. Most batches of guinea pig complement—either fresh or lyophilized serum—are optimally effective at a 1:10 final dilution if DEAE-dextran is present in the Bacto agar at a concentration of 0.3–0.5 mg/ml and a 1:20 final dilution in Cunningham chambers. A tenfold higher concentration of GPC often agglutinates the red cells and decreases the number of detectable plaques. The following are recommended sources of complement to be used with certain lymphoid cells and/or erythrocytes:

guinea pig complement—mouse lymphoid cells, sheep red cells;
rabbit complement—mouse lymphoid cells, rat red cells;
human complement—mouse lymphoid cells, hamster red cells; hamster lymphoid cells, mouse red cells; rat lymphoid cells, mouse red cells;
chicken complement—chicken lymphoid cells, sheep red cells.

B. Concentration of Red Cells

The optimal final red cell concentration is 1% (0.1 ml of a 20% red cell suspension in 2 ml of the top layer). At lower red cell concentrations larger plaques are obtained, but there is no increase in the number detected.

C. Conditions of Incubation

Prolonged incubation prior to or after the addition of complement only marginally affects the plaque size and number. Incubation temperatures of from 37° to 40°C reveal approximately the same number of plaques. Temperatures below 37°C cause a reduction in plaque numbers.

D. False Plaques

Plaques must appear only after the addition of complement. Microscopic examination must reveal the antibody-releasing cell in the center of a plaque.

1. Small air bubbles can be easily identified by their sharp-edged appearance.

2. Tissue fragments at the center of a plaque can be easily detected by the naked eye.

3. An individual batch of sheep red cells will rarely contain plaque-forming elements, possibly due to autohemolytic antibody-forming cells in

certain sheep. Such plaques can be identified when the sheep red cells are plated alone.

4. Red cells used as antigen in cultures may bind such a high number of antibody molecules that, when the lymphoid cell sample is plated, antibody shed by red cells induces the formation of false plaques. Such plaques are very small.

E. Total Number of Plaques Counted

It is a widespread habit to count plaques on a single sample even if the actual number of plaques is exceedingly low. The Poisson component for low plaque count may cause a major error. PFC counts below 10 PFC per sample lead to highly unreliable results. The convenient range of PFC per sample is 30–100 PFC, leading to a sampling error between ±20 and 10%, respectively.

F. Indirect Plaques

If PFC's for nonhemolytic classes of antibody have to be revealed, developing serum is added to the samples (Dresser and Wortis, 1965; Šterzl and Říha, 1965). The optimal dilution of developing serum to be used must be determined empirically. Basically two approaches can be used: (1) The developing serum is added together with complement and the total number of "direct" and "indirect" plaques is counted. (2) Complement is added alone, the mixture is incubated, "direct" plaques are counted, the complement is poured off, and then developing serum and fresh complement are added and incubated and newly developed "indirect" plaques are counted.

This can be done for both the petri dish technique and the slide technique, whereas in Cunningham's technique (Cunningham and Szenberg, 1968) the developing serum must be added together with the lymphoid cell mixture and the complement. Antisera specific for individual classes of immunoglobulins of several species are commercially available.

REFERENCES

Cunningham, A. J. (1965). *Nature* (*London*) **207**, 1106.
Cunningham, A. J., and Szenberg, A. (1968). *Immunology* **14**, 599.
Dresser, D. W., and Wortis, H. H. (1965). *Nature* (*London*) **208**, 859.

Jerne, N. K., and Nordin, A. A. (1963). *Science* **140,** 405.
Jerne, N. K., Nordin, A. A., and Henry, C. (1963). *In* "Cell-Bound Antibodies" (B. Amos and H. Koprowski, eds.), p. 109. Wistar Inst. Press, Philadelphia, Pennsylvania.
Jerne, N. K., Henry, C., Nordin, A. A., Fuji, H., Koros, A. M. C., and Lefkovits, I. (1974). *Transplant. Rev.* **18,** 130.
Šterzl, J., and Říha, I. (1965). *Nature (London)* **208,** 858.

20

Plaquing and Recovery of Individual Antibody-Producing Cells

Marc Shulman

I. OBJECTIVE

The method described here, in which antibody-secreting cells are plated in methyl cellulose, permits efficient recovery of the individual plaque-forming cells and their subsequent growth into large cultures.

Usually plaque formation is done in agar or agarose (Jerne and Nordin, 1963), between glass slides (Cunningham and Szenberg, 1968), or in carboxymethyl cellulose (Nossal *et al.*, 1970). Under such conditions it is difficult to recover and grow the individual plaque-forming cells. In this method the red blood cells are plated in agarose, thus providing a firm support in which the red cells cannot diffuse and aggregate. On top of the red cell–agar mixture are plated the plaque-forming cells in methyl cellulose. Used at a concentration of 1%, the methyl cellulose is sufficiently viscous that the plaque-forming cells are adequately immobilized and it is sufficiently liquid to be easily mixed and pipetted. After plaque formation, the individual plaque-forming cell is transferred with a micropipette to ordinary liquid medium.

The cells used to develop this method were the IgM-producing hybridoma cell lines Sp1 and Sp7 described by Köhler and Milstein (1976). Sp1 antibody is directed against a normal constituent of sheep red cells; Sp7 antibody binds TNP, so that it can lyse sheep red cells to which the hapten

IMMUNOLOGICAL METHODS
Copyright © 1979 by Academic Press, Inc.
All rights of reproduction in any form reserved.
ISBN 0-12-442750-2

TNP has been attached. Presumably this method would work for any antibody–antigen combination that produces plaques under the ordinary agar conditions.

II. MATERIALS

RH medium (2× concentrated = 2× RH) (Wabl *et al.*, 1978)
2.08 gm of H18 (Gibco) powder (RPMI 1640)
40 ml of fetal calf serum (Gibco)
2 ml of a penicillin–streptomycin solution (10,000 U/ml)
    (Gibco)
6 ml of 1 M Hepes (Flow Laboratories)
5.32 ml of 7.5% $NaHCO_3$ (Gibco)
Distilled H_2O to a 120-ml final volume; sterilize by filtration
Methyl cellulose
Agarose
Sheep red cells
Trinitrophenyl (TNP)

Methyl cellulose 4000 (Hoffman-LaRoche) was added to boiling water to give a concentration of 2% methyl cellulose and removed from heat. The mixture was stirred overnight at 4°C and centrifuged for 2 hr at 10,000 g. For plating, methyl cellulose was used at a final concentration of 1%; that is, the 2% methyl cellulose solution was mixed with an equal volume of 2× RH. To measure the amount of the viscous methyl cellulose solutions accurately, a syringe rather than a pipette was used.

Indubioise A37 (agarose, L'Industrie Biologique Francaise) was dissolved by boiling in H_2O. Solutions containing indubiose at 1 and 0.6% were mixed with equal volumes of 2× RH.

Sheep red cells were haptenated with TNP as described by Rittenberg and Pratt (1969). Packed cells were diluted fourfold in phosphate-buffered saline before using.

III. PROCEDURE

The following procedure was used to obtain plaques in 35-mm plastic dishes (Falcon). A 1-ml layer containing 0.5% Indubiose in RH medium was used to give a flat surface in the dish. Then 0.2 ml of 0.3% Indubiose in RH medium containing 10 μl of complement (lyophilized guinea pig complement, Oray, Behringwerke) and 10 μl of sheep red cells was overlaid.

Finally 1 ml of 1% methyl cellulose in RH medium containing the antibody-secreting cells was overlaid.

Plaques appeared after 2 hr. The 1% methyl cellulose layer is sufficiently liquid that the upper portion of this layer can flow if the plate is tipped, thus moving the plaque-forming cells away from their plaque. Therefore, it is better to incubate the plates undisturbed overnight so that the plaque-forming cells settle onto the agarose layer. Cells used here yielded plaques about 1 mm in diameter (see Fig. 1).

The plaque-forming cells were then transferred with a micropipette. The cells used here, Sp1 and Sp7, were transferred to microtiter plates containing a feeder layer of 3T3 fibroblasts that had been killed by irradiation (3300 rad) and in which the fibroblast medium had been replaced with 15 μl of RPMI 1640 medium supplemented with 30 mM Hepes. When the Sp cells had grown substantially they were transferred to 0.1 ml of fresh medium, and as the cells grew the amount of medium was increased.

We obtained microcultures from single cells in about 50% of the transfers.

The Sp cells used here formed colonies in the methyl cellulose, and after several days the plaques were somewhat larger than after the first day.

To test the efficiency with which plaque-forming cells are detected in the presence of large numbers of non-plaque-forming cells we have plated about 100 plaque-forming cells in the presence of 0, 10^4, 10^5, or 10^6 non-plaque-

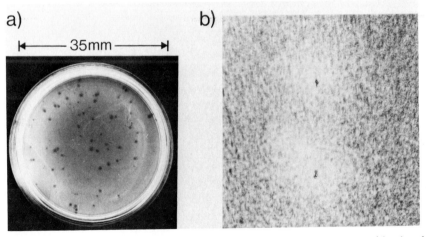

Fig. 1. Plaques in methyl cellulose. The cell line Sp 7 was plated for plaques and incubated overnight at 37°C. (a) A plate at 1.2× magnification. (b) Individual plaques, each with two cells that had divided during the overnight incubation.

forming cells. Plaques are perceived under these different conditions at about the same efficiency, although at high cell concentrations the non-plaque-forming cells impart a turbid background and the particular plaque-forming cell cannot be recognized. Under such conditions the entire area about the plaque should be picked, grown, and replated at a lower cell density.

REFERENCES

Cunningham, A. J., and Szenberg, A. (1968). *Immunology* **14,** 599.
Jerne, N. K., and Nordin, A. A. (1963). *Science* **140,** 405.
Köhler, G., and Milstein, C. (1976). *Eur. J. Immunol.* **6,** 511.
Nossal, G. J. V., Bussard, A. E., Lewis, H., and Mazie, J. C. (1970). *J. Exp. Med.* **131,** 894.
Rittenberg, M. B., and Pratt, K. L. (1969). *Proc. Soc. Exp. Med.* **132,** 575.
Wabl, M., Forni, L., and Loor, F. (1978). *Science* **199,** 1078.

21

Assay for Specific Alloantigen-Binding T Cells Activated in the Mixed Lymphocyte Reaction

Bruce E. Elliott,[1] Zoltán Nagy, and Markus Nabholz

[1] Research Fellow of the National Cancer Institute of Canada.

IMMUNOLOGICAL METHODS
Copyright © 1979 by Academic Press, Inc.
All rights of reproduction in any form reserved.
ISBN 0-12-442750-2

I. OBJECTIVE

The technique reported here was designed to determine the specificity of individual T cells activated *in vitro* during a mixed lymphocyte reaction (MLR).

II. PRINCIPLE OF THE METHOD

Responder blasts generated in primary MLR cultures with B-depleted responder cells carry surface-bound stimulator alloantigens that appear to be bound via specific receptors. These surface-bound stimulator alloantigens can be detected by anti-stimulator alloantibodies followed by indirect immunofluorescence. The responder cells seem to be "monospecific" in the sense that, among T blasts responding to a mixture of two stimulators with different allogeneic determinants, most of the responder cells carry antigens from only one or the other type of stimulator cell (Nagy *et al.*, 1976a,b).

We have shown that the surface-bound stimulator alloantigens can be removed from MLR-activated blasts by trypsin treatment and that these cells are, after a recovery period, able to specifically bind fresh stimulator cell material (Elliott *et al.*, 1977).

III. CELLS AND ALLOANTISERA

A. Cell Preparation and Culture Procedures

Cell preparation and culture procedures are described in detail elsewhere (see Chapter 15; see also Nabholz *et al.*, 1974; Julius *et al.*, 1973). However, several important points will be discussed here.

1. Media

The culture medium was Hepes-buffered (30 mM) RPMI 1640 (Grand Island Biological Co., Grand Island, New York) supplemented with L-glutamine (2 mM final concentration), streptomycin (100 μg/ml), penicillin (100 IU/ml), 5% human serum, and 2-mercaptoethanol (3×10^{-5} M final concentration).

The medium used for the preparation of cell suspensions and washing of cells was the same except that it did not contain 2-mercaptoethanol. In the absence of serum, Hepes was found to be toxic; therefore, a minimum of 2.5% human serum was present during all washing procedures.

Human serum rather than fetal calf serum (FCS) was used because it was found to yield lower background proliferation of responder cells cultured with irradiated syngeneic cells (control). Human serum was prepared as follows: Blood from pretested donors was aseptically collected directly into sterile conical tubes (Falcon Plastic 2070, 50 ml) and allowed to clot for 2–3 hr at room temperature. The serum was transferred to fresh tubes and centrifuged for 15 min at 2000 g to remove red cells and platelets. The sera were collected separately, assayed for sterility, pooled, heat-inactivated, fractioned, and stored at $-20°C$.

2. Cell Preparation for MLR Cultures

Unless otherwise indicated, all centrifugations were carried out at 4°C and at 150 g for 15 min. Inguinal, axillary, cervical, and mesenteric lymph nodes and/or spleens were removed aseptically and placed in cold medium. They were then cut into pieces with scissors. The lymphocytes were released by gentle grinding with a loose-fitting Teflon homogenizer in a plastic tube. To remove clumps and debris, the cell suspensions were passed through a 10-ml syringe filled halfway with loosely packed nylon or cotton wool. The cells were forced through with the plunger, and another 5–8 ml of medium was used to wash out the remaining cells. (Note: This procedure is distinct from the preparation of B-depleted lymph node cells described in Section III,A,3). The pooled cells were then spun down, the fatty supernatant was carefully removed, and the cells were resuspended in 10 ml of fresh medium. This procedure was repeated twice more before the cells were finally resuspended to the required concentration. Viable and total nucleated cells were counted before the last spin, after mixing a cell sample with an equal volume of 1% eosin Y (in PBS). Viability was between 78 and 93%.

3. Nylon-Wool Column Separation

In most experiments responder cells were enriched for T cells by passing normal lymph node cells over nylon-wool columns according to the method of Julius *et al.* (1973) modified as follows. Nylon wool (Leuko-Pak leukocyte filter, Fenwall Laboratories, Division of Travenol Laboratories, Inc., Deerfield, Illinois) was dispersed by hand to remove knots or clumps and autoclaved in a glass beaker for 20 min at 110°C. Preboiling the wool was found to be unnecessary for primary MLR cultures. The columns were packed in a 10-ml plastic (or glass) syringe plugged with a No. 18 needle (in its case) to stop the flow of medium. Five to ten milliliters of medium (PBS with 5% heat-inactivated FCS) was present during the packing of the column to prevent the formation of air pockets. With long forceps, small pieces (1 to 2 cm in length) of nylon wool were packed into the column to the 6-ml mark. The flow rate (without the needle) was adjusted by additional packing to 150–200 drops per minute with a 2-ml head of medium on the column. The final volume of the column was kept to 6 ml. The column was washed with 20 ml of medium, plugged with the needle (in its case), and incubated in an upright position with a 2-ml head at 37°C for at least 1 hr. A sterile paper or plastic cover was used to maintain sterility. Prior to adding the cells, the needle was removed and the excess medium was drained.

The optimal cell number to be loaded on the column was found to be 1×10^8. The cells were resuspended in 2 ml of medium and added dropwise by a Pasteur pipette evenly over the surface of the column. An additional 1.5 ml of medium was added to spread the cells into the column. The eluted medium was discarded. The column was plugged and incubated in an upright position for 45 min at 37°C. The needle was then removed, and nonadherent cells were eluted from the column (in an upright position) by dropwise administration of fresh medium (20 ml) at 37°C. The temperature of the column (and the medium) was kept at 37°C during the elution of cells from the column by holding the column near to the low flame of a Bunsen burner. The majority of the nonadherent T cells (more than 90%) were recovered in the first 10-ml fraction.

Of the nonadherent cells, 97–99% were T cells (as tested by anti-Thy 1.2 serum plus guinea pig C); between 50 and 90% of the T cells loaded on the column were recovered. B-cell contamination (Ig^+ by immunofluorescence) was 0.5–2.5%.

4. MLR

Unidirectional MLR cultures were set up as follows. The responder cells either were untreated or were lymph node cells separated on a nylon-wool column. The concentration of responder cells was adjusted to $5 \times 10^6/ml$, that of stimulator cells to $1 \times 10^7/ml$. Stimulator cells were X-irradiated (3300 R, Phillips RT 305 at 300 kV, 10 mA, and 100 rpm). Two milliliters of responder (R) cell suspension was mixed with an equal volume of stimulator (S) cell suspension (R to S ratio, 1:2) in a Falcon 30-ml plastic bottle (No. 3012, Falcon Plastics, Division of BioQuest, Oxnard, California). The bottle was incubated in an upright position in a 5% CO_2/95% air humidified atmosphere for 4 days. After 3 days, 40 μCi of [^{3}H]thymidine (2 Ci/mmole; The Radiochemical Centre, Amersham, England) was added and [^{3}H]thymidine incorporation was determined on day 4 of culture by processing a 0.2-ml sample from each bottle as described in Chapter 15. The stimulation index (SI) was calculated as the ratio of counts per minute in allogeneic cultures to that in syngeneic cultures. In most experiments, parallel cultures with 100 μl of responder cells mixed with 100 μl of stimulator cells were set up in Microtest II tissue culture plates (No. 3040, Falcon Plastics) for determination of [³H]thymidine incorporation.

B. Preparation of Alloantisera

The following procedure was found to be optimal for the production of hyperimmune antisera. A first injection (subcutaneous in the axillary regions, and intraperitoneal) of 2–3 × 10⁸ spleen and lymph node cells (prepared and washed in PBS without serum) from the appropriate strain was followed 10 days later by a boost of 3 × 10⁶ cells ip and at least two additional weekly injections (3 × 10⁶, ip). Seven days after the last injection, the mice were bled and the sera were collected.

In addition to antisera prepared as described above, the following hyperimmune anti-H-2 sera used in our experiments (Nagy *et al.*, 1976a,b; Elliott *et al.*, 1977) were generously supplied by Dr. D. C. Shreffler, Department of Genetics, Washington University School of Medicine, St. Louis, Missouri: (B10×A)F₁ anti-A.SW, A.TL anti-A.AL, A.TH anti-A.TL, and A.TL anti-A.TH. All the antisera were heat-inactivated (56°C, 30 min), fractioned, and stored at −70°C until use.

Anti-stimulator sera were absorbed with cells from the responder and third party strains as follows. Spleen and lymph node cells from each strain required were prepared in PBS without serum and mixed together in equal numbers. Two volumes of antiserum was mixed with one volume of packed spleen and lymph node cells in Eppendorf 1-ml plastic tubes (No. 39/10A, Sarstedt) and incubated for 30 min at 0°C. The cells were removed by centrifugation for 1 min in an Eppendorf centrifuge (No. 3300). The absorption was carried out once with responder cells and two or three times with cells from the third party strain. After the final absorption, sera were spun at 20,000 *g* and stored at −70°C.

The cytotoxic titer and the degree of cross-reactivity of each antiserum were determined by a dye exclusion microcytotoxicity test (Frelinger *et al.*, 1974) using lymph node target cells from the appropriate strains.

C. Immunofluorescent Reagents

Sheep anti-mouse Ig and sheep anti-rabbit Ig sera were prepared and conjugated with fluorescein isothiocyanate (FITC) and tetramethylrhodamine isothiocyanate (TRITC), respectively, as described in Chapter 9. Protein concentrations, measured by spectrophotometry, were adjusted to 0.5 mg/ml; sodium azide (10 m*M*) was added, and the reagents were stored at 4°C.

Immunofluorescent reagents were kindly provided by L. Forni (Basel Institute for Immunology).

IV. DETECTION OF T-CELL MARKERS AND STIMULATOR ANTIGENS ON RESPONDER BLASTS

A. Preparation of Blasts and Incubation with Alloantisera

On day 4, the cultured cells were resuspended and the entire 4 ml was transferred to a Falcon tube (No. 3033). A 2-ml Ficoll (Pharmacia, Uppsala, Sweden)–Urovison (Schering, Berlin) mixture (density, 1.077 gm/cm^3) was gently introduced under the cell suspension by Pasteur pipette. After centrifugation at 600 g for 15 min at room temperature, the cells (at least 98% viable) were recovered and washed three times in RPMI medium plus 5% heat-inactivated FCS and 15 mM Hepes. The recovery of viable cells after Ficoll treatment was 5–44% of the original number of responder cells cultured. On the average, 50% of the viable cells recovered were large- and medium-sized blasts. We define blast cells as cells with a diameter at least twice that of a small lymphocyte, with a distinctly smaller nuclear to cytoplasmic ratio and with a nonsegmented nucleus (in distinction from nonlymphoid cells).

All incubations with alloantiserum were performed in plastic tubes (No. TPS-55, Milian Plastics) for 45 min at 0°C. The cells (not more than 2.5×10^5 per tube) were resuspended in 50 μl of RPMI plus 5% FCS and 15 mM Hepes, to which 50 μl of the appropriate antiserum diluted to two times the required final concentration in RPMI medium without FCS or Hepes was added. Before use in each experiment, alloantisera were diluted and centrifuged at 20,000 g for 20 min in 0.5-ml conical plastic centrifuge tubes (No. EET-23P, Milian Plastics) to remove any precipitates formed during freezing.

B. Immunofluorescence

After incubation with alloantiserum, cells were washed three times in the same tubes (see Section IV,A) with Hanks' balanced salt solution (Flow Laboratories Ltd., Irvine, Scotland) containing 5% heat-inactivated FCS, 15 mM Hepes, and 10 mM sodium azide at 4°C and were kept throughout in this medium. Cells (no more than 2.5×10^5 per group) were resuspended carefully in 50 μl of medium to which 50 μl of the appropriate fluorescent reagent was added (at a predetermined dilution), incubated at 4°C for 30 min, and washed once between each incubation with antiserum.

Ig^+T^+ blasts were detected by treating the cells in three stages: first with rabbit Ig anti-mouse T (Sauser *et al.*, 1973) (a gift from Dr. C. Bron, Institut de Biochimie, Université de Lausanne, Switzerland), second with TRITC–sheep anti-rabbit Ig, and third with FITC–sheep anti-mouse Ig. This combination of reagents was chosen because there is no significant cross-reaction between sheep and rabbit Ig's.

In some experiments, cells were stained indirectly with rabbit anti-mouse μ detected by TRITC–sheep anti-rabbit Ig or directly with FITC–goat anti-mouse μ or FITC–goat anti-mouse γ.

After the final antiserum treatment, cells were washed twice, counted, washed once more, and resuspended to 2.5×10^5/ml. This concentration was found to yield preparations with good cell density. Clumps were minimized by carefully resuspending the pellet after each wash, before adding fresh medium. Approximately 15 min before use, the cytocentrifuge (Shandon–Elliott) was loaded with clean labeled slides and primed as follows: 25 μl of medium was introduced into each well and spun at 800 rpm for 10 min.

The cells (50 μl per tube) were introduced into each well and centrifuged at 800 rpm for 10 min at room temperature. The preparations were air-dried for 5 min, fixed in 100% ethanol or methanol for 5 min, and washed two times in PBS (3 min each). Methanol fixative was found to yield preparations with better preserved morphology than ethanol.

Without drying after the last wash, the slides were placed face up on absorbent paper. One drop of a PBS–glycerol solution (60 ml of glycerol, 10 ml of 10× PBS, 30 ml of distilled H_2O, 1 ml of 1 N NaN_3, pH 7.2) was placed onto the center of a glass coverslip, which was then gently laid over the cell smear. Excess fluid was removed by *gently* pressing the top of the coverslip with absorbent paper. The coverslips were sealed with nail polish. Care was taken not to move the coverslip on the slide during this step.

C. Scoring of Preparations

Preparations were scored under a Leitz Orthoplan fluorescence microscope with an Osram HBO-100 mercury vapor lamp and an Opak Fluor Ploem vertical illuminator (E. Leitz GmbH, Wetzlar, Germany) with filter blocks N (for TRITC excitation) and I (for FITC excitation).

With filter block I, some (5–10%) TRITC excitation is also observed. However, in most situations, the pattern of FITC fluorescence is clearly different from that of TRITC. In doubtful cases, filter block L can be used to view FITC excitation under conditions in which all TRITC excitation is excluded. This block is not used routinely because it also excludes 30% of the FITC excitation.

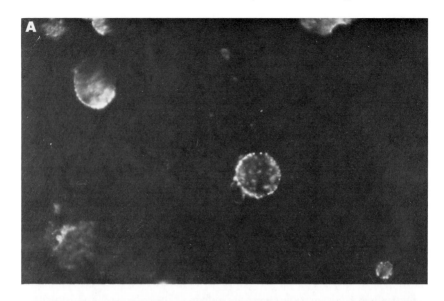

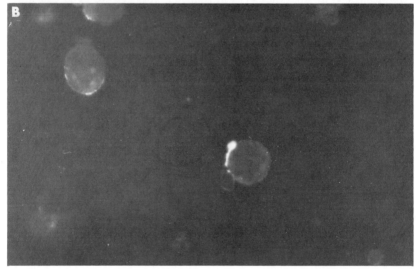

Fig. 1. B-depleted CBA responders were activated in MLR against SJL stimulators. T blasts were treated with anti-H-2^s serum (1/20), followed by a double-staining procedure with rabbit anti-T serum (detected by TRITC-labeled sheep anti-rabbit Ig) and FITC-labeled sheep anti-mouse Ig as described in the text. The same cells were viewed under illumination for rhodamine or fluorescein. (A) TRITC-positive blast and small lymphocytes (T cells); (B) FITC-positive blast (Ig$^+$) in the same field; (C) phase-contrast view of cell preparation under low-power magnification. (From Nagy *et al.*, 1976a.)

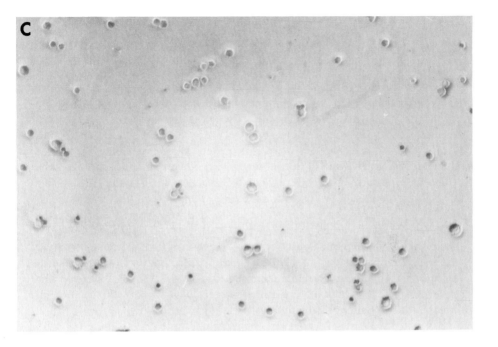

Fig. 1—*Continued*

The preparations were viewed throughout with a Leitz water-immersion objective of 50× magnification to obtain optimal resolution of fluorescent spots. The field was first viewed under phase-contrast illumination for counting total blasts. Cells scored should not be in contact with other cells and should be morphologically intact.

Double-stained preparations were next scored under fluorescent illumination with filter block N to detect cells labeled with TRITC–sheep anti-rabbit Ig. Each TRITC-positive cell was then individually viewed with filter block I to detect membrane-bound FITC–sheep anti-mouse Ig. An example of a field viewed under phase-contrast, TRITC, and FITC illuminations is shown in Fig. 1. The quality of fluorescence observed is discussed further in Section VI,B.

At least 200 blasts per preparation were scored and the percentage of T^+Ig^+ blasts was determined.

V. ASSAY FOR ALLOANTIGEN-BINDING CELLS

A. Trypsin Treatment

To detect alloantigen binding by MLR-activated blasts, it was first necessary to remove surface-bound stimulator alloantigens on the responder cells with trypsin. In all experiments dead cells were removed prior to trypsin treatment to standardize the enzyme reaction with a constant viable cell concentration. To obtain good recovery of both blasts and small lymphocytes, the dead cells were removed by centrifuging the entire 4-ml culture over 2 ml of Ficoll (density, 1.09 gm/ml) in a Falcon tube (No. 3033) according to the method of Davidson and Parish (1975). After centrifugation at 2000 g for 15 min at room temperature, the cells (at least 95% viable) were recovered from the interface and from the upper half-volume of Ficoll, washed twice in RPMI with 15 mM Hepes and 5% heat-inactivated FCS, counted, washed once more in RPMI without serum or Hepes, and resuspended in Hanks' balanced salt solution (Flow Laboratories, Glasgow, Scotland) to a concentration of 2 × 10^7 cells/ml. The recovery of viable cells after Ficoll treatment was 37–63% of the original number of responder cells cultured.

To 0.2 to 1 ml of each cell suspension, an equal volume of PBS containing 5 mg/ml of tosyl-L-phenylalanine chloromethyl ketone (TPCK)-treated trypsin (Merck, Darmstadt) was added, and the mixture was incubated at 37°C for 30 min. At least once during the incubation, the cells were mixed by shaking. To end the reaction, ice-cold RPMI (10 ml) with 15% FCS was added; the cells were counted, washed three times, and cultured overnight at 37°C in fresh MLR culture medium with 5% human serum at a concentration of no more than 5 × 10^5 cells/ml in a Falcon flask (No. 3012 for volumes 2.5 to 6 ml; No. 3024 for greater than 6 ml). Recovery of viable cells after trypsin treatment and overnight incubation was 40–88%.

B. Preparation of Stimulator Cell Material for Binding Studies

Membrane vesicles were prepared from stimulator cells as follows. Fresh spleen and lymph node cells from the appropriate stimulator strains were prepared as described in Section III,A,2, except the medium was PBS containing 5% FCS. When viability was less than 85%, dead cells were removed by filtration in low ionic strength medium through cotton wool (von Boehmer and Shortman, 1973). This procedure gave optimal cell yields when large numbers of cells had to be prepared. The remaining cells were counted and prepared for disruption by nitrogen cavitation by the method of Ferber *et al.* (1972) modified as follows.

Buffer solutions for cell disruption consisted of solution A [0.002 M MgCl$_2$, 0.13 M NaCl, 0.02 M Hepes (pH 7.4)] and solution B (0.5 M sucrose). On the day of use, a protease inhibitor, phenylmethylsulfonyl fluoride (PMSF; Schwarz–Mann, Toronto, Ontario, Canada) (stored in propanol, 10^{-1} M), was dissolved (by dropwise addition while stirring) in each solution at a final concentration of 10^{-3} M, and the solutions were passed through a Millipore filter (0.45 μm) to remove any precipitated PMSF.

The cells were resuspended in solution A to 6.0 $\times$ 10^7 nucleated cells/ml. To this cell suspension (5–50 ml), an equal volume of solution B was added dropwise with continuous stirring using a magnetic stirrer. The cells were introduced in a 20- or 50-ml beaker into a pressure homogenizer (Parr Instrument Co., Moline, Illinois), which had been cooled on ice. (To prevent bacterial contamination, the tubing was washed before use with detergent and rinsed with 70% ethanol followed by distilled water.) While stirring continued, pressurized nitrogen was administered for 10 min at 800 psi, released slowly (over a period of 1.5–2 min), and administered at the same pressure for a further 15 min. The cells were disrupted by forcing the cell suspension dropwise through a fine nozzle into a beaker covered with Parafilm to avoid squirting. A sample of the lysate was counted in the same medium under a phase-contrast microscope, and the recovery of nuclei and whole cells was determined. This two-stage treatment resulted in optimal yields of membrane vesicles from normal lymphocytes, while leaving the majority of nuclei intact. Optimal pressure and time must be determined empirically for each cell source (e.g., blasts or cultured cells may require only a single 15-min pressurization period).

The cell lysate was centrifuged at 750 g for 20 min to remove nuclei, the pellet was resuspended in a 1:1 mixture of solutions A and B, and the centrifugation was repeated. The pooled supernatants were centrifuged at 20,000 g for 15 min, and the pellet was discarded. The supernatant from this step was centrifuged at 120,000 g for 60 min with a fixed-angle rotor, and the pellet containing membrane vesicles was resuspended in 1 ml of RPMI tissue culture medium without serum (to avoid foaming) by forcing it repeatedly through a No. 26 needle with a 1-ml syringe. This preparation was stable for at least 1 day at 4°C. For long-term storage (i.e., several months), the membrane vesicles were suspended in 0.25 M sucrose, 1 mM Hepes (pH 8.2) and frozen at −70°C. The material contained serologically detectable H-2 antigen activity as determined by its capacity to specifically inhibit antibody-mediated complement-dependent cell lysis in a dye exclusion microcytotoxicity test (Frelinger *et al.*, 1974). The recovery of antigen activity compared to an equivalent number of whole cells was 50–85%.

Prior to use, the concentration of the material was adjusted to be equivalent to 1.2×10^8 cells/ml with RPMI tissue culture medium (with 5% FCS or human serum, and supplements), and the preparation was centrifuged at 250 *g* for 10 min to remove large aggregates. Material that had been frozen as described above was dialyzed against RPMI in a collodion bag (SM 13200, Sartorius–Membranefilter GmbH, Goettingen, Germany) before dilution.

C. Exposure of Trypsin-Treated Blasts to Stimulator Cell Material and Detection of Bound Alloantigens

After the overnight incubation, the trypsin-treated cells were counted, washed once, and resuspended to 1.5×10^6 viable cells/ml; 0.3-ml aliquots of this cell suspension were incubated for an additional time period with 0.7 ml of fresh tissue culture medium (complete) or with medium containing stimulator cell material. Afterward, the cells were counted again; dead cells were removed by centrifugation over Ficoll–Urovison [density, 1.09 gm/ml (Davidson and Parish, 1975)]. Recovery of cells after incubation with stimulator material for 2–4 hr ranged between 90 and 100%. Allogeneic cell material bound by the recovered responder cells was detected by indirect immunofluorescence after incubating the cells first with anti-stimulator alloantiserum and then with FITC-labeled anti-mouse sheep Ig as described above.

VI. CRITICAL APPRAISAL: APPLICATIONS AND LIMITATIONS

A. Summary of Results and Applications

The methods described above have yielded the following results.

1. After allogeneic stimulation, a large proportion (24–44%) of T blasts derived from unfractionated lymph node cells carry immunoglobulin on their surface. Depletion of B cells from the responder cells prior to stimulation, by filtration through nylon-wool columns, reduced this fraction to 3 to 6% (Nagy *et al.*, 1976a).

2. Most or all activated T blasts from nylon-wool-fractionated responder cells carry surface-bound stimulator alloantigens that can be detected by anti-stimulator serum and indirect immunofluorescent reagents. This material is bound via specific T-cell receptors, since among blasts activated

against a mixture of two stimulators most or all cells carry material derived from one stimulator only (Nagy *et al.*, 1976a).

3. Similar results are obtained when T cells are activated against a mixture of *H-2I* region and of *H-2K* region incompatible stimulators. In this case, most or all of the K-region product-binding cells express Ly-2 but not Ly-1 alloantigens, whereas the cells binding material from the I-region incompatible stimulators express the Ly-1 but not Ly-2 phenotypes (Nagy *et al.*, 1976b).

4. Trypsin treatment removes the bound stimulator alloantigens from the activated blasts. The trypsin-treated blasts can, after an overnight recovery period, specifically bind fresh stimulator cell material obtained from MLR supernatants or from fresh cells disrupted by nitrogen cavitation (Elliott *et al.*, 1977).

All of the above results were obtained with unprimed responder cells after 4 days of MLC, at a time when these cultures contained the maximum percentage of blasts. We have been unable to detect antigen binding by small lymphocytes from the same cultures. Antigen binding by cells cultured in MLC for shorter periods has not yet been thoroughly investigated. However, a significant proportion of small lymphocytes (12–18%) surviving after long-term MLR cultures, which yield cell populations highly enriched for cells reacting to the "priming" stimulator (Fathman *et al.*, 1976), bind specifically detectable amounts of stimulator cell membrane fragments (B. E. Elliott, unpublished result).

While the assay described here should be potentially applicable to an analysis of any T-cell population containing a sufficiently high proportion of cells of known specificity, certain limitations, discussed in Section VI,B, should be kept in mind.

B. Technical Comments

1. Scoring

To obtain satisfactory results, good preparations are essential. Double staining with an anti-T-cell reagent as described above facilitates scoring greatly because it allows screening each field for cells with the uniform spotty fluorescence characteristic for T blasts, each of which is then scored for staining with the anti-Ig reagent, used to detect anti-stimulator alloantibody.

The fluorescence due to bound alloantigen is usually faint, spotty, and concentrated at one pole of the cell. Since the background and the strength of the specific fluorescence may vary from one experiment to another (even with the same strain combinations) and with different antisera, it is essential to include all appropriate controls in every experimental group and to score slides blind. Although almost all (94.4%) of the blast cells in these preparations are responder cells, a few percent of stimulator blast cells (3.8%) can sometimes be found (Table I). They are easily distinguishable because they are brightly fluorescent over their whole surface.

In cultures with B-depleted responder cells, the background (i.e., without alloantiserum treatment) of Ig^+ responder T blasts was in most experiments a few percent (1.7–5.2). Two possible explanations for this background are (1) that contaminating B blasts (0.5–2.9%) secrete Ig, which binds to T blasts either specifically or otherwise, and (2) that the fluorescent reagent itself recognizes some other specificity on the T cells or, alternatively, binds to them nonspecifically.

After treatment with alloantisera directed against a strain unrelated to either stimulator or responder, this background usually increased slightly (by an additional 2–4%), even after extensive absorption with cells of the latter two strains. This is most likely due either to some residual cross-reactivity with the stimulator antigens or to nonspecific uptake of immunoglobulin from the serum. Despite this overall background of 6.9% (maximum), the proportion of T blasts stained with hyperimmune anti-stimulator serum ranged between 9.2 and 11.8 times greater than that stained with an unrelated antiserum with both responder and stimulator cells.

In contrast, unabsorbed or incompletely absorbed sera often stained a significant fraction of the cells. The possible interpretations of such "cross-reactivity" are considered in Section VI,C.

2. Reproducibility and Sensitivity

While the qualitative reproducibility of the assay is good, the quantitative reproducibility is less so. We have observed specific antigen binding with several different responder–stimulator combinations and using many different alloantisera (Nagy *et al.*, 1976a). However, the number of antigen-binding T blasts detected varies considerably from experiment to experiment. Most likely this is due to variation in the amount of stimulator antigen bound. This variation and the observation that the alloantibody concentration, even when kept as high as feasible, is limiting suggest that one is working at the limit of the sensitivity of this type of system. Nevertheless, in many experiments, close to 100% of all blasts carried detectable amounts of stimulator material (Nagy *et al.*, 1976a).

3. Experimental Design

The limitations discussed in the preceding paragraph impose an experimental design that allows conclusions not based on absolute values. The simplest and most certain way to ensure an unambiguous interpretation is

TABLE I

Example of Indirect Immunofluorescent Staining of MLR-Activated T Blasts with Anti-Stimulator or Anti-Responder Alloantibodies

Strain combination		Incubation with antiserum (dilution)	T^+Ig^+ blast/total blast			T^-Ig^+ blast/total blast (%)	Percentage total blast
R^a	S		Bright (%)	Spotted (%)	Percentage total		
A(kkdd)[b]	B6(bbbb)[b]	— (—)	5/181 (2.8)	0/181 (0)	2.8	1.80 (0.6)	54.7
A(kkdd)	B6(bbbb)	αK^k [c] (1/20)	170/184 (94.4)	0/184 (0)	94.4	Not done (—)	
A(kkdd)	B6(bbbb)	αB6[d] (1/50)	9/213 (3.8)	9/236 (41.9)	45.7	Not done (—)	

[a] Responder cells, nylon-wool-passaged nonadherent lymph node cells.

[b] H-2 haplotypes (lowercase letters refer to allelic origin of K, I, S, and D regions, respectively).

[c] αK^k: A.TL αA.AL absorbed twice with B6 spleen and lymph node cells.

[d] αB6: CBA αB6 absorbed twice with A/J and SJL spleen and lymph node cells.

to use one form or another of so-called criss-cross experiments, as shown, for example, in the following tabulation.

Culture		Cells stained with	Percentage of T^+Ig^+ blasts per total blasts
Responder	Stimulator		
A	B	—	
		αB	
		αC	
A	C	—	
		αB	
		αC	

To avoid cross-reactivity of the alloantisera, each anti-stimulator serum must be thoroughly absorbed with cells from the third party and responder strains as described in Section III,C.

This protocol can easily be applied when the T blasts are activated against normal allogeneic cells, but may be more difficult to achieve in other potential applications of the assay (e.g., tumor antigens, haptens, or binding by putative antigen-specific T-cell lines).

C. The Nature of the "Antigen"

Although we have not investigated this point sufficiently, many experiments indirectly suggest that the stimulator cell material bound by, and detected in, our assay on the activated responder cells does not consist of single molecules, but more likely of membrane fragments of considerable and possibly very heterogeneous size. The following two observations led us to this conclusion.

1. When responder cells were stimulated with cells incompatible for the entire *H-2* region, the sum of the fractions of cells stained with anti-stimulator *I*-region and with anti-stimulator *K*-region antisera separately was much higher than the fraction stained by a mixture of the two antisera (Nagy *et al.*, 1976a). This was not the case in similar experiments where responder cells were stimulated with a mixture of *I*-region incompatible and *K*-region incompatible cells (Nagy *et al.*, 1976b).

2. The stimulator cell material from MLR supernatants, which is bound by previously trypsinized T blasts, can be sedimented by centrifugation at 100,000 *g* for 60 min. While this suggests that some of the stimulator cell material bound by the activated T cells is in the form of membrane fragments, it is entirely possible that they also bind single molecules; but this is quite likely below the sensitivity of the assay in its present form (Nagy *et al.*, 1976a). The implication of these findings is that the

alloantibodies bound by the responder cells are not necessarily directed against the same molecules, let alone the same determinants as are recognized by the presumptive endogenous receptors of this cell. [In passing it might be pointed out that, presumably, the sites through which a stimulator cell fragment is bound by the responder cell are not available to the added alloantibody.] Thus, in the absence of any data on the size of, and the antigen distribution among, the bound membrane fragments, we do not know whether there is any relationship between the specificities of the responder cell receptors and the alloantibody bound by them: The alloantisera serve, at this stage, only as a means to detect stimulator cell material bound by the responder cells.

This point can be illustrated with an example: When stimulator antigens are removed, by trypsinization, from CBA cells activated against B6, many of these cells will rebind fresh B6 cell material, but some, albeit fewer, will also bind SJL cell material (Elliott *et al.*, 1977). This latter is detected with an anti-SJL alloantibody that has been absorbed with B6 (and CBA)! While this might at first suggest that the binding of SJL material must be nonspecific, assuming monospecificity of *H-2*-reactive T cells, it is also entirely compatible with the possibility that some of the B6-responsive cells carry receptors cross-reacting with SJL determinants, because the bound SJL material will not be detected through the determinants shared with B6 but through others present on the same membrane fragment. This type of argument would, of course, even apply if the bound material were monomolecular, because of the multiple determinants on a single MHC-antigen molecule.

VII. CONCLUSION

The assay described here is a very significant step forward in the characterization of specific antigen binding by T cells. It allows, for the first time, identification of MHC-reactive T cells, not through their functional activity (proliferation, target cell lysis), but through visualization of specific antigen binding of individual cells. While the assay has already contributed significantly to an understanding of various aspects of specific antigen recognition by MHC-reactive cells, there are a number of parameters that have yet to be sufficiently explored. We hope that this chapter will stimulate other investigators to contribute to the relevant analyses.

ACKNOWLEDGMENTS

We wish to thank Dr. D. Shreffler for his generous gifts of hyperimmune anti-H-2 sera and recombinant mouse strains, Ms. L. Forni for her generous gift of immunofluorescent reagents, and Dr. V. Miggiano and Dr. B. Pernis for helpful advice and discussions. Ms. B. Hausmann and Ms. A. M. Rynbeck provided expert technical assistance.

REFERENCES

Davidson, W. F., and Parish, C. R. (1975). *J. Immunol. Methods* **7,** 291.

Elliott, B. E., Nagy, Z., Nabholz, M., and Pernis, B. (1977). *Eur. J. Immunol.* **7,** 287.

Fathman, C. G., Collavo, D., Davies, S., and Nabholz, M. (1976). *J. Immunol.* **118,** 1232.

Ferber, E., Resch, K., Wallach, D. F. H., and Imm, W. (1972). *Biochim. Biophys. Acta* **266,** 494.

Frelinger, J. A., Niederhuber, J. E., David, C. S., and Shreffler, D. C. (1974). *J. Exp. Med.* **140,** 1273.

Julius, M., Simpson, E., and Herzenberg, L. A. (1973). *Eur. J. Immunol.* **3,** 645.

Nabholz, M., Vives, J., Young, H. M., Meo, T., Miggiano, V., Rijnbeck, A., and Shreffler, D. C. (1974). *Eur. J. Immunol.* **4,** 378.

Nagy, Z., Elliott, B. E., Nabholz, M., Krammer, P., and Pernis, B. (1976a). *J. Exp. Med.* **143,** 648.

Nagy, Z., Elliott, B. E., and Nabholz, M. (1976b). *J. Exp. Med.* **149,** 1545.

Sauser, D., Anckers, C., and Bron, C. (1973). *J. Immunol. Methods* **2,** 293.

von Boehmer, H., and Shortman, K. (1973). *J. Immunol. Methods* **2,** 293.

22

Assay for Antigen-Specific T-Cell Proliferation in Mice

Şefik Ş. Alkan

I. OBJECTIVE

While lymphocyte proliferative responses to allogeneic cells or to mitogens in the mouse can be readily measured (Thorpe and Knight, 1974; see also Chapter 15), the reliable assay of antigen-induced T-lymphocyte proliferation in culture has proved to be substantially more difficult to establish. In the past, several methods have been described (Tyan, 1972; Lonai and McDevitt, 1974; Phanuphak *et al.*, 1974; Osborne and Katz, 1973a) and used with varying degrees of success. The uncontrolled nature of proliferation and the contribution of B-cell responses (Osborne and Katz, 1973a,b; Moorhead *et al.*, 1973) have made these methods of questionable value as a T-cell assay. Schwartz and co-workers (1975) have described

IMMUNOLOGICAL METHODS
Copyright © 1979 by Academic Press, Inc.
All rights of reproduction in any form reserved.
ISBN 0-12-442750-2

another system, which measures the response of murine T lymphocytes. There are, however, some difficulties with this method. First, it requires an elaborate lymphocyte purification procedure from the peritoneal exudates of primed mice. Second, the yield of lymphocytes per mouse is so low (3×10^5) that a large number of mice is required for any single experiment.

The purpose of this chapter is to outline a recently developed short-term microculture method (Alkan, 1978) that eliminates these difficulties and provides a reliable assay for antigen-induced responses of murine T lymphocytes. The novel features of the method are the use of only draining lymph node cells of primed mice instead of spleen cells and the use of horse serum in the culture medium instead of fetal calf serum.

II. PRINCIPLE OF THE METHOD

Only draining lymph node cells rich for antigen-reactive cells are used. Animals are sensitized by injecting antigen into the tail or footpads, the draining lymph nodes are removed, the cells are cultured in microculture plates in the presence or absence of antigens (and/or mitogens), and proliferation is measured by [³H]thymidine uptake. This technique can be used for several antigens, such as monovalent antigens (azobenzene–arsonate–L-tyrosine), protein antigens (human γ-globulin, ovalbumin), hapten-carrier conjugates (arsonate–keyhole limpet hemacyanin) (Alkan, 1978), and many others (Schwartz *et al.*, 1975).

III. MATERIALS

Balanced salt solution (BSS)
Phosphate-buffered saline (PBS)
Purified protein derivative from tuberculin (PPD, preservative free, Statens Serum Institute, Copenhagen)
Lipopolysaccharide (LPS, Difco)
Concanavalin A (Con A, Pharmacia)
Millipore filters
Teflon pestle (ϕ 13 mm)
Complete and/or incomplete Freund's adjuvant (Difco)
RPMI 1640 with $NaHCO_3$ (Gibco)
Penicillin–streptomycin (Gibco)
L-Glutamine (Gibco)
Hepes (Calbiochem)
2-Mercaptoethanol (Merck)

Horse serum (Gibco)
Microculture plates (Falcon Plastics Microtest 3040
  or flat-bottom Cooke trays)
[³H]Methylthymidine TRA-310, 2 Ci/mmole (Amersham)

IV. PROCEDURE

A. Preparation of Antigen

The antigen is dissolved in PBS or BSS and the pH is adjusted to 7.5. The solution is sterilized by passing it through a 0.45-μm Millipore filter and stored at 4°C.

For injection, equal amounts of antigen solution are mixed with Freund's adjuvant (complete or incomplete depending on the antigen). The mixing should be done in a glass vial and a glass syringe should be used for emulsification. The sample is cooled on ice, and the emulsification is repeated. The emulsion is kept at 4°C. The amount of antigen to be injected usually varies berween 10 to 100 μg per mouse depending on the antigen.

B. Immunization

Mice can be immunized either in the tail subcutaneously or in the hind footpads. The injection of emulsion is made by a 1- to 2-ml glass syringe fitted with a 26-guage needle. The emulsion (40–50 μl) is injected subcutaneously in the base of the tail. During the injection one should be able to see the emulsion entering under the tail skin. For footpad injection, 25 μl of emulsion into each hind footpad is sufficient.

C. Preparation of Culture Medium

The basic medium is RPMI 1640 (Gibco) supplemented as described in Table I.

D. Collecting Lymph Nodes

One to four weeks after the immunization, the mice are killed by cervical dislocation, dipped into 70% ethanol, and prepared for excision of the lymph nodes. If the immunization is performed via the tail, the two inguinal and two or three periaortic lymph nodes are removed. If the mouse was immunized by footpad injection, only the popliteal lymph nodes are removed. The lymph nodes are placed in a petri dish containing cold PBS or BSS (supplemented) and are then freed from fat.

TABLE I

Supplements of Culture Medium and of Washing Solution[a]

Supplement	Stock solution	Storage temperature (°C)	Final concentration in culture medium
Hepes[b]	2 M	4	10 mM
L-Glutamine	0.2 M	−20	2 mM
2-Mercaptoethanol[c]	14 M	4	0.028 mM
Penicillin	10^4 U/ml	−20	100 U/ml
Streptomycin	10^4 μg/ml	−20	100 μg/ml
Horse serum[d]		−20	5%

[a] Phosphate-buffered saline or BSS (as a washing solution) is supplemented with penicillin (100 U/ml), streptomycin (100 μg/ml), and horse serum (2.5%).

[b] Hepes, 25 gm, is dissolved in 1 N NaOH and RPMI medium is added up to 105 ml; the mixture is then sterilized through a Millipore filter.

[c] The dilution is always made fresh: First, a 1000-fold dilution in BSS is made (14 mM); from this, 0.2 ml is added to 100 ml of medium.

[d] Should be inactivated at 56°C for 30 min before storage at −20° or −70°C.

E. Preparation of Lymph Node Cell Suspension

The lymph nodes are transferred to a 15-ml tube (Falcon Plastics), placed onto the inside wall of the tube, and minced with sterile scissors. PBS (supplemented, 1–2 ml) is added and the lymph nodes are disrupted by squeezing with a loose-fitting Teflon pestle. PBS (supplemented, 10 ml) is added to the tube, mixed, and allowed to stand on ice for 5 min. The suspension is transferred to another 15-ml tube, with the clumps left behind.

The cells are washed in cold PBS (supplemented,) twice at 150 *g* for 10 min. After the first spin, there will be a fat layer on the top of the PBS, which should be removed by pipetting. This removal of the fat layer is important and should be done before pouring off the supernatant.

The cells are then washed once more in culture medium, and a sample for counting is taken from the cell suspension just before the last spin.

F. Culture Conditions

First the antigens and/or mitogens are distributed into wells of micro-culture plates in replicates. Medium or PBS is added to two or three wells for control. Then, 20 μl of antigen solution in PBS at the appropriate concentration and 0.2 ml of cell suspension (2×10^6/ml) are placed into each well. [For most antigens it was found that optimal concentrations ranged between 10 and 400 μg/ml of culture (Alkan, 1978). Optimal cell input per well is around $5 \pm 1 \times 10^5$ cells.]

The culture trays are then covered with a loose-fitting lid and incubated at 37°C for 2–4 days in a CO_2 incubator. The peak proliferative response may vary for different antigens from 2 to 4 days in this system.

For pulsing the cells, 16–24 hr before the termination of culture, 2 μCi of [³H]thymidine is added to each well. This is done as follows. The [³H]thymidine stock label is first diluted in RPMI 1640 to give 40 μCi/ml. Then one drop (50 μl) of the isotope is added to each well.

Harvesting the culture is performed using a semiautomated sample collector. Cells from each row are collected and washed on a strip of glass filter paper and dried on a hot plate, and each disk from the strip is placed in a scintillation vial to which 10 ml of scintillation fluid is added. The incorporation of radioactive thymidine is then determined by liquid scintillation spectrophotometry.

Stimulation values are expressed either as *indexes*, that is, ratios between the mean counts per minute incorporated into experimental and control cultures, or as *deltas*, that is, the differences in the mean counts per minute of increments of experimental and control cultures. For larger experiments, a computer program is used to make all the required calculations.

G. Controls

1. To ensure that culture conditions, cells, and medium are satisfactory, one should include mitogens as control stimulants. In the present system, optimal doses for LPS and Con A are 500 and 10–20 μg/ml, respectively. Note that these mitogen concentrations are about 10 times higher in this system (RPMI + horse serum) than in culture systems using fetal calf serum.

2. PPD can serve as an excellent internal control if the animals are immunized with an antigen–CFA mixture. PPD (50 μg/ml) induces a substantial thymidine incorporation in cultures of lymph nodes from all CFA-injected animals.

3. When unprimed lymph node cells are used, some antigens induce a response, whereas others are toxic. To avoid the latter possibility, it is advantageous to check all antigens also with nonimmunized or only CFA-injected mouse lymph node cells.

4. To make sure that antigen does not stimulate proliferation of B cells in culture, the following controls should be included: (a) pretreatment of lymph node cells with anti-Thy 1.2 serum plus complement (thymidine incorporation is expected not to exceed the background level); (b) assay for antigen-specific plaque-forming cells in culture (negligible background level is expected); (c) staining of stimulated cells with fluorescein-conjugated anti-mouse Ig (proliferating cells are expected to be Ig⁻).

V. CRITICAL APPRAISAL

Although this method has been found to be applicable for many antigens (including synthetic, semisynthetic, and natural antigens) (Alkan, 1978, also unpublished observations), critical variables such as (1) antigen dose and time after immunization, (2) optimal antigen concentration in culture, and (3) duration of culture should be evaluated to optimize the system for each antigen.

Most culture systems described previously are not suitable for antigen-induced cell responses due to the high level of [³H]thymidine uptake in unstimulated cultures, usually associated with the use of fetal calf serum. This problem is eliminated with the use of 5% horse serum in the present assay. Moreover, the low background level in the presence of horse serum is not confined to a particular batch of serum. We obtained similar results with two other batches from Gibco. One batch, kept at $-20°C$ for over a year, was used successfully. Fetal calf serum (selected for low mitogenicity) and some human sera have also been tried, but all were found to give much lower stimulation indexes than cultures containing horse serum.

Although flat-bottom plates were found to be the most convenient, U- and V-shaped culture plates can also be used for some purposes. However, cell density requirements as well as changes in other parameters of the response must be established for these plates. Usually the cell density must be lowered and the culture period shortened.

It should be noted that immunization into the tail is done subcutaneously, *not intravenously*. This is facilitated by using a standard restrainer and injecting the antigen between the veins close to the base of the tail.

The cell yield from periaortic and inguineal lymph nodes in a mouse immunized in the tail varies between 10 and 40×10^6 lymph node cells per mouse, which is enough to perform a full experiment. Furthermore, cells from syngeneic mice can be pooled, since there is little variation between the mean of individual assays and the results using pooled lymph node cells.

We have recently demonstrated that this method measures antigen-specific T-lymphocyte responses to a number of antigens, and we have also shown that B-cell participation is minimal or nonexistent (Alkan, 1978). However, for a given antigen, to rule out the possibility of B-cell participation, the following criteria should be fulfilled: (1) Treatment of lymph node cells with anti-Thy 1.2 and complement prior to culture should abolish the proliferative response. (2) The number of antigen-specific plaque-forming cells should not increase at the peak of the proliferative response. (3) The number of B cells detected by surface staining should not increase after antigenic stimulation in culture. For further information about this last point, see Schwartz *et al.* (1975) and Alkan (1978).

ACKNOWLEDGMENT

I am grateful to Dr. G. Corradin for pointing out the intratail sensitization method and for sending a copy of his manuscript prior to its publication.

REFERENCES

Alkan, S. S. (1978). *Eur. J. Immunol.* **8**, 112.
Lonai, P., and McDevitt, H. O. (1974). *J. Exp. Med.* **140**, 977.
Moorhead, J. W., Walters, C. S., and Claman, H. N. (1973). *J. Exp. Med.* **137**, 411.
Osborne, D. P., Jr., and Katz, D. H. (1973a). *J. Immunol.* **111**, 1164.
Osborne, D. P., Jr., and Katz, D. H. (1973b). *J. Immunol.* **111**, 1176.
Phanuphak, P., Moorhead, J. W., and Claman, H. N. (1974). *J. Immunol.* **112**, 115.
Schwartz, R. H., Jackson, L., and Paul, W. E. (1975). *J. Immunol.* **115**, 1330.
Thorpe, P. E., and Knight, S. C. (1974). *J. Immunol. Methods* **5**, 387.
Tyan, M. L. (1972). *J. Immunol.* **108**, 65.

NOTE ADDED IN PROOF

Recently, I have shown that pretreatment of lymph node cells with sheep anti-mouse Ig plus complement had no effect on antigen-induced proliferation, although LPS responsiveness was eliminated.

While this chapter was in press, a paper by G. Corradin, H. M. Etlinger, and J. M. Chiller appeared in *J. Immunol.* (1977) **119**, 1048.

23

Antigen-Specific Helper T-Cell Factor and Its Acceptor

Michael J. Taussig

I. INTRODUCTION

The T-cell factors are soluble mediators of lymphocyte interaction. Their effect on the immune response may be either to enhance ("helper" factors) or to inhibit ("suppressor" factors) and may be either antigen specific or nonspecific (Taussig, 1974; Munro and Taussig, 1975; Katz and Benacerraf, 1976; Taussig et al., 1974; Taussig and Finch, 1977; Luzzati et al., 1976; Mozes, 1976; Taniguchi et al., 1976). Some of these factors are coded, at least partially, by genes in the major histocompatibility complex (MHC). There is considerable interest in the specific MHC-derived factors, because they may be the soluble expression of the T-cell antigen-recognition system, thereby providing a useful means of studying the strangely indeterminable T-cell receptor. Furthermore, the presence in the mouse of Ia determinants

317

IMMUNOLOGICAL METHODS
Copyright © 1979 by Academic Press, Inc.
All rights of reproduction in any form reserved.
ISBN 0-12-442750-2

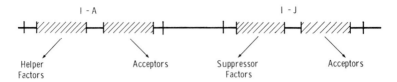

Fig. 1.   Cell interaction molecules of the *I* region of the mouse H-2 complex.

on these factors has illuminated the role of *I*-region products in cell interaction. Briefly, it appears that two types of gene products are coded for by the *I* region, namely, the factors and their lymphocyte acceptors, the latter being the molecules that react with the factors and transmit their signals to the cell. An interaction "set" of a factor and its acceptor is coded by a pair of closely linked *I*-region genes. For the helper factors, these genes have so far been located only in the *I-A* subregion of H-2, whereas for the specific suppressor factors and their acceptors the genes are found in the *I-J* subregions, as shown in Fig. 1.

Both the specific helper and suppressor factors have a demonstrable binding site for antigen, yet are not immunoglobulins (Ig's). The specific helper factor is a glycoprotein of molecular weight ~50,000 and lacks antigenic determinants of both *V* and *C* regions of Ig (Taussig *et al.*, 1976). On the other hand, it can be absorbed with either antigen or anti-Ia adsorbents. It has been suggested that the *I* region may contain genes coding for variable regions of T-cell factors, though this is at present an open question.

The acceptor for the helper factor is located on B lymphocytes and carries Ia specificities of the *I-A* subregion, in addition to the site at which factor is received. Both factors and acceptors are likely to be the products of immune response (*Ir*) genes, since (1) either may be absent in low responder mice and (2) they carry Ia antigens.

II. PRINCIPLE OF THE METHOD

The specific helper factor is prepared by short-term *in vitro* culture of T cells specifically educated (primed) to the antigen in question. The factor is tested by its ability to cooperate with B cells *in vivo*. The acceptor is detected by the ability of B lymphocytes to absorb the factor (i.e., to remove its activity).

III. MATERIALS

The antigens that are used most frequently are the synthetic poly-peptides poly(Tyr,Glu)-poly(DLAla)--poly(Lys), abbreviated as (T,G)-A--L; poly(Phe,Glu)-poly(DLAla)--poly(Lys), (Phe,G)-A--L and poly(Tyr,Glu)-poly(Pro)--poly(Lys), (T,G)-Pro--L. These antigens have been synthesized by Dr. Edna Mozes (Department of Chemical Immunology, Weizmann Institute of Science, Rehovot, Israel). However, sheep and horse eryth-rocytes have also been used, as have hapten–protein conjugates. For cultures of murine educated T cells, minimal Eagle's medium is used and is not supplemented by serum. The cultures are plated in 50-mm petri dishes, supplied by Sterilin (P122). However, the importance of a particular type of culture dish is debatable, and other dishes have been found to give satisfactory results.

IV. PROCEDURE

A. T-Cell Factor

The preparation of factors is shown in Fig. 2a. Mouse T cells are primed to the antigen by injecting 10^8 thymocytes into a lethally irradiated recipient mouse, antigen being given ip in CFA. The strain of mouse chosen is dictated by several considerations, such as the antigen under test and the susceptibility of the strain to irradiation. For (T,G)-A--L, the strains of

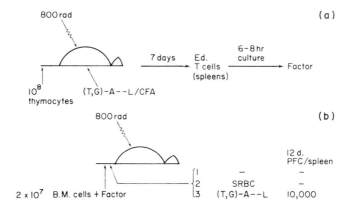

Fig. 2. Preparation of antigen-specific T-cell factor. (a) Production of factor from educated T cells; (b) test of factor in irradiated recipients.

choice are C57Bl, BALB/c, and C3H [although C3H is a low responder to (T,G)-A--L, it can nevertheless make the T-cell factor]. Similarly, the dose of antigen required for priming T cells, the optimal day for harvesting the cells, etc., very much depend on the antigen and the animal. For sheep erythrocytes, 10^8 T cells are primed by 0.1 ml of 10% SRBC and are obtained in the spleens of recipients at 5 days; for (T,G)-A--L, the dose is 10 μg in CFA and cells are taken at 7 days. At this time, the spleens of the recipient mice should contain educated T cells specific for the antigen used. The yield is between 1 and 5×10^6 cells/spleen. It is essential to control for education by transferring cells from these spleens together with bone marrow cells into a second irradiated recipient. Educated T cells ($1-2 \times 10^6$) transferred together with 2×10^7 bone marrow cells should give responses to the antigen which are significantly raised compared with bone marrow controls. If they do not give such responses, it may be assumed that T-cell priming has failed.

When conditions for reproducible priming of T cells have been established, the preparation of factor can proceed. A suspension of the spleen cells containing educated T cells is prepared without washing the cells, in minimal Eagle's medium containing glutamine. If the T cells must be washed, or purified by nylon-wool separation, adding fetal calf serum (10%) to the medium is necessary. The cells are brought to a density of 10^7/ml and antigen is added. The optimal amount of antigen must be determined by experimentation; for (T,G)-A--L, it is 1 μg/ml of culture and for SRBC 0.1 ml of a 0.1% solution/ml of culture. Petri dishes containing 2-3 ml of the cell suspensions are incubated under 5% CO_2/95% air at 37°C for about 8 hr; once again, the optimal time of culture is empirical. It is recommended that the viability of educated T cells be assessed with trypan blue at the beginning and end of culture; no more than 20-30% of the cells should die during this culture period. If viability is satisfactory, the cells are removed by centrifugation and supernatant is used as the source of T-cell factor.

The presence and activity of the factor are assayed by transferring the factor plus bone marrow cells and antigen into irradiated recipient mice as shown in Fig. 2b. It is not necessary for the factor to be syngeneic in origin with the bone marrow cells; the helper factor has been found to function equally well in syngeneic and allogeneic combinations (Munro and Taussig, 1975; Taussig et al., 1974). The efficacy of T–B cooperation must first be established in vivo by transfer of normal or educated thymus and bone marrow cells, since the assay for factor is essentially one of its specific T-cell-replacing activity. The supernatant, containing factor, is mixed with bone marrow cells and antigen prior to transfer and inoculated into the tail vein of lethally irradiated recipient mice. The proportions of factor and cells are adjusted so that each recipient receives 0.5–1 spleen equivalent of factor (one spleen equivalent is the amount produced by cells of one spleen in culture) and 2×10^7 bone marrow cells. The optimal amount of antigen must be determined by experimentation; for synthetic polypeptides, 10 μg per mouse is a suitable dose and for erythrocytes it is 0.1 ml of a 10% suspension. In addition to the test group of animals receiving factor, antigen, and B cells, it is essential to set up controls receiving B cells and antigen and, as a specificity control, a group receiving factor, B cells, and a non-cross-reacting antigen. In addition, groups receiving T cells, B cells, and the test antigens should be included for comparison. Eight to fourteen days after transfer, depending on the antigen and strain, the animals are bled out and their spleens are removed. It is useful to perform both serum antibody titration and plaque-forming cell assays. Antibody titers and spleen PFC are determined by standard methods, using indicator erythrocytes coated with the test antigen. For synthetic polypeptides, using chromic chloride ($CrCl_3$) to coat the SRBC is the method of choice. The conditions for optimal coating vary depending on the erythrocytes and the antigen and must be determined in advance. In general, equal volumes of packed red cells, antigen (range, 1–10 mg/ml), and $CrCl_3$ (1–10 mg/ml) are mixed in that order; all reagents must be in saline without phosphate buffer. After 5 min at room temperature, excess phosphate-buffered saline is added and the cells are washed thoroughly. If there is excessive hemolysis, the $CrCl_3$ level must be reduced. Coating of the cells is ascertained immediately by agglutination with a standard antiserum. In most cases, the erythrocytes are coated with the same antigen used in immunization. However, in the case of (T,G)-A--L, the PFC are usually determined using (T,G)-Pro--L-coated indicator cells, which tends to give plaques that are more easily read.

B. Acceptor

The stimulation of a response in B cells by the factor is an indication of the presence of an acceptor site for the factor on the cells. However, the acceptor is most easily demonstrated by absorption. The T-cell factor is mixed with the test cells in the cold (4°C) for at least 30 min. For B cells of a "responder" animal, 10^7 normal bone marrow cells absorb 1 spleen equivalent of factor in this time in the absence of added antigen. The effectiveness of absorption is determined by testing the supernatant for factor activity before and after absorption. Removal of factor, when it occurs, is usually complete. Using this test it is possible to distinguish (1) different cells types on the basis of the presence or absence of acceptor and (2) acceptor positive or negative strains of mice (high and low absorbers, respectively). For the helper factor, allogeneic B cells can be used for absorption, and xenogeneic absorptions have also been successfully accomplished (Taussig and Finch, 1977). For example, for (T,G)-A--L, factor produced by a responder strain can be tested against different low responders to detect which of the latter are defective in the B-cell acceptor site. Furthermore a mouse factor can be used across species as in the mouse–man studies of immune response genes (Taussig and Finch, 1977; Luzzati *et al.*, 1976).

The nature of the acceptor site can be studied with antiserum by pretreating B cells with the serum prior to absorption of factor, that is, testing for blocking of the acceptor site. In such experiments, it is important to avoid sera that possess reactivity against the factor.

V. CALCULATIONS

It is usual to set up at least 5–10 animals per group and to calculate the geometric mean PFC response of the group. Standard errors or deviations are computed and the usual statistical tests for significance are applied.

VI. CRITICAL APPRAISAL

The method described here for production and test of the antigen-specific helper factor has been used successfully for some years both in the author's laboratory (Taussig, 1974; Munro and Taussig, 1975) and elsewhere (Mozes, 1976; Isac and Mozes, 1977; Mozes *et al.*, 1976). Nevertheless, the method is subject to a significant failure rate, and it is therefore important to consider the causes of failure and possible means for improving the technique. There are three main stages at which difficulties arise, namely: (1) preparation of educated T cells *in vivo*, (2) culture of educated T cells to stimulate release of factor, and (3) test for factor activity in irradiated recipients. These will be considered in turn.

A. Preparation of Educated T Cells *in Vivo*

The priming of thymocytes in irradiated recipients has often been successfully used for erythrocytes and protein antigens. However, high levels of educated T cells may well be less easily achieved for molecules of low immunogenicity, such as (T,G)-A--L and other synthetic polypeptides of interest. The effectiveness of priming must therefore be established by testing the educated T cells either by transferring them with bone marrow cells into irradiated recipients or by culturing them *in vitro* with a source of

B cells. While some workers have reported satisfactory priming of T cells using the method described here as a preliminary to producing factors to human and rabbit γ-globulin and bovine serum albumin (Shiozawa *et al.*, 1977), others have turned to *in vitro* priming for (T,G)-A--L, L-glutamic acid[60]-L-alanine[30]-L-tyrosine[10] (GAT), and proteins (Howie *et al.*, 1977; Howie and Feldmann, 1977). For *in vitro* T-cell priming, the method of choice is the Diener–Marbrook tissue culture system, in which unfractionated spleen or lymph node cells or nylon-wool-fractionated T cells are cultured with antigen in the inner chamber for 4 days. The results obtained with synthetic polypeptides (Howie *et al.*, 1977; Howie and Feldmann, 1977) and protein antigens (McDougal and Gordon, 1977a,b) suggest that this may well be a reliable means of preparing specifically primed T cells capable of releasing T-cell factors.

B. Culture of Educated T Cells to Stimulate Release of Factor

Another potential source of difficulty in the technique is the culture of primed T cells *in vitro*, for release of T-cell factor. Clearly, the precise conditions of cell concentration, antigen level, culture medium, time of incubation, culture vessel, and so on will be empirically determined by the investigator in each case. It has been suggested that the successful production of helper factor by incubation in serum-free medium is due to the death of cells in culture and their release of internally stored factor. Although extensive cell death is not a prerequisite for the appearance of factor in culture supernatants, some workers have successfully released specific helper factors by cell lysis, either by homogenization (Shiozawa *et al.*, 1977) or by sonication (Tada *et al.*, 1976). It may be that *in vitro* culture, especially in the absence of serum, encourages proteolysis of factor after its release and that this is avoided in the rapid release of factor by lytic methods. The destruction of factor by enzymatic degradation may well be a significant source of failure to detect factor in culture supernatants and may be responsible for the rapid decline in its activity when it is stored. Other workers have modified the conditions for factor production in culture. For example, Kindred and Corley (1977) have cultured MLC-activated thymocytes for 4 hr in serum-free medium to produce a helper factor specific for histocompatibility antigens. Howie and Feldmann (1977), working with (T,G)-A--L, cultured 1.5×10^7 helper T cells and 1 μg of (T,G)-A--L per milliliter in medium containing 10% fetal calf serum in Diener–Marbrook flasks for various times. They found that the supernatants were most active after 24 hr of culture. McDougal and Gordon (1977b) found activity in supernatants in which the T cells had been primed for 4 days, in the same culture system. Thus, a considerable number of permutations on the method for encouraging T cells to relinquish their active molecules are possible.

C. Test for Factor Activity in Irradiated Recipients

The final stage in the method is the factor assay. In the author's experience and that of others (Taussig, 1974; Mozes, 1976; Feldmann *et al.*, 1977), the transfer of factor with a source of B cells into irradiated recipients is a satisfactory method, provided the problems inherent in dealing with irradiated mice can be overcome. A major drawback is a high rate of disease and death among the animals, even after bone marrow reconstitution. Reducing the dose of irradiation to the minumum required to abolish host responsiveness is one expedient, though this inevitably leads to a question of significant T-cell survival in the irradiated hosts. The most important single factor is probably the cleanliness of the available animal facilities, because the mice are sensitive to infection after irradiation. Nude mice have been used as satisfactory replacements for irradiated, recon-stituted recipients (Kindred and Corley, 1977). To avoid *in vivo* testing altogether is another alternative and here a variety of *in vitro* methods for generating antibody responses in culture are available and have been used to test helper factor (Shiozawa *et al.*, 1977; Howie and Feldmann, 1977; McDougal and Gordon, 1977a,b).

The T-cell factors, particularly those capable of specific antigen recog-nition, are a powerful means by which both the T-cell recognition system and cellular interactions, may be studied. Examples of the type of information that can be obtained can be found in the references. Among the

TABLE I

Cellular Defects in the Antibody Response to (T,G)-A--L

H-2	Strain	Response	T-cell factor	B-cell acceptor
b	B10	High	Yes	Yes
d	B10.D2	High	Yes	Yes
	BALB/c			
k	B10.Br	Low	Yes	No
	C3H			
j	I/St	Low	Yes	No
f	B10.M	Low	No	Yes
s	SJL	Low	No	No
s	A.SW	Low	No	Yes

useful studies that can be carried out is cellular analysis of the function of immune response genes. Table I shows the results obtained in screening (T,G)-A--L low responder strains for the presence of factor and acceptor. This principle is not confined to the mouse, since, by making use of the ability of factors to react xenogeneically, the *Ir* genes of different species can be approached, including those of man (Taussig and Finch, 1977).

REFERENCES

Feldmann, M., Baltz, M., Erb, P., Howie, S., Kontiainen, S., Woody, J., and Zvaifler, N. (1977). *In* "The Immune System: Genes and the Cells in Which They Function" (E. Sercarz, L. Herzenberg, and C. F. Fox, eds.), ICN–UCLA Symposia on Molecular and Cellular Biology, Vol. VIII. Academic Press, New York.

Howie, S., and Feldmann, M. (1977). *Eur. J. Immunol.* 7, 417.

Howie, S., Feldmann, M., Mozes, E., and Maurer, P. H. (1977). *Immunology* 32, 291.

Isac, R., and Mozes, E. (1977). *J. Immunol.* 118, 584.

Katz, D. H., and Benacerraf, B., eds. (1976). "The Role of Products of the Histocompatibility Gene Complex in Immune Responses." Academic Press, New York.

Kindred, B., and Corley, R. B. (1977). *Nature (London)* 268, 531.

Luzzati, A. L., Taussig, M. J., Meo, T., and Pernis, P. (1976). *J. Exp. Med.* 144, 573.

McDougal, J. S., and Gordon, D. S. (1977a). *J. Exp. Med.* 153, 676.

McDougal, J. S., and Gordon, D. S. (1977b). *J. Exp. Med.* 145, 693.

Mozes, E. (1976). *In* "The Role of Products of the Histocompatibility Gene Complex in Immune Responses" (D. H. Katz and B. Benacerraf, eds.), p. 485. Academic Press, New York.

Mozes, E., Isac, R., Givol, D., Zakut, R., and Beitsch, D. (1976). *In* "Immune Reactivity of Lymphocytes" (M. Feldmann and A. Globerson, eds.), p. 397. Plenum, New York.

Munro, A. J., and Taussig, M. S. (1975). *Nature (London)* 256, 103.

Shiozawa, C., Singh, B., Rubinstein, S., and Diener, E. (1977). *J. Immunol.* 118, 2199.

Tada, T. M., Taniguchi, M., and David, C. S. (1976). *Cold Spring Harbor Symp. Quant. Biol.* 41, 119.

Taniguchi, M., Tada, T., and Tokuhisa, T. (1976). *J. Exp. Med.* 144, 20.

Taussig, M. J. (1974). *Nature (London)* 248, 234.

Taussig, M. J., and Finch, A. P. (1977). *Nature (London)* 270, 151.

Taussig, M. J., Finch, A. P., and Kelus, A. S. (1976). *Nature (London)* 264, 776.

Taussig, M. J., Mozes, E., and Isac, R. (1974). *J. Exp. Med.* 140, 301.

24

In Vitro Immunization of Dissociated Murine Spleen Cells

Max H. Schreier

I. OBJECTIVE

A culture of unprimed lymphoid cells capable of responding to antigens seems to be a priori the most appropriate tool for the detailed study of induction and regulation of a humoral immune response. Ideally, in such an *in vitro* system, every constituent of the culture medium should be defined and the cell populations should be under the control of the experimenter. At present there is no system that meets these demands.

Two culture systems have been in use since the late 1960s to study the humoral immune response *in vitro*. The most widely used technique was originated in 1966 by Mishell and Dutton. Under conditions defined in detail (Mishell and Dutton, 1967), the culture of spleen cells in small petri

IMMUNOLOGICAL METHODS

dishes leads to the antigen-dependent appearance of antibody-forming cells, in numbers and at rates similar to those obtained *in vivo*. In another culture system developed by Marbrook (1967), the spleen cell suspension, together with antigen, is placed on a dialysis membrane attached to the end of a glass tube and immersed in a larger vessel containing culture medium.

Here we describe in detail two minor modifications of the culture method of Mishell and Dutton (1967), designated system A and system B, respectively (Schreier and Nordin, 1977). In terms of total response and kinetics, both systems give similar results. System A differs only by a slightly modified medium and feeding schedule from the original procedure. System B is more convenient because it requires no feeding and will work with some batches of fetal bovine serum unsuited to other techniques. Both systems gave rise to consistently more PFC whenever they were compared to the exact original procedure.

II. PRINCIPLE OF THE METHOD

A spleen cell suspension (or an appropriate combination of "purified" cells) is cultured in plastic petri dishes at high cell density (5 to 20×10^6 cells/ml) in the presence of antigen (mostly SRBC). The culture medium is supplemented with selected batches of fetal bovine serum (FBS). The cultures are incubated under low oxygen tension and with gentle agitation for a period of 4 to 6 days.

III. MATERIALS

A. Mice

Young adult C57BL/6J, C57BL/6J × A/J, or C57BL/6J × DBA/2 are most frequently used for the induction of an anti-SRBC response. The health status of the mouse is of critical importance for the outcome of *in vitro* immunization. We keep SPF (specific pathogen free) animals in germfree isolators in cages of five.

B. Salt Solutions and Media

Earle's balanced salt solution (BSS) without sodium bicarbonate as a $10\times$ stock solution is prepared as follows: 68.0 gm of NaCl, 4.0 gm of KCl, 1.4 gm of $NaH_2PO_4 \cdot H_2O$, 2.0 gm of $MgSO_4 \cdot 7H_2O$, 10.0 gm of $D(+)$-glucose, and 0.1 gm of phenol red, made up to 1 liter with glass-distilled water. The solution is sterilized by passing it through a 200-nm-pore filter pad. A $100\times$ $CaCl_2$ solution containing 2.0 gm of anhydrous $CaCl_2$ per 100 ml is autoclaved. For use, BSS is prepared by combining 890 ml of triple-distilled water with 100 ml of $10\times$ BSS and 10 ml of $100\times$ $CaCl_2$ solution. The pH is adjusted to 7.2 by adding 0.5 M NaOH (about 1.5 ml/liter).

Eagle's minimal essential medium (MEM) with Earle's salts, which we use for culture system A, is modified from the original formula (Eagle, 1959). Sodium chloride is reduced to 100 mM and the bivalent cations to 0.5 mM. It is prepared from two concentrates and all other supplements are commercially available (e.g., Gibco, Flow).

Concentrate 1 ($10\times$) contains, per liter, 58.44 gm of NaCl, 3.73 gm of KCl, 1.38 gm of $NaH_2PO_4 \cdot H_2O$, 21.2 gm of $NaHCO_3$, and 9.0 gm of glucose. Concentrate 2 ($100\times$) contains, per 100 ml, 1.016 gm of $MgCl_2 \cdot 6$ H_2O and 0.735 gm of $CaCl_2 \cdot 2$ H_2O. The MEM is prepared from the following constituents:

100 ml of concentrate 1
10 ml of concentrate 2
10 ml of $100\times$ vitamin solution
20 ml of $50\times$ essential amino acid solution
10 ml of $100\times$ nonessential amino acid solution
10 ml of sodium pyruvate solution, 100 mM
10 ml of Hepes buffer, pH 7.3, 1.0 M
1 ml of phenol red, 0.5%
Triple-distilled water to a final volume of 1 liter

RPMI 1640 is commercially available or can be prepared from instant tissue culture powder.

The nutritional mixture, slightly modified from Mishell and Dutton (1967), is prepared from the following stock solutions:

7 ml of concentrate 1
0.7 ml of concentrate 2
5.0 ml of L-glutamine (200 mM)
2.5 ml of $100\times$ nonessential amino acids
5.0 ml of $50\times$ essential amino acids
2.0 ml of D-glucose (500 mg/ml)
12.5 ml of $NaHCO_3$ (7.5%)
Triple-distilled water to a final volume of 100 ml

C. Fetal Bovine Serum

Fetal bovine serum, pretested for its supportive activity for an immune response *in vitro*, can be ordered from several companies as "serum contract approved lot" for a slightly higher price than random batches of

FBS. These sera are regularly supportive in culture system A. Their incidence in random test samples, made available by some companies, is about 15% (Shiigi and Mishell, 1975). After adding 2-mercaptoethanol, the score is significantly higher. FBS batches supportive for culture system B are more frequently found (up to 75% of tested samples). Highly supportive batches for either culture system are rare.

D. Sheep Red Blood Cells

Since the antigenicity of SRBC can vary widely between different sheep, an appropriate donor must be selected from several animals (Mishell and Dutton, 1967). The same sheep can be bled over several years (50 ml/week) and the same source of SRBC is used for *in vitro* immunization and the plaque assay. The blood, collected in Alsever's solution, is distributed in aliquots equivalent to 5 ml of packed cells and supplemented with sodium azide to a final concentration of 0.08%. It can be stored for up to 3 months. Prior to use, the SRBC are washed three times in sterile BSS.

E. Incubation Boxes and Rocker Platform

To establish an atmosphere of 7% O_2, 10% CO_2, and 83% N_2, the culture dishes are placed in airtight incubation boxes and the boxes are perfused with the gas mixture (Mishell and Dutton, 1967). The models we use are made from Lucite and they accommodate 75 (small box) and up to 150 cultures (large box). They are commercially available from Biotec, CH-4124 Schoenenbuch, Switzerland. Gentle agitation is achieved by placing the incubation box on a rocker platform (Bellco Glass, Inc., Vineland, New Jersey) as described by Mishell and Dutton (1967).

IV. PROCEDURE

A. Preparation of a Spleen Cell Suspension

Mice are killed by neck dislocation, and their spleens are removed aseptically and transferred into a bacteriological-type plastic petri dish containing 10 ml of BSS. The cells are teased from the capsule with a spatula. Clumps of cells are further dispersed by pipetting up and down with a 10-ml plastic pipette. The suspension is transferred to a 15-ml polycarbonate tube, in which clumps are allowed to settle for 2 to 3 min. The cell suspension is decanted into another tube and centrifuged for 15 min at 170 g at 4°C. The cells are resuspended in BSS and, after a second centrifugation, are resuspended in complete culture medium (about 0.5 ml per spleen to give a final concentration of 2×10^8 cells/ml). An aliquot of the cells is counted (20 μl + 1 ml of trypan blue solution). The viability is consistently above 95%.

B. Initiation of Cultures

The complete culture medium is prepared by supplementing the respective media with L-glutamine, penicillin–streptomycin, 2-mercaptoethanol, and a preselected batch of non-heat-inactivated fetal bovine serum:

Culture system A
  Modified MEM, 93.0 ml
  L-Glutamine (200 mM), 1.0 ml
  Penicillin–streptomycin, 0.5 ml
  2-Mercaptoethanol (0.01 M), 0.5 ml
  FBS, 5.0 ml
Culture system B
  RPMI 1640, 78.0 ml
  L-Glutamine (200 mM), 1.0 ml
  Penicillin–streptomycin, 0.5 ml
  2-Mercaptoethanol (0.01 M), 0.5 ml
  FBS, 20.0 ml

One milliliter of complete culture medium is pipetted into 3.5-cm plastic petri dishes (e.g., Falcon 3001 or 1008). Any cell-free additions (such as drugs, mediators, or serum fractions) in a volume of up to 100 μl are pipetted onto the bottom of the dish beforehand. Washed SRBC, 50 μl of a 1% solution in medium or BSS, are added to the cultures, which are then transferred to the Lucite box for gassing. Exposure of the lymphoid cells to alkaline pH is thus avoided. Finally, spleen cells in a volume of 50 μl are added with an Eppendorf pipette.

The Lucite boxes are then gassed again for 3 to 5 min and placed in a 37°C incubator on a rocker platform, set to about 6–8 Hz (Mishell and Dutton, 1967).

In culture system A, 100 μl of the nutritional mixture is added after 24 and 48 hr, whereas, in culture system B, the cultures need no further feeding until harvesting.

C. Cell Harvest

After 4, 5, and 6 days, duplicate cultures are harvested by gently scraping the culture dishes with a rubber policeman. The contents of each dish are transferred into 10 ml of BSS in graduated 15-ml glass tubes. They are pelleted by centrifugation for 15 min at 170 *g* and resuspended in an appropriate volume of BSS so that 50 to 100 μl gives a convenient number of PFC in the hemolytic plaque assay. The number of viable cells recovered is about 20 to 40% of the cell input.

V. CRITICAL APPRAISAL

Injection of mice with an immunogenic dose of SRBC leads to a quite predictable induction of PFC, as far as both numbers and early kinetics are concerned. *In vitro* immunization, as judged from the literature and the results of individual investigators over a prolonged period of time, can vary quantitatively by at least three orders of magnitude. More disturbing are qualitative differences, which have led to numerous controversies concerning cellular requirements or substitution of cell functions by cell lines, their products, or defined chemical compounds.

In view of the complexity of the system, such controversies are not surprising. At least four cell types, namely, adherent cells (macrophages), helper T cells, suppressor T cells, and B cells, are cocultured at high cell density. Their subpopulations may have different requirements for induction. Through cell cooperation or release of cell products, these cells interact in a positive or negative way depending on the circumstances. The net outcome is habitually measured by a single parameter: the relative number of antibody-forming cells appearing at a given time after initiation of the culture. Induction, proliferation, and maturation cannot be individually controlled.

The cellular cooperation and humoral interactions involved in the response to a given antigen can be influenced by numerous parameters. Some variables have been outlined by Schreier and Nordin (1977), although many more remain to be understood and controlled.

Any approach aiming at a better defined culture system will focus primarily either on the constituents of the medium and general culture conditions or on an exact definition of the cell populations cultured in a given medium. Neither approach has so far led to a satisfactory solution.

The least defined constituent of the medium is the fetal bovine serum, an absolute requirement for the efficient induction of antibody-forming cells *in vitro*. In the original system of Mishell and Dutton, only 15% of the marketed batches of FBS are sufficiently supportive (Shiigi and Mishell, 1975). As pointed out in Section III,C in the modified culture system B, the incidence of satisfactory batches is much higher (up to 75%). The basis of the difference between supportive and nonsupportive batches has been the subject of numerous investigations. Evidence for (and in part against) the mandatory presence of B-cell mitogenic, T-cell mitogenic, and macrophage-replacing activity has been reported.

Rigorous investigation of serum components, to establish their requirements and mechanisms of action, demands a constant source of defined lympoid cells. The cell source, however, must change from experiment to experiment and is most likely to be the major source of variability (Schreier and Nordin, 1977). This applies not only to different strains of mice, but also to the same strain over a prolonged period of time. Any changes in the health or immune status of the mouse will give rise to much greater variation *in vitro* than *in vivo*.

The major obstacle in achieving better defined cell populations is the absolute requirement of high cell density (close to 10^7 cells/ml) for successful *in vitro* immunization. Cross-contamination in highly purified (98% pure) or depleted cell populations can readily prevent analysis. The use of irradiated spleen cells as filler cells (Osoba, 1969) can be useful for some experimental designs, but the release of cell products from these irradiated cells is still uncontrolled. We never found it beneficial to use thymocytes as filler cells.

The first cell type that becomes limiting upon dilution seems to be the adherent cell population. This limitation can to some extent be compensated by the inclusion of mercaptoethanol in the culture medium (Click *et al.*, 1972), which fully or partly replaces, or enhances, the macrophage function (Chen and Hirsch, 1972). The cell type that is clearly never limiting at these cell densities is the specific B-cell precursor. These considerations and other lines of evidence (Schreier and Nordin, 1977) led us to conclude that it is the generation of helper T cells or the accumulation of a sufficient concentration of their product(s) that makes the high cell density mandatory for successful *in vitro* immunization. The experimental evidence that the system becomes dependent on exogenous (*in vivo*) activated T cells, if cocultured under nonsupportive culture conditions, is in line with this view.

The induction of suppressive cells during *in vitro* immunization has passed unnoticed for a long time. Spleen cells of mice immunized *in vivo* 4 days earlier can be readily restimulated *in vitro* with the same antigen, even under culture conditions that would not support the induction of a primary response (Mishell and Dutton, 1967). Spleen cells that have been immunized *in vitro* for 4 days cannot be restimulated with the same antigen. These precultured cells can even abolish the induction of PFC if added to primary cultures. Few cells (10^4 to 10^5) are required to induce this suppressive effect. The suppressive cell, which is induced in the absence of antigen, is a nonadherent θ-positive blast (Schreier and Lefkovits, 1978). Antigen-specific suppressor cells have also been described (Eardley and Gershon, 1976). The presence or induction of suppressive cells might, to a large extent, be responsible for the wide variation of *in vitro* results.

When interpreting the results of an *in vitro* immunization, absolute quantitative considerations are almost consistently ignored by experimenters. The same number of PFC described by one author as a negligible or extremely low background is presented by others as an "optimal response." This raises the question of how many PFC we should expect from 10^7 *in vitro* immunized spleen cells. By analogy to *in vivo* results, we should expect about 10^4 PFC per culture. If we consider, however, the lack of recruitment from the recirculating lymphocyte pool or the evasion of significant control mechanisms that are relevant *in vivo*, this estimate can well be either too high or too low. Under the culture conditions described above, using C57BL/6J mice, we regularly find 30,000 to 40,000 PFC per culture at the peak of the response. Over a period of several years, this response has periodically decreased or increased by a factor of 2 to 3, without obvious reason.

A more valid basis for quantitative considerations may be the frequency of antigen-specific precursors. If the highest estimates, as determined in mitogen-stimulated, low cell density cultures (Andersson *et al.*, 1977), turn out to be valid for antigen-induced responses, we might have up to about 1500 SRBC-specific B-cell precursors in 10^7 spleen cells. Since a clone size of about 10^2 can be readily anticipated, it becomes obvious that in inefficient *in vitro* systems only a small fraction of precursors is triggered to respond. Plainly, the behavior of a minor fraction of B-cell precursors cannot be a sound basis for speculations on the mechanism of induction and regulation of a humoral immune response.

REFERENCES

Andersson, J., Coutinho, A., and Melchers, F. (1977). *J. Exp. Med.* **145,** 1520.
Chen, C., and Hirsch, J. G. (1972). *Science* **176,** 60.
Click, R. E., Benck, L., and Alter, B. J. (1972). *Cell. Immunol.* **3,** 264.
Eagle, H. (1959). *Science* **130,** 432.
Eardley, D. D., and Gershon, R. K. (1976). *J. Immunol.* **117,** 313.
Marbrook, J. (1967). *Lancet* **2,** 1279.
Mishell, R. I., and Dutton, R. W. (1966). *Science* **153,** 1004.
Mishell, R. I., and Dutton, R. W. (1967). *J. Exp. Med.* **126,** 423.
Osoba, D. (1969). *J. Exp. Med.* **129,** 141.
Schreier, M. H., and Lefkovits, I. (1978). *Immunology* (in press).
Schreier, M. H., and Nordin, A. A. (1977). *In* "B and T cells in Immune Recognition" (F. Loor and G. E. Roelants, eds.), pp. 127–152. Wiley, New York.
Shiigi, S. M., and Mishell, R. I. (1975). *J. Immunol.* **115,** 741.

Induction of a Secondary Antibody Response in Vitro with Rabbit Peripheral Blood Lymphocytes

Alma L. Luzzati

I. OBJECTIVE

The utilization of blood lymphocytes for studies of antibody formation *in vitro* allows the investigator to perform repeated experiments with the cells of a given animal at different stages of immunization. This is of particular importance when outbred animals, such as rabbits or monkeys,

IMMUNOLOGICAL METHODS
Copyright © 1979 by Academic Press, Inc.
All rights of reproduction in any form reserved.
ISBN 0-12-442750-2

are used. In addition, this method opens up interesting possibilities for an approach to studies of the immune response in man.

II. PRINCIPLE OF THE METHOD

The leukocytes from the peripheral blood of immunized rabbits, after removal of the erythrocytes and of a population of adhering suppressor cells (Luzzati and Lafleur, 1976), are cultured in the presence of the specific antigen (Luzzati *et al.*, 1973a).

Two types of cultures can be performed: (1) regular 1-ml cultures and (2) microcultures (see Chapter 27). The occurrence of an immune response is determined at different intervals, in the first type of culture by enumerating the direct (IgM) and indirect (IgG) plaque-forming cells (PFC) and in the second type of culture by spot test or by counting the PFC.

The supernatant of the positive microcultures often contains enough antibody for immunochemical characterization.

III. MATERIALS

A. Antigen: Sheep Red Blood Cells (SRBC)

The sheep blood is collected in Alsever's solution (1 vol of blood in 1 vol of Alsever's solution) and is allowed to age for at least 1 week before use.

The red cells are pelleted by centrifugation at 2500 rpm for 10 min and washed twice, taking care to remove the buffy coat. The washing is usually performed in saline (0.15 M NaCl) when the erythrocytes are used for *in vivo* immunization or as indicator cells, whereas it is performed in sterile Hanks' BSS when they are used as antigen *in vitro*.

B. Pig Skin Gelatin

A 3% solution of pig skin gelatin (Eastman Kodak Co., Rochester, New York, No. 5242) is freshly made in saline (0.15 M NaCl). The gelatin is allowed to dissolve at 40°–50°C (boiling must be avoided). The solution is filtered through a Nalgene 0.45-μm filter (Nalge, Sybron Corp., Rochester, New York).

C. Nylon Wool

A synthetic fiber sold by a local dealer as cushion filling (Coop, Basel, Switzerland, No. 609.002) is used in this laboratory. The wool is soaked overnight in detergent (7×) and rinsed under running tap water for 24 hr and then in several changes of distilled water. The washed wool is then dried, teased, and packed in weighed amounts into plastic syringes (see the tabulation below), which are then autoclaved.

Syringe	Nylon (gm)	Blood[a] (ml)
10-ml	0.6	4
20-ml	1.2	8
50-ml	3.0	20

[a] The volume of blood that can be accommodated on a given amount of nylon.

D. Culture Medium

RPMI 1640 medium (Microbiological Associates, Bethesda, Maryland, No. 12–702) containing 10% fetal calf serum and 50 U/ml of both streptomycin and penicillin (Microbiological Associates, No. 17603F) is used.

The fetal calf serum must be carefully selected. Some sera support a good IgM response, whereas others are able to induce IgG responses also. A few batches do not support effectively any kind of response. We have successfully used several batches of Rehatuin (Reheis Chemical Co., Chicago, Illinois) and a contract approved serum from Gibco (Grand Island Biological Co., Grand Island, New York).

E. Hanks' Balanced Salt Solution (Hanks' BSS)

This can be obtained from Microbiological Associates, Bethesda, Maryland (No. 10-508).

F. Eagle's Minimum Essential Medium (MEM)

This can be obtained from Grand Island Biological Co., Grand Island, New York.

G. Agar for Enumeration of PFC (0.7% Bacto Agar)

A 1.4% solution of agar (Bacto agar, Difco, Detroit, Michigan) in distilled water, freshly made every day, is diluted 1:1 with twice-concentrated MEM (prewarmed at 45°C) and placed in a 45°C water bath.

H. Agar for Allotype Assay (2% Noble Agar)

A 4% solution of agar (Noble agar, Difco, Detroit, Michigan) in distilled water is diluted 1:1 with 0.05 M Veronal buffer, pH 8.6, containing 0.5 gm of sodium azide per liter. The 2% agar solution is distributed in bottles and can be kept in the refrigerator for up to 2 months. Before use the agar is melted in boiling water.

I. Complement

Reconstituted lyophilized guinea pig complement (Behringwerke A.G., Marburg-Lahn, West Germany) is absorbed twice, in the cold, with SRBC (0.3 ml of packed SRBC/10 ml of complement). Absorbed complement is stored at $-70°C$.

IV. PROCEDURE

A. Preparation of the Cells and Setting Up the Cultures

1. The rabbits are bled from the central artery of the ear and the blood is collected into heparinized bottles.

2. Nylon-wool-packed syringes are accommodated on a rack specially designed to hold them in a vertical position. The plunger is removed and the wool is made compact by pushing it down with the aid of a pipette. Measured aliquots of blood are then distributed on top of the wool. The optimal ratio between amount of wool and volume of blood in a given syringe was given earlier (see the tabulation).

With the aid of the syringe plunger, the blood is forced into the wool until it reaches the far end, care being taken that it does not flow out of the wool.

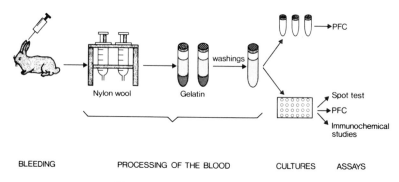

Fig. 1. Flow diagram of the procedure.

The syringe nozzle is then sealed. The distribution of the blood in the wool is made even by gently tapping the syringe. The filled syringes are placed in a humidified CO_2 incubator at 37°C for 30 min. At the end of this period, the blood is squeezed out of the syringes and the wool is rinsed twice with warm (37°C) Hanks' BSS, each time with a volume equal to half the initial volume of blood. Both the blood and the washing fluids are squeezed out of the wool by pushing the syringe plunger down as far as possible.

3. The nylon-wool-filtered blood added with the washing fluids is mixed with the 3% pig skin gelatin solution (2 vol of blood + 1 vol of gelatin). The mixture is distributed into conical plastic tubes (Falcon Plastics, type 2070), which are put in a vertical position in a CO_2 incubator at 37°C. After 30 min the tubes are rotated 180° around their axis, so that red cell clumps sticking to the walls detach and settle with the rest of the erythrocytes. After another 15 min the leukocyte-rich supernatant is collected and spun at 1500 rpm for 10 min at 20°C.

4. The pellet is washed twice with Hanks' BSS (by centrifugation; 1100 rpm for 10 min) and then suspended in tissue culture medium at a concentration of 4×10^6 cells/ml.

5. Antigen is added in the form of 0.05 ml of 2% sheep red blood cells in Hanks' BSS per milliliter of cell suspension.

6. The cell suspension is distributed in 1-ml aliquots in plastic tubes (Falcon Plastics, type 2003) for regular cultures and in 10-μl aliquots in the wells of tissue culture trays (Falcon Plastics, type 3034) for microcultures. Both types of cultures are then incubated in a humidified 5% CO_2 incubator without any further treatment until assayed.

B. Assay of Plaque-Forming Cells (PFC)

At the time of harvesting, duplicate 1-ml cultures are pooled, and the cells are washed once in Hanks' BSS and resuspended in 0.5 ml of MEM. The number of direct (IgM) and indirect (IgG) PFC is assayed using a modification of the gel hemolysis method described in Chapter 19.

Portions of 0.5 ml of 0.7% Bacto agar in MEM are distributed in 50×8-mm glass tubes and kept in a 45°C water bath. Twenty microliters of a 10 mg/ml solution of DEAE-dextran (Pharmacia, Uppsala, Sweden), 20 μl of 20% SRBC, and from 10 to 50 μl of the lymphoid cell suspension are added to the tubes. When high activity is expected, 10 μl of one or more fivefold dilutions of the lymphocyte suspension should be tested. The mixture is spread on glass microscope slides precoated with agar.

After the agar has solidified, the slides are inverted on special Lucite racks provided with a shallow well that allows the application of constant amounts of incubation medium (about 1 ml per slide). The slides are incubated in a CO_2 incubator at 37°C, first for 1 hr with MEM and then, after transfer to clean racks, for 2.5 hr with a 1:30 dilution of SRBC-absorbed guinea pig complement or with sheep anti-rabbit Ig diluted in 1:30 guinea pig complement. The dilution of the developing anti-Ig serum must be one that gives the maximum number of indirect plaques with no inhibition of direct plaques.

Counting the plaques is performed with an automated colony counter by holding the slides under a magnifying lens in indirect light. Counting is most reliable with 40 to 150 plaques per slide. The number of IgG-producing cells is determined by subtracting the number of IgM-producing cells from the total number of PFC developed with the anti-Ig serum.

Tests for PFC in individual microculture wells are performed in essentially the same way.

C. Studies on the Antibody Released in the Culture Fluid

In the culture fluid of regular 1-ml cultures, antibody accumulates in sufficient amounts for qualitative and quantitative studies only when a high enough number of PFC (more than 2000–3000/ml) is active for several days. However, positive microcultures very often contain high concentrations of specific antibody. The anti-SRBC antibody of the culture fluids can be determined quantitatively by performing a hemagglutination or hemolysis titration.

When cells from rabbits heterozygous at the *b* locus of the light chains of Ig are cultured, the clonal nature of the antibody released in single microculture wells can be verified by testing for allotype. Only one allele should be expressed in each clone. For this purpose, a sensitive method is required, one that can be performed on very minute amounts of specific antibody. We describe here the inhibition of diffusion method (Luzzati *et al.*, 1973b).

Agar-coated microscope slides are layered with 1 ml of 2% Noble agar in barbital buffer. After the agar has solidified triplets of wells are dug in the agar (Fig. 2) with the aid of a stainless steel gel cutter attached to a water pump. The diameter of the wells is 1.5 mm and the center-to-center distance between the wells in a triplet is 5 mm. The volume of the wells is about 2 μl.

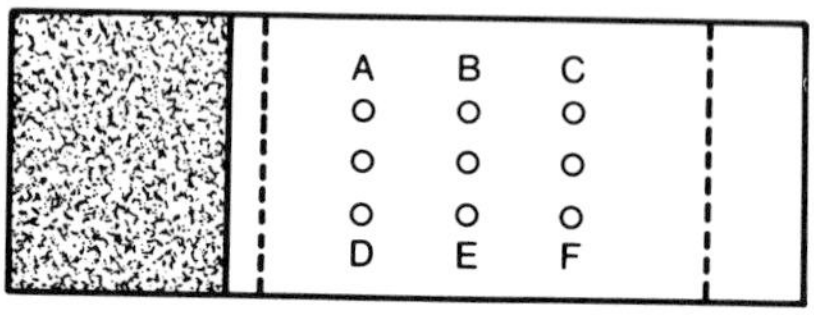

Fig. 2. Pattern of wells for the inhibition of diffusion method.

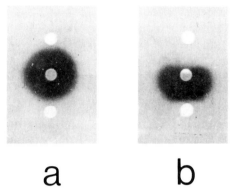

Fig. 3. Test for allotype of the anti-SRBC antibody produced in a microculture of cells from a *b4/b4* homozygote. (a) Central well, culture fluid; outer wells, normal rabbit serum; (b) central well, culture fluid; top well, anti-b4 serum; bottom well, anti-b6 serum. (From Luzzati *et al.*, 1973b.)

Culture fluids from microcultures scored as positive with the spot test are placed in the central wells of the triplets, and the outer wells are filled with undiluted anti-allotype sera. The anti-allotype sera used in this test should be non-cross-reacting among themselves; that is, for a heterozygous *b4,b6* rabbit, anti-b4 and anti-b6 sera made in *b9* rabbits should be used. The antisera are heat-inactivated (56°C for 30 min) and SRBC-absorbed.

The slides are left overnight at room temperature in a moist chamber.

The following day the slides are rinsed for 5–15 min in 0.15 M NaCl. The excess saline is drained, the lateral edges of the agar are cut with a razor blade (see the dotted lines in Fig. 2), and the slides are placed on a warm surface. The following mixture, prepared in 0.5 × 8-mm glass tubes kept in a 45°C water bath, is then immediately poured on each slide: 0.25 ml of 0.7% Bacto agar in MEM, 20 μl of DEAE-dextran (10 mg/ml), and 20 μl of 20% SRBC.

The slides are transferred to a cold surface and allowed to stand for 1–2 min; they are then inverted on special Lucite racks. The racks are filled with SRBC-absorbed guinea pig complement diluted 1:10 in MEM.

After 2.5 hr of incubation in a humidified CO_2 incubator, the position of lysis is recorded.

A complete circle of lysis around the central well means that no inhibition occurred. A lytic zone in the shape of a half-circle means that the anti-SRBC antibody was blocked by the anti-allotype serum placed in the well on the side with no lysis; hence, it is expressing that particular allotype (Fig. 3)

Lack of inhibition may occur because (a) the antibody present in the fluid does not carry the allotype being tested or (b) the antibody present in the fluid is a mixture of two populations of molecules: one carrying the particular allotype and hence blocked by the antiserum, the other expressing another allele and therefore not blocked and still able to give complete lysis. In the second case, a mixture of the two antibodies directed against the two allelic allotypes, when placed in one of the outer wells, will cause complete inhibition of lysis.

Although the sensitivity of this technique is difficult to evaluate precisely, its reliability in detecting "contaminant" antibodies produced by other clones was tested by performing artificial mixtures of antibodies of the two allelic allotypes (*b4* and *b6*). Fifteen of such mixtures were tested and in all instances the two alleles were detected.

V. COMMENTS

The induction of a secondary antibody response *in vitro* to SRBC with rabbit peripheral blood lymphocytes (PBL) is usually very reproducible. Rarely can a significant response be observed before day 5. The number of PFC then slowly increases, reaching a maximum between days 10 and 20. This maximum number of PFC can be maintained for several days or even weeks.

Although there is a great difference from animal to animal in the height and in the kinetics of the response, repeated experiments performed with samples of blood taken from the same animal over a period of several weeks can give strikingly similar results. This is mainly true if the animal has been primed *in vivo* at least a year previously. Recently primed animals tend to give poorer responses.

Control cultures, performed without antigen, usually give a very low number of plaques and/or a small number of positive wells in the microculture system (low background).

The ratio of direct to indirect plaques obtained *in vitro* is highly contingent on the animal and on the time elapsed from the priming as well as on the batch of fetal calf serum used (and probably also on other as yet unidentified culture and/or cell separation variables).

The method described here for the response to SRBC has been successfully applied to studies on the *in vitro* antibody response to streptococcal-group polysaccharide antigens (Read and Braun, 1974; Braun *et al.*, 1976) and to studies on the early inductive phase of the *in vitro* antibody response (Pawlita *et al.*, 1978).

Attempts to extend this method to studies with human blood have encountered great difficulties, probably due to the fact that the human donors have not been primed with the antigen and the induction of a primary response *in vitro* with blood lymphocytes may present different problems. On the other hand, the possibility cannot be excluded that human lymphocytes are more difficult to stimulate *in vitro* with antigen than rabbit lymphocytes. However, with the help of additional stimulatory agents and with a modification of the method described here (Luzzati *et al.*, 1976, 1977), *in vitro* immunization of human PBL has been obtained. In fact, antibody responses to SRBC, HRBC, and (T,G)-A--L have been elicited with the help of an antigen-specific mouse T-cell factor (Luzzati *et al.*, 1976). Responses to SRBC and HRBC have been induced in human PBL cultured with the specific antigen in the presence of Epstein Barr virus (Luzzati *et al.*, 1977).

REFERENCES

Braun, D. G., Quintáns, J., Luzzati, A. L., Lefkovits, I., and Read, S. E. (1976). *J. Exp. Med.* **143,** 360.

Luzzati, A. L., and Lafleur, L. (1976). *Eur. J. Immunol.* **6,** 125.

Luzzati, A. L., Lefkovits, I., and Pernis, B. (1973a). *Eur. J. Immunol.* **3,** 632.

Luzzati, A. L., Lefkovits, I., and Pernis, B. (1973b). *Eur. J. Immunol.* **3,** 636.

Luzzati, A. L., Taussig, M. J., Meo, T., and Pernis, B. (1976). *J. Exp. Med.* **144,** 573.

Luzzati, A. L., Hengartner, H., and Schreier, M. H., (1977). *Nature (London)* **269,** 419.

Pawlita, M., Andersen, V., Lefkovits, I., and Braun, D. G. (1978). *Scand. J. Immunol.* **7,** 221.

Read, S. E., and Braun, D. G. (1974). *Eur. J. Immunol.* **4,** 422.

26

Induction of Immune Responses with Clonal Dominance at High Antibody Levels

Dietmar G. Braun

I. INTRODUCTION

A standard immune response is the sum of many clonal responses. However, the study of clonal expression itself or an analysis of its products requires separation of clones. One approach to this goal is the generation of responses where one or a few clones make up the bulk of the antibody population.

The success of this approach rests on the homogeneity of the immunogen. Bacterial cell walls, carrying regularly spaced polysaccharide structures on their surface, meet this demand: They are known to induce antibody responses of predictable clonal patterns. Given the uniqueness of epitopes

IMMUNOLOGICAL METHODS

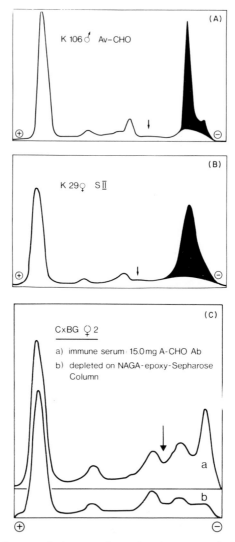

Fig. 1. Densitometric scans of microzone electrophoretic patterns of rabbit and mouse hyperimmune sera to bacterial polysaccharide antigens. (A) Rabbit anti-streptococcal group A-variant antiserum before and after absorption. (B) Rabbit anti-pneumococcal type II antiserum before and after absorption. (C) Mouse anti-streptococcal group A antiserum before and after absorption.

on identical carriers, clonal dominance reflects established hierarchies among immunocytes and is thus a regulatory phenomenon (Braun *et al.*, 1976).

II. PRINCIPLE OF THE METHOD

In rabbits, optimal conditions for eliciting dominant clonotypes with anti-polysaccharide specificity are achieved by intraveneous immunization with streptococcal or pneumococcal vaccines (Braun *et al.*, 1969; Pincus *et al.*, 1970). In certain inbred mouse strains both intraperitoneal and intravenous immunizations are successful in inducing large amounts of restricted antibody (Braun *et al.*, 1972; Briles and Krause, 1972; Eichmann, 1972). Two conditions are required to achieve this with streptococcal vaccines: (1) The genetic background of rabbits and of mice must be considered, and (2) the dead bacterial vaccine must be prepared such that, for example, the streptococcal group polysaccharide constitutes the outer layer. The topography of the group polysaccharide is of considerable importance.

In the following sections I shall describe the methods used currently for the *in vivo* induction of large amounts of restricted antibody to bacterial cell wall moieties (Fig. 1), and I shall give reference to systems that use hapten–carrier conjugates.

Antigens Used

β-Hemolytic streptococci: strains J17A4 (group A), A486,M – (group A variant), 090R (group B), and C74 (group C); all of these strains are from the collection of Dr. R. C. Lancefield, The Rockefeller University, New York

Pneumococci: Types II, III, and VIII were obtained from the American Type Culture Collection, Atlanta, Georgia

Peptidoglycan of β-hemolytic streptococci (Schleifer and Krause, 1971)

Micrococcus leisodeikticus (Strosberg *et al.*, 1974)

D-Ala–D-Ala–group A streptococci (Kolb, 1976)

DNP–gramicidin S (Montgomery *et al.*, 1975)

p-Azobenzoate (Appella *et al.*, 1974)

III. VACCINE PREPARATION

Here I shall describe only the preparation of streptococcal and pneumococcal vaccines as examples.

A. Streptococci

For a large batch of vaccine the following procedure is used. Of a 16-hr Todd–Hewitt broth culture (Difco, Detroit), 1500 ml at 37°C is centrifuged twice at 7000 *g* for 20 min. The bacterial sediment is collected, washed twice with sterile saline, resuspended in 30 ml of sterile saline, heat-killed at 56°C for 45 min, centrifuged twice at 7000 *g* for 20 min, resuspended in 30 ml of saline, and adjusted to pH 2 with HCl. Seventy-five milligrams of pepsin is added, and digestion is carried out for 2 hr at 37°C. The bacterial suspension is neutralized with 2 *M* NaOH to pH 7 and centrifuged, the supernatant is discarded, and the sediment is washed twice in saline. The sediment is resuspended in 100 ml of sterile saline and adjusted to an optical density (650 nm) of 3.15/ml. This density of streptococci is associated with approximately 400 μg of group polysaccharide/ml of vaccine. The vaccine is checked for sterility by plating on blood agar.

B. Pneumococci

Pneumococci are grown for 16 hr in Todd–Hewitt medium under conditions the same as those described for streptococci. Growth is terminated by heat-killing (see Section III,A). Cells are washed three times in cold formalinized saline (containing 0.25% formalin) and adjusted to an optical density (590 nm) of 5.95, representing 4×10^9 cells/ml. While streptococcal vaccines are stable at this point, pneumococcal vaccines must be washed once before immunization to remove the capsular-type polysaccharide dissociated into the supernatant. This free polysaccharide will otherwise cause tolerance rather than induction of high and restricted antibody levels.

IV. IMMUNIZATION

A. Streptococcal Vaccines

Rabbits for restricted high response must first be searched for (random frequency is between 1 and 10% depending on the source of rabbits and the streptococcus taken) and can then be bred selectively for this trait (Braun *et al.*, 1969, 1973; Eichmann et al., 1971).

Alternative schedules (A + B) of immunization of rabbits against streptococcal group polysaccharide (Braun *et al.*, 1969, 1973; Davie *et al.*, 1968; Eichmann *et al.*, 1970, 1971; Fleischman *et al.*, 1968; Miller *et al.*, 1967; Osterland *et al.*, 1966) are shown in the following tabulation.

Week	A			B	
	Day	Amount/ml	Route	Day	Amount/ml
1	Monday	0.25	iv	Monday	0.5
	Tuesday	0.25	iv	Tuesday	0.5
	Wednesday	0.25	iv	Wednesday	0.5
	Thursday	0.25	iv		
	Friday	0.25	iv		
	Saturday	0.25	iv		
2	Monday	0.5	iv	Monday	1.0
	Tuesday	0.5	iv	Tuesday	1.0
	Wednesday	0.5	iv	Wednesday	1.0
	Thursday	0.5	iv		
	Friday	0.5	iv		
	Saturday	0.5	iv		
3	Monday	1.0	iv	Monday	1.0
	Tuesday	1.0	iv	Tuesday	1.0
	Wednesday	1.0	iv	Wednesday	1.0
	Thursday	1.0	iv		
	Friday	1.0	iv		
	Saturday	1.0	iv		
4				Monday	1.0
				Tuesday	1.0
	Wednesday	Bleed 60–70 ml	iv	Wednesday	1.0
	Friday	Bleed 50–70 ml	iv		
5	Monday	Bleed 50–70 ml		Monday	Bleed 50–70 ml
	Wednesday	Bleed 50–70 ml		Wednesday	Bleed 50–70 ml
	Friday	Bleed 50–70 ml		Friday	Bleed 50–70 ml

Bleeding is continued for the following 2 weeks every second or third day, depending on the condition of the rabbit and on the level of antibody, checked by microzone electrophoresis and quantitative precipitation with the isolated group polysaccharide (Braun *et al.*, 1969). Bleeding is always done from the central ear artery. Xylene should be avoided to induce hyperemia; its use results in scarring. Gentle warming of the ears is more effective. An alternative way of collecting large amounts of blood is exchange transfusion of rabbits (for details, see Greenblatt *et al.*, 1973).

This primary immunization course may be followed by a secondary immunization course after a rest of 6 months (Braun *et al.*, 1969). In this case, the rabbits are only immunized for 2 weeks and bleeding is started 5 days after the last injection in the third week. A considerable number of rabbits will only respond after a secondary immunization (Braun *et al.*, 1969). A secondary immunization course may be followed by a tertiary immunization course after another 6 months. Generally, clonal persistence is observed, which allows up to 10–15 gm of antibody to be collected over the course of 18 months (Cramer and Braun, 1975b).

Alternative schedules of immunization for inbred mouse strains [A/J, BALB/c, and SWR are restricted high responders (see Braun *et al.*, 1972; Briles and Krause, 1972; Cramer and Braun, 1974, 1975a; Eichmann, 1972, 1973)] are shown in the following tabulation.

Week	Day	Amount/ml	Route
1	Monday	0.05	ip
	Tuesday	0.05	ip
	Wednesday	0.05	ip
2	Monday	0.1	ip
	Tuesday	0.1	ip
	Wednesday	0.1	ip
3	Monday	0.1	ip
	Tuesday	0.1	ip
	Wednesday	0.1	ip
4	Monday	0.1	ip
	Tuesday	0.1	ip
	Wednesday	0.1	ip
5	Monday		
	Wednesday		
	(bleed from tail vein)		
	Friday		
1	Monday	0.1	iv
	Tuesday	0.1	iv
	Wednesday	0.1	iv
2	Monday	0.1	iv
	Tuesday	0.1	iv
	Wednesday	0.1	iv
3–6	Rest period		
7	Monday	0.1	iv
	Tuesday	0.1	iv
	Wednesday	0.1	iv
8	Monday	0.1	iv
	Tuesday	0.1	iv
	Wednesday	0.1	iv
9	Bleed two or three times from tail vein or venous eye plexus		

B. Pneumococcal Vaccines

Inbred mouse strains do not produce large amounts of IgG antibodies in response to pneumococcal type III vaccines. The immunization schedule shown in the following tabulation is only valid for rabbits immunized with type II, III, or VIII vaccines (Chen *et al.*, 1973; Kimball *et al.*, 1971; Pincus *et al.*, 1970, 1973).

Week	Day	Amount/cells	Route
1	Monday	10^8	iv
	Tuesday	10^8	iv
	Wednesday	10^8	iv
2	Monday	5×10^8	iv
	Tuesday	5×10^8	iv
	Wednesday	5×10^8	iv
3	Monday	10^9	iv
	Tuesday	10^9	iv
	Wednesday	10^9	iv
4	Monday	10^9	iv
	Tuesday	10^9	iv
	Wednesday	10^9	iv
5	Three bleeds		
	Monday, Wednesday, and Friday		

If sera contain high amounts of restricted antibody at this time, bleeding is continued for another 2–3 weeks followed by a rest period of 4 weeks. Immunization is then continued with 5×10^9 cells three times for the first week and twice for the following 4 weeks. Bleeds are taken 5 days after the last injection. Testing of antisera for restricted antibodies is performed by microzone electrophoresis; the amount of specific antibody is determined by quantitative precipitin analysis.

V. SERIAL TRANSFER OF LIMITED SPLEEN CELL NUMBERS

Briles and Krause (1972) and Eichmann (1972, 1973) have adopted continuing serial transfer of spleen cells into irradiated mice, developed by Askonas *et al.*, (1970) for anti-DNP-forming clones, for the production of large amounts of single clonal products. Spleen cells ($2-10 \times 10^6$) of mice with single dominating group A polysaccharide-specific clonotypes, identified by isoelectric focusing, were transferred into syngeneic mice irradiated with 600 R. These reconstituted mice received four times 0.1 ml of streptococcal group A vaccines iv within 2 weeks. A rest period of 4 weeks was followed by a regular secondary immunization course lasting 2 weeks.

VI. CRITICAL APPRAISAL

There was some controversy in the past whether immune responses with restricted heterogeneity and high antibody levels leading to clonal dominance were under genetic control. For the rabbit model, developed in response to streptococcal group polysaccharides, the heritable trait is beyond doubt. This trait is independent of heavy- and light-chain allotypes and is also independent of the light-chain isotype. A rabbit line has been developed that lacks the expression of κ light chains (Kelus and Weiss, 1977), yet a high proportion of these closely related, partly inbred rabbits respond to the streptococcal group A-variant polysaccharide with high and restricted antibody levels (Weiss *et al.*, 1977). Two rabbit lines have been established in the past 8 years, and in both lines as many as 90% of the offspring of some families were restricted high responders (D. G. Braun, unpublished).

Inbred mouse strains are either restricted high, intermediate, or low responders to the streptococcal group A polysaccharide (Cramer and Braun, 1975a). This response is under autosomal control, is not linked to the H-2 complex as are responses to a great many other antigens, and shows a close association (at least three genes are involved in the regulation of this immune response) to the *Ig* locus that controls subclass expression (Braun *et al.*, 1978). This situation has much in common with high responses to other polysaccharide antigens, for example, dextran (Hansburg *et al.*, 1976) and lipopolysaccharide antigens of gram-negative bacteria (R. di Pauli, personal communication). Certain inbred rat strains may show similar responses to the streptococcal group A polysaccharide. Again, there is no linkage to the major histocompatibility locus of the rat (Stankus and Leslie, 1976). Hence, there are similar patterns of responsiveness in members of at least three different species.

SUGGESTED READING

Braun, D. G., and Jaton, J.-C. (1974). Homogeneous antibodies: Induction and value as probe for the antibody problem. *Curr. Top. Microbiol. Immunol.* **66,** 29–76.

Haber, E. (1971). Homogeneous elicited antibodies: Induction, characterization, isolation and structure. *Ann. N.Y. Acad. Sci.* **190,** 283–304.

Kindt, T. J., Thundberg, A. L., Mudgett, M., and Klapper, D. G. (1974). A study of V region genes using allotypic and idiotypic markers. *In* "The Immune System: Genes, Receptors,

Signals" (E. E. Sercarz, A. R. Williamson, and C. F. Fox, eds.), pp. 69–88. Academic Press, New York.

Krause, R. M. (1970a). Factors controlling the occurrence of antibodies with uniform properties. *Fed. Proc., Fed. Am. Soc. Exp. Biol.* **29,** 59–65.

Krause, R. M. (1970b). The search for antibodies with molecular uniformity. *Adv. Immunol.* **12,** 1–16.

REFERENCES

Appella, E., Roholt, O. A., Chersi, A., Radzinski, G., and Pressman, (1974). *Biochem. Biophys. Res. Commun.* **53,** 1122.

Askonas, B. A., Williamson, A. R., and Wright, B. E. G. (1970). *Proc. Natl. Acad. Sci. U.S.A.* **67,** 1398.

Braun, D. G., Eichmann, K., and Krause, R. M. (1969). *J. Exp. Med.* **129,** 809.

Braun, D. G., Kindred, B., and Jacobson, J. B. (1972). *Eur. J. Immunol.* **2,** 138.

Braun, D. G., Kjems, E., and Cramer, M. (1973). *J. Exp. Med.* **138,** 645.

Braun, D. G., Huser, H., and Riesen, W. F. (1976). *In* "The Generation of Antibody Diversity: A New Look" (A. J. Cunningham, ed.), p. 31. Academic Press, New York.

Braun, D. G., Schalch, W., and Schmid, I. (1978). *In* "Streptococcal Diseases and the Immune Response" (M. McCarty and J. B. Zabriskie, eds.). Academic Press, New York (in press).

Briles, D. E., and Krause, R. M. (1972). *J. Immunol.* **109,** 1311.

Chen, F. W., Strossberg, A. D., and Haber, E. (1973). *J. Immunol.* **110,** 98.

Cramer, M., and Braun, D. G. (1974). *J. Exp. Med.* **139,** 1513.

Cramer, M., and Braun, D. G. (1975a). *Eur. J. Immunol.* **5,** 823.

Cramer, M., and Braun, D. G. (1975b). *Scand. J. Immunol.* **4,** 63.

Davie, J. M., Osterland, C. K., Miller, E. J., and Krause, R. M. (1968). *J. Immunol.* **100,** 814.

Eichmann, K. (1972). *Eur. J. Immunol.* **2,** 301.

Eichmann, K. (1973). *J. Exp. Med.* **137,** 603.

Eichmann, K., Lackland, H., Hood, L., and Krause, R. M. (1970a). *J. Exp. Med.* **131,** 207.

Eichmann, K., Braun, D. G., Feizi, T., and Krause, R. M. (1970b). *J. Exp. Med.* **131,** 1169.

Eichmann, K., Braun, D. G., and Krause, R. M. (1971). *J. Exp. Med.* **134,** 48.

Fleischman, J. B., Braun, D. G., and Krause, R. M. (1968). *Proc. Natl. Acad. Sci. U.S.A.* **60,** 134.

Hansburg, D., Briles, D., and Davie, J. M. (1976). *J. Immunol.* **117,** 569.

Greenblatt, J. J., Bernstein, D., Bokisch, V. A., and Krause R. M. (1973). *J. Immunol.* **110,** 862.

Kelus, A. S., and Weiss, S. (1977). *Nature (London)* **265,** 156.

Kimball, J. W., Pappenheimer, A. M., and Jaton, J.-C. (1971). *J. Immunol.* **106,** 1177.

Kolb, H. (1976). *J. Immunol.* **117,** 1711.

Miller, E. J., Osterland, C. K., Davie, J. M., and Krause, R. M. (1967). *J. Immunol.* **98,** 710.

Montgomery, P. C., Rockey, J. H., Kahn, R. L., and Skandera, C. A. (1975). *J. Immunol.* **115,** 904.

Osterland, C. K., Miller, E. J., Karakawa, W. W., and Krause, R. M. (1966). *J. Exp. Med.* **123,** 599.

Pincus, J. H., Jaton, J.-C., Bloch, K. J., and Haber, E. (1970). *J. Immunol.* **104,** 1143.

Pincus, J. H., Mage, R. G., Alexander, C., and Chase, N. M. (1973). *Eur. J. Immunol.* **3,** 435.

Schleifer, K.-H., and Krause, R. M. (1971). *Eur. J. Biochem.* **19**, 471.

Stankus, R. P., and Leslie, G. A. (1976). *Immunogenetics* **3**, 65.

Strosberg, A. D., Hamers-Easterman, C., Van der Loo, H. W., and Hamers R. (1974). *J. Immunol.* **113**, 1313.

Weiss, S., Kelus, A. S., and Braun, D. G. (1977). *J. Exp. Med.* **146**, 1195.

27

Limiting Dilution Analysis

Ivan Lefkovits

IMMUNOLOGICAL METHODS

I. OBJECTIVE

The objective of the microculture technique is to analyze the frequency of rare cells involved in the immune response. The precursors of antibody-forming cells (B cells), helper T cells, and suppressor T cells are considered rare cells. The microculture assay further allows the assessment of the average clone size of the progeny of precursors, the class, the allotype, and other characteristics of the products of B cells.

II. PRINCIPLE OF THE METHOD

Many small aliquots of lymphoid cells are cultured in the presence of antigen. The number of cells in each aliquot is chosen so that a considerable fraction of cultures will not contain any precursor cell. From the fraction of nonresponding cultures, using the Poisson formula, it is possible to calculate the frequency of precursor cells (Lefkovits, 1972; Quintáns and Lefkovits, 1973).

The analysis of the fraction of nonresponding cultures is performed, as a rule, on the culture fluid. Samples of culture fluid are removed by an automated replicator and deposited on an assay plate (Lefkovits and Kamber, 1972). Complement-dependent zones of lysis mark the cultures that have produced antibody.

Often the analysis is extended to cells; in this case, PFC's are estimated from each individual culture. In most instances the plain fluctuation test at a single cell concentration is difficult to interpret, and a more complex analysis, called "limiting dilution analysis," is used. This analysis is conducted within a range of lymphoid cell dose where it can be ensured that only the "titrated" type of cells is limited.

III. MATERIALS

A. Media

1. Preparation Medium

Eagle's minimal essential medium, with Earle's salts, without bicarbonate [Grand Island Biological Co. (Gibco), 109S]

2. Culture Medium

Medium A
   100 ml of MEM for suspension cultures, MA (Microbiological Associates, Bethesda, Maryland) 12126

1 ml of L-glutamine (200 mM), MA 17605F

1 ml of nonessential amino acids (100×), MA 13114

1 ml of sodium pyruvate (100 mM), MA 13115

1 ml of a streptomycin–penicillin mixture (5000 U/ml each), MA 17603F

2 ml of Hepes buffer (1 M), MA 17737

0.3 ml of 2-mercaptoethanol (14 mM), Merck

5.5 ml of fetal calf serum, Reheis Co., Armor Pharmaceutical Co., Kanakee, Illinois

Medium B

80 ml of RPMI 1640, MA 12702

1 ml of L-glutamine, MA 17605F

1 ml of a streptomycin–penicillin mixture (5000 U/ml each), MA 17603F

0.3 ml of 2-mercaptoethanol (14 mM), Merck

20 ml of fetal calf serum, Reheis Co. or Gibco

3. Maintenance Medium (Nutritional Cocktail)

15 ml of Eagle's MEM, Gibco 109S

2 ml of essential amino acids (50×), MA 13606

1 ml of nonessential amino acids (100×), MA 13114

1 ml of L-glutamine (200 mM), MA 17605F

3 ml of sodium bicarbonate (7.5%), MA 17613

0.4 ml of glucose (50%), Difco 0973-60-0

10 ml of fetal calf serum, Reheis Co.

B. Antigens

Red cells (50 μl of a 1% red cell suspension/ml of a lymphoid cell suspension)

Streptococcal vaccines (3 μg of rhamnose/ml of a lymphoid cell suspension)

Pneumococcus vaccines (10^6 heat-killed rough *Pneumococcus* strain R36A/ml of lymphoid cell suspension)

C. Indicator Red Cells

Red cells aged for about 1 week (kept in Alsever's solution), washed three times by centrifugation, and resuspended in PBS or BSS

D. Complement

Oray 20 (Behringwerke AG, Marburg-Lahn) diluted 1:10 in Dulbecco's PBS

E. Plastic and Glass Material

Tissue culture trays (Falcon Plastics, Type 3034)
Tissue culture dishes (Falcon Plastics, Types 3001 and 3002)
Tubes (Falcon Plastics, Types 2006 and 2070)
Petri dishes, 10 cm (Falcon Plastics, Greiner, or Sterilin)

F. Multi-Syringe Dispensers (Fig. 1)

Hamilton No. 83729: six syringes holding 500 μl each and delivering 10 μl
at a time
Hamilton No. 83726: six syringes holding 50 μl each and delivering 1 μl
at a time

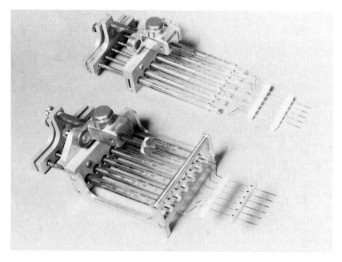

Fig. 1. The Hamilton multi-syringe dispenser with six syringes assembled in a row. Each syringe holds 500 μl and delivers 10 μl at a time. Two modifications of the instrument are shown. Careful washing of the syringes with sterile medium (filling and emptying the dispenser 10–15 times) satisfies the requirements for sterile work.

G. Replicator (Fig. 2)

The replicator is produced in small series by Biotec (Basel, Switzerland); it simultaneously removes 60 samples from a tissue culture tray and releases them onto an assay plate or into a sampling rack (Lefkovits and Kamber, 1972).

The replicator consists of four main parts: vacuum chamber, calibrated

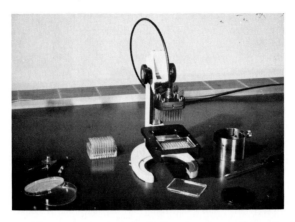

Fig. 2. Replicator. The instrument can simultaneously remove all samples from a 60-well tissue culture tray and release them on an assay plate that contains agar with embedded indicator cells (red cells). Tissue culture tray sampling racks and assay plate are also shown.

dosage plate, rubber membrane, and dispensing unit. The calibrated dosage plate is exchangeable. The volume of a "pocket" determines the volume of the sample drawn into the corresponding needle. The four components are locked together by four easily removable screws. The replicator is attached to a microscope stand, with a stage for the microculture tray. The vacuum chamber is connected through a vacuum pedal to a vacuum pump. The replicator is connected to a pulse generator, which takes care of rinsing the replicator by applying a preselected number of vacuum pulses. (This pulse generator is not available commercially, and it is not of crucial importance.)

When samples are to be removed from a microculture tray, the tray is placed on the stage, and the replicator needles are lowered and immersed into the culture fluid in the wells. Vacuum is then applied by pressing the vacuum pedal, and 60 samples are withdrawn into the needles of the dispensing unit. The replicator is lifted, an agar plate or a sampling rack is placed beneath the dispensing unit, the vacuum is released, and the agar (or the sampling rack) is gently touched with the droplets on the tips of the replicator. The dispensing unit is then lowered into a container with PBS and the pulse generator is operated to rinse the replicator.

H. Sampling Rack

A rack containing 60 disposable plastic tubes (diameter 8 mm) is used. The tubes touch each other; metal rods at the bottom of the rack hold the tubes in position even when the rack is not completely filled.

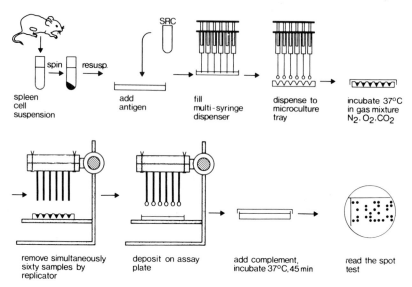

Fig. 3. Flow diagram of the basic operations of the microculture technique.

IV. METHODS (FIG. 3, FLOW DIAGRAM)

A. Setting Up the Microcultures

The preparation of cell suspensions is identical to that described in the chapter on Mishell–Dutton cultures (Chapter 24). Briefly, mice are killed by cervical dislocation. Their spleens are removed aseptically and placed into a sterile 60-mm culture dish containing 3 ml of chilled preparation medium per spleen. The cells are gently teased, using a pair of surgical forceps. The medium is then transferred into a test tube for 5 min. At the end of this period, when most of the clumps have settled, the supernatant is transferred to a centrifuge tube and the cells are spun at 500 g for 10 min. The cells are taken up in a small volume of culture medium, counted, and brought to a final concentration of $1-2 \times 10^7$ cells/ml.

Antigen is added in the form of about 50 μl of a 1% heterologous red cells per milliliter of spleen suspension (or 50 μl of another kind of antigen, such as *Streptococcus* vaccine, *Pneumococcus* heat-killed bacteria, or soluble protein) and the mixture is drawn into a multi-syringe dispenser. Then, 10 μl is dispensed into each of the 60 wells of a tissue culture tray, about 0.4 ml of medium is pipetted into the peripheral groove to maintain the humidity, and the plates are covered. The incubation box is first perfused with a mixture of 83% N_2, 10% CO_2, and 7% O_2 and then sealed and incubated at 37°C.

B. Maintenance of Cultures

A standard experiment takes 4–6 days. If the microcultures are performed in MEM, daily feeding with maintenance medium (nutritional cocktail) is necessary. Cultures performed in RPMI medium do not need to be fed. Feeding is done through a sterile multi-syringe dispenser. One microliter of the maintenance medium is added to each well by lowering the droplets onto the surface of the microculture. The incubation box is regassed after feeding and further incubated at 37°C. Too frequent opening is to be avoided, as some of the medium in the wells will evaporate.

C. Determination of the Response

1. Hemolytic Spot Test

A plate containing a layer of agar is predried for 1 hr at 37°C (bottom layer) and is then overlaid with an agar top layer containing red cells (for a detailed description of the preparation of the agar bottom and top layers, see Chapter 19). Samples of the medium are taken with the replicator and released onto the plate (volume of the droplets, 2 μl). When the droplets have soaked in, 2 ml of complement is added and the plates are incubated for 45 min at 37°C. Zones of lysis mark the cultures that have produced

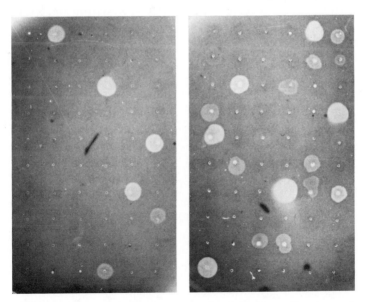

Fig. 4. Hemolytic spot test for antibody response in microcultures. Complement-dependent zones of lysis mark the cultures that have produced antibody. (From Lefkovits, 1974, Precommitment in the Immune System, *Curr. Top. Microbiol. Immunol.* **65**, 21.)

antibody (Fig. 4). The plates may be fixed by covering them with 5 ml of 0.25% glutaraldehyde in PBS.

2. PFC Test

a. Rough Estimate. The microculture tray is spun down (500 *g* for 5 min) and the tray is flooded with BSS. The excess BSS is removed, and the cells are dispersed by pulsing the replicator five to ten times. Aliquots are transferred to a plate containing bottom agar. The droplets are allowed to soak in and are then overlaid with top agar containing red cells and incubated for 1 hr at 37°C. Then 2 ml of complement is added and the test is read after a further 45-min incubation at 37°C. The number of plaques in each sample is recorded.

b. Assay of Individual Wells. The microculture tray is spun down (500 *g* for 5 min) and the tray is flooded with BSS. The excess BSS is removed and samples from each well are assayed using Cunningham's modification of Jerne's plaque assay (see Chapter 19).

D. Limiting Dilution Analysis

The result of a typical microculture experiment is that only a certain fraction of microcultures respond. Because there are three cell populations—B cells, T cells, and macrophages—involved in the response, it is by no means certain that a nonresponding microculture lacks the specific cell that is being titrated. To estimate the frequency of B precursor cells with confidence, it is necessary to manipulate separately the cells involved, so as to ensure that only the B precursor cells are limiting. The following strategy is used to ensure that nonresponding wells will correspond to those microcultures that lack only the B precursor cell specific to SRC.

1. Spleen cells from nude mice are the source of B cells. They are titrated over the range 1×10^4–1.8×10^5 nude spleen cells per microculture.

2. A functional excess of T-cell activity is ensured either by allogeneic complementation or by adding helper factor. The number of allogeneic spleen cells is kept constant: 2–4×10^4 cells per microculture. [If the contribution of B cells to the response present among the allogeneic cells should be prevented, irradiation of allogeneic cells (1200 rad) is performed.]

3. Constant cell density is maintained by compensating the titrated active nude spleen cells with irradiated nude spleen cells. Since macrophages are thought to be radioresistant, the constant cell density ensures a constant number of macrophages.

E. Protocol for B-Cell Titration (Fig. 5).

Two protocols for B-cell titration are shown in Table I.

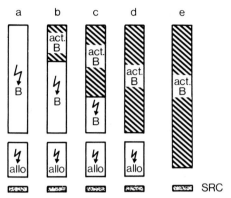

Fig. 5. Protocol for B-cell titration. Representation of the mixing proportions of the three cell suspensions (nude spleen cells, irradiated nude spleen cells, and irradiated allogeneic spleen cells); a, b, c, d, and e refer to the five groups shown in Table I.

TABLE I

Two Protocols for B-Cell Titration[a]

Group	Irradiated allogeneic cells (ml)	Irradiated nude cells (ml)	Active nude cells (ml)	SRC (drops)	Active nude cells per 10 μl of culture
a	0.5	1.5	—	2	0
b	0.5	1	0.5	2	5×10^4
c	0.5	0.5	1	2	1×10^5
d	0.5	—	1.5	2	1.5×10^5
e	—	—	2	2	2×10^5

Group	Helper factor (ml)	Irradiated nude cells (ml)	Active nude cells (ml)	SRC (drops)	Active nude cells per 10 μl of culture
a	1	1	—	2	0
b	1	0.75	0.25	2	5×10^4
c	1	0.5	0.5	2	1×10^5
d	1	0.25	0.75	2	1.5×10^5
e	—	—	1 ml + 1 ml of medium	2	2×10^5

[a] *Top protocol:* The cell density for all three stock cell suspensions is 2×10^7/ml. The final cell density for all five groups is 2×10^7/ml. Group e is the control group. *Bottom protocol:* The cell density for both stock cell suspensions is 4×10^7/ml. The final cell density for all five groups is 2×10^7/ml. Group e is the control group. The amount of the helper factor can be easily varied. Usually allogeneic factor is less active than Con A helper factor. In the above protocol, a 1:1 addition is considered. If Con A factor is used, often a 1:5 dilution is satisfactory. A preliminary test of activity is advisable.

F. The Semilogarithmic Plot

If B cells are randomly and independently distributed throughout the wells, the number of precursors per well follows a Poisson distribution. The mean number of precursor cells can be calculated from the observed proportion of negative cultures using the Poisson formula,

$$F_r = \frac{u^r}{r!} \cdot e^{-u}$$

where F_r is the fraction of cultures containing r precursor cells, u is the mean number of precursor cells per well, and r is the actual number of precursor cells in a microculture well $(0, 1, 2, 3, \ldots)$.

The zero term of the Poisson equation is

$$F_0 = e^{-u}$$

The logarithms of the equation are

$$\ln F_0 = -u$$
$$\ln F_0 = u$$

which means that the negative logarithm of the fraction of nonresponding cultures is linearly proportional to the mean number of precursor cells per well.

If we plot on the y-axis the negative logarithm of the fraction of nonresponding cultures $(-\ln F_0)$ and on the x-axis on linear scale the cell input, the experimental points are expected to fit a straight line.

The above equation simplifies for $u = 1$:

$$F_0 = e^{-1} = 0.37$$

Thus, when the mean number of precursor cells per well is one, 37% of the wells will remain negative.

Figure 6 shows the plot of a limiting dilution analysis of B cells. This is an example of the semilogarithmic plot. Interpolating at the level of 0.37 we read 3×10^4. Thus, 3×10^4 B cells contain, on average, *one* precursor B cell. The frequency of precursor cells is $1/(3 \times 10^4) = 3.3 \times 10^{-5}$.

G. Protocol for T-Cell Titration

The principle for the T-cell titration (shown in Table II) is the same as that for the B-cell titration. There is, however, one major difference. In the T-cell titration, each microculture well contains more than one B precursor cell, and the T cells are limiting (Waldmann *et al.*, 1975). Often there is a considerable background response in the absence of any external T-cell

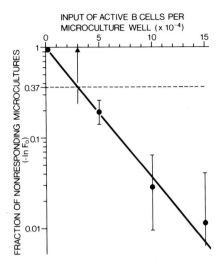

Fig. 6. Limiting dilution of B cells. All microcultures contained a constant number of irradiated allogeneic cells (5×10^4 per microculture). Irradiated and nonirradiated (active) nude spleen cells were mixed at different ratios to give 1.5×10^5 total nude spleen cells per well. The abscissa indicates the input of active nude spleen cells per microculture. The ordinate indicates the fraction of nonresponding microcultures ($-\ln F_0$). Each point is based on spot tests from three trays (180 microcultures). About 3×10^4 active B cells correspond to 37% negative microcultures (frequency, $f = 3.3 \times 10^{-5}$).

TABLE II

Protocol for T-Cell Titration[a]

Group	Active nude cells (ml)	Medium (ml)	Helper T cells (ml)	SRC (drops)	Helper T cells per 10 μl of culture
a	1	1	—	2	0
b	1	0.8	0.2	2	2×10^4
c	1	0.6	0.4	2	4×10^4
d	1	0.4	0.6	2	6×10^4

[a] The cell density of the nude spleen cell suspension is 1.5×10^7/ml. The cell density of the T-cell stock cell suspension is 1×10^7/ml. The final cell density is not constant (range, 1.5×10^7–2.1×10^7). Irradiated T cells cannot be used for keeping the cell density constant, because irradiation does not abolish the helper activity and irradiated cells would contribute to T-cell help.

influence. This background response is not observed in all experiments, but, if it happens, it might be a considerable obstacle in analyzing the results.

H. Protocol for Suppressor-Cell Titration

The protocol is essentially the same as that for T-cell titration. The only change is that a constant volume of helper factor is added to the cultures.

The results are plotted again in a semilogarithmic fashion; it should be noted that not F_0 but F_+ is plotted, because here the zero term is based on cultures that do not contain a suppressor cell, with the consequence that such cultures do respond.

The results of a suppressor cell titration are shown in Fig. 7. The frequency of suppressor cells here is 1 in 10^4, thus 10^{-4}.

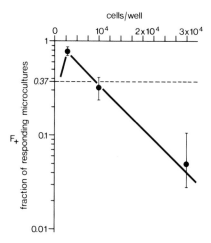

Fig. 7. Limiting dilution of suppressor cells. All microcultures contained a constant number of nude spleen cells (10^5 per microculture) and adequate helper activity. Suppressor cells were added, but the cell density was not corrected for. The abscissa indicates the input of suppressor cells per microculture. The ordinate indicates the fraction of responding microcultures; note that the fraction of *responding* cultures is plotted here, whereas in the limiting dilution of B cells the fraction of *nonresponding* cultures is plotted. (Data shown were obtained in an experiment performed in collaboration with Ron Corley and Bernice Kindred.)

I. Clone Size Estimation

To calculate the clone size, the value of u, the mean number of precursor cells per well, must be known. This value is calculated from the Poisson formula or read from a titration curve. The theoretical number of clones

(N) is then $N = wu$, w being the number of wells assayed for plaque-forming cells. The average clone size, $\bar{c}$, is given by

$$\bar{c} = (\Sigma \text{PFC})/N$$

where ΣPFC is the total number of PFC found in w wells (Quintáns and Lefkovits, 1974).

V. LIMITATIONS AND SENSITIVITY

A. Spot Test

If clones of a very small size are expected (two to five plaque-forming cells), false negative spots might be obtained. In such an instance, a PFC test from individual wells must be performed. This is of crucial importance when the response to certain thymus-independent antigens is measured. With "normal" thymus-dependent antigens, there is no problem with false negatives, except when the response on day 2 or 3 is measured. In this case again a PFC test from individual wells is recommended.

B. Deviation from Linearity

For the purpose of calculating the frequency of precursor cells, only the results that conform to a single-hit kinetics (straight line on a semi-logarithmic plot) can be interpreted unambiguously. Where multi-hit or multi-target kinetics is obtained, I suggest not to attempt to compute the frequency of precursor cells.

If plotted points deviate considerably from linearity, the only conclusion that can be drawn at present is that (a) more than one cell type is limiting, (b) more than one cell is needed for a response, or (c) more than one cell is needed to detect a response.

In many *in vitro* systems the range of cell density in which antibody response can be obtained is very narrow; alternatively, saturation with one kind of cells cannot be achieved. This is, for example, the case with rabbit lymphocytes (see Chapter 25). If a full titration with graded numbers of lymphoid cells cannot be performed, the calculated frequencies are called "frequency of responding units" rather than "frequency of precursor cells."

C. 95% Confidence Limits (Table III)

The number of cultures for each experimental point should never be less than 60. Whenever possible, 120 or even 180 cultures should be used. The

TABLE III

Calculation of Confidence Limits[a]

		$W_T = 60$				$W_T = 120$				
		95% confidence limits				95% confidence limits				95% confidence limits
w_R	F_0	Lower	Upper	w_R	F_0	Lower	Upper	w_R	F_0	Lower Upper
0	1	0.94	–1	0	1	0.97–1				
1	0.98	0.91	–1	1	0.99	0.95–1		61	0.49	0.40 –0.58
2	0.97	0.88	–1	2	0.98	0.94–1		62	0.48	0.39 –0.58
3	0.95	0.86	–0.99	3	0.98	0.93–0.99		63	0.48	0.38 –0.57
4	0.93	0.84	–0.98	4	0.97	0.92–0.99		64	0.47	0.38 –0.56
5	0.92	0.82	–0.97	5	0.96	0.90–0.99		65	0.46	0.37 –0.55
6	0.90	0.79	–0.96	6	0.95	0.89–0.98		66	0.45	0.36 –0.54
7	0.88	0.77	–0.95	7	0.94	0.88–0.98		67	0.44	0.35 –0.54
8	0.89	0.75	–0.94	8	0.93	0.87–0.97		68	0.43	0.34 –0.53
9	0.85	0.73	–0.93	9	0.93	0.86–0.97		69	0.43	0.34 –0.52
10	0.83	0.71	–0.92	10	0.92	0.85–0.96		70	0.42	0.33 –0.51
11	0.82	0.70	–0.90	11	0.91	0.84–0.95		71	0.41	0.32 –0.50
12	0.80	0.68	–0.89	12	0.90	0.83–0.95		72	0.40	0.31 –0.49
13	0.78	0.66	–0.88	13	0.89	0.82–0.94		73	0.39	0.30 –0.49
14	0.77	0.64	–0.87	14	0.88	0.81–0.93		74	0.38	0.30 –0.48
15	0.75	0.62	–0.85	15	0.88	0.80–0.93		75	0.38	0.29 –0.47
16	0.73	0.60	–0.84	16	0.87	0.79–0.92		76	0.37	0.28 –0.46
17	0.72	0.59	–0.83	17	0.86	0.78–0.92		77	0.36	0.27 –0.45
18	0.70	0.57	–0.81	18	0.85	0.77–0.91		78	0.35	0.27 –0.44
19	0.68	0.55	–0.80	19	0.84	0.76–0.90		79	0.34	0.26 –0.43
20	0.67	0.53	–0.78	20	0.83	0.75–0.89		80	0.33	0.25 –0.43
21	0.65	0.52	–0.77	21	0.83	0.74–0.89		81	0.33	0.24 –0.42
22	0.63	0.50	–0.75	22	0.82	0.74–0.88		82	0.32	0.24 –0.41
23	0.62	0.48	–0.74	23	0.81	0.73–0.87		83	0.31	0.23 –0.40
24	0.60	0.47	–0.72	24	0.80	0.72–0.87		84	0.30	0.22 –0.39
25	0.58	0.45	–0.71	25	0.79	0.71–0.86		85	0.29	0.21 –0.38
26	0.57	0.43	–0.69	26	0.78	0.70–0.85		86	0.28	0.21 –0.37
27	0.55	0.42	–0.68	27	0.78	0.69–0.85		87	0.28	0.20 –0.36
28	0.53	0.40	–0.66	28	0.77	0.68–0.84		88	0.27	0.19 –0.36
29	0.52	0.38	–0.65	29	0.76	0.67–0.83		89	0.26	0.18 –0.35
30	0.50	0.37	–0.63	30	0.75	0.66–0.82		90	0.25	0.18 –0.34
31	0.48	0.35	–0.62	31	0.74	0.65–0.82		91	0.24	0.17 –0.33
32	0.47	0.34	–0.60	32	0.73	0.64–0.81		92	0.23	0.16 –0.32
33	0.45	0.32	–0.58	33	0.73	0.64–0.80		93	0.23	0.15 –0.31
34	0.43	0.31	–0.57	34	0.72	0.63–0.79		94	0.22	0.15 –0.30
35	0.42	0.29	–0.55	35	0.71	0.62–0.79		95	0.21	0.14 –0.29
36	0.40	0.28	–0.53	36	0.70	0.61–0.78		96	0.20	0.133–0.28
37	0.38	0.26	–0.52	37	0.69	0.60–0.77		97	0.19	0.126–0.27
38	0.37	0.25	–0.50	38	0.68	0.59–0.76		98	0.18	0.119–0.26
39	0.35	0.23	–0.48	39	0.68	0.58–0.76		99	0.18	0.112–0.26
40	0.33	0.22	–0.47	40	0.67	0.57–0.75		100	0.17	0.105–0.25
41	0.32	0.20	–0.45	41	0.66	0.57–0.74		101	0.16	0.098–0.24
42	0.30	0.19	–0.43	42	0.65	0.56–0.73		102	0.15	0.092–0.23
43	0.28	0.17	–0.41	43	0.64	0.55–0.73		103	0.14	0.085–0.22
44	0.27	0.16	–0.40	44	0.63	0.54–0.72		104	0.133	0.078–0.21
45	0.25	0.15	–0.38	45	0.63	0.53–0.71		105	0.125	0.072–0.20
46	0.23	0.134	–0.36	46	0.62	0.52–0.70		106	0.117	0.065–0.19
47	0.22	0.120	–0.34	47	0.61	0.51–0.70		107	0.108	0.059–0.18
48	0.20	0.110	–0.32	48	0.60	0.51–0.69		108	0.100	0.053–0.17
49	0.18	0.095	–0.30	49	0.59	0.50–0.68		109	0.092	0.047–0.16
50	0.17	0.083	–0.29	50	0.58	0.49–0.67		110	0.083	0.041–0.15
51	0.15	0.071	–0.27	51	0.58	0.48–0.66		111	0.075	0.035–0.138
52	0.133	0.060	–0.25	52	0.57	0.47–0.66		112	0.067	0.029–0.128
53	0.117	0.048	–0.23	53	0.56	0.46–0.65		113	0.058	0.024–0.117
54	0.100	0.038	–0.21	54	0.55	0.46–0.64		114	0.050	0.018–0.106
55	0.083	0.028	–0.18	55	0.54	0.45–0.63		115	0.042	0.013–0.095
56	0.067	0.018	–0.16	56	0.53	0.44–0.62		116	0.033	0.009–0.083
57	0.050	0.010	–0.14	57	0.53	0.43–0.62		117	0.025	0.005–0.071
58	0.033	0.004	–0.115	58	0.52	0.42–0.61		118	0.017	0.002–0.059
59	0.017	0.001	–0.089	59	0.51	0.42–0.60		119	0.008	0. –0.046
60	0	0	–0.060	60	0.50	0.41–0.59		120	0	0 –0.030

[a] W_T, number of microculture wells tested;

W_R, number of responding microcultures;

F_0, fraction of nonresponding microcultures.

Adopted from Documenta Geigy (K. Diem, ed.), Basel.

			$W_T = 180$					
		95% confidence limits			95% confidence limits			95% confidence limits
w_R	F_r	Lower Upper	w_R	F_0	Lower Upper	w_R	F_0	Lower Upper
0	1	0.98–1						
1	0.99	0.97–1	61	0.66	0.59–0.73	121	0.33	0.26 –0.40
2	0.99	0.96–1	62	0.66	0.58–0.72	122	0.33	0.26 –0.40
3	0.98	0.95–1	63	0.65	0.58–0.72	123	0.32	0.25 –0.39
4	0.98	0.94–0.99	64	0.64	0.57–0.71	124	0.31	0.24 –0.38
5	0.97	0.94–0.99	65	0.64	0.56–0.71	125	0.31	0.24 –0.38
6	0.97	0.93–0.99	66	0.63	0.56–0.70	126	0.30	0.23 –0.37
7	0.96	0.92–0.98	67	0.63	0.55–0.70	127	0.29	0.23 –0.37
8	0.96	0.91–0.98	68	0.62	0.55–0.69	128	0.29	0.22 –0.36
9	0.95	0.91–0.98	69	0.62	0.54–0.69	129	0.28	0.22 –0.36
10	0.94	0.90–0.97	70	0.61	0.54–0.68	130	0.28	0.21 –0.35
11	0.94	0.89–0.97	71	0.61	0.53–0.68	131	0.27	0.21 –0.34
12	0.93	0.89–0.97	72	0.60	0.52–0.67	132	0.27	0.20 –0.34
13	0.93	0.88–0.96	73	0.59	0.52–0.67	133	0.26	0.20 –0.33
14	0.92	0.87–0.96	74	0.59	0.51–0.66	134	0.26	0.19 –0.33
15	0.92	0.87–0.95	75	0.58	0.51–0.66	135	0.25	0.19 –0.32
16	0.91	0.86–0.95	76	0.58	0.50–0.65	136	0.24	0.18 –0.31
17	0.91	0.85–0.94	77	0.57	0.50–0.64	137	0.24	0.18 –0.31
18	0.90	0.85–0.94	78	0.57	0.49–0.64	138	0.23	0.17 –0.30
19	0.89	0.84–0.94	79	0.56	0.49–0.63	139	0.23	0.17 –0.30
20	0.89	0.83–0.93	80	0.56	0.48–0.63	140	0.22	0.16 –0.29
21	0.88	0.83–0.93	81	0.55	0.47–0.62	141	0.22	0.16 –0.28
22	0.88	0.82–0.92	82	0.54	0.47–0.62	142	0.21	0.15 –0.28
23	0.87	0.81–0.92	83	0.54	0.46–0.61	143	0.21	0.15 –0.27
24	0.87	0.81–0.91	84	0.53	0.46–0.61	144	0.20	0.14 –0.27
25	0.86	0.80–0.91	85	0.53	0.45–0.60	145	0.19	0.14 –0.26
26	0.86	0.80–0.90	86	0.52	0.45–0.60	146	0.19	0.135–0.25
27	0.85	0.79–0.90	87	0.52	0.44–0.59	147	0.18	0.130–0.25
28	0.84	0.78–0.89	88	0.51	0.44–0.59	148	0.18	0.125–0.24
29	0.84	0.78–0.89	89	0.51	0.43–0.58	149	0.17	0.120–0.24
30	0.83	0.77–0.88	90	0.50	0.42–0.58	150	0.17	0.116–0.23
31	0.83	0.76–0.88	91	0.49	0.42–0.57	151	0.16	0.111–0.22
32	0.82	0.76–0.87	92	0.49	0.41–0.56	152	0.16	0.106–0.22
33	0.82	0.76–0.87	93	0.48	0.41–0.56	153	0.15	0.101–0.21
34	0.81	0.75–0.87	94	0.48	0.40–0.55	154	0.14	0.097–0.20
35	0.81	0.75–0.86	95	0.47	0.40–0.55	155	0.14	0.092–0.20
36	0.80	0.74–0.86	96	0.47	0.39–0.54	156	0.133	0.087–0.19
37	0.79	0.73–0.85	97	0.46	0.39–0.54	157	0.128	0.083–0.19
38	0.79	0.73–0.85	98	0.46	0.38–0.53	158	0.122	0.078–0.18
39	0.78	0.72–0.84	99	0.45	0.38–0.53	159	0.117	0.074–0.17
40	0.78	0.71–0.84	100	0.44	0.37–0.52	160	0.111	0.069–0.17
41	0.77	0.70–0.83	101	0.44	0.37–0.51	161	0.106	0.065–0.16
42	0.77	0.70–0.83	102	0.43	0.36–0.51	162	0.100	0.060–0.15
43	0.76	0.69–0.82	103	0.43	0.36–0.50	163	0.094	0.056–0.15
44	0.76	0.69–0.82	104	0.42	0.35–0.50	164	0.089	0.051–0.14
45	0.75	0.68–0.81	105	0.42	0.34–0.49	165	0.083	0.047–0.134
46	0.74	0.67–0.81	106	0.41	0.34–0.49	166	0.078	0.043–0.127
47	0.74	0.67–0.80	107	0.41	0.33–0.48	167	0.072	0.039–0.121
48	0.73	0.66–0.80	108	0.40	0.33–0.48	168	0.067	0.035–0.114
49	0.73	0.66–0.79	109	0.39	0.32–0.47	169	0.061	0.031–0.107
50	0.72	0.65–0.79	110	0.39	0.32–0.46	170	0.056	0.027–0.100
51	0.72	0.64–0.78	111	0.38	0.31–0.46	171	0.050	0.023–0.093
52	0.71	0.64–0.78	112	0.38	0.31–0.45	172	0.044	0.019–0.086
53	0.71	0.63–0.77	113	0.37	0.30–0.45	173	0.039	0.016–0.079
54	0.70	0.63–0.77	114	0.37	0.30–0.44	174	0.033	0.012–0.072
55	0.69	0.62–0.76	115	0.36	0.29–0.44	175	0.028	0.009–0.064
56	0.69	0.62–0.76	116	0.36	0.29–0.43	176	0.022	0.006–0.056
57	0.68	0.61–0.75	117	0.35	0.28–0.42	177	0.017	0.004–0.048
58	0.68	0.60–0.74	118	0.34	0.28–0.42	178	0.011	0 –0.040
59	0.67	0.60–0.74	119	0.34	0.27–0.41	179	0.006	0 –0.031
60	0.67	0.59–0.73	120	0.33	0.27–0.41	180	0	0 –0.020

greater the number of cultures, the narrower the 95% confidence limits, thus enabling the experimenter to obtain a better analysis of the data. The titration curve shown in Fig. 6 is based on 180 cultures per experimental point, and it can be seen that the range of 95% confidence limits for some points is still quite wide. Tests based on 10 cultures are so are by no means acceptable.

D. Efficiency of Stimulation

We know very little about the efficiency of our culture system. We know only that we can detect most of the clones that are "switched on," but the percentage of precursor cells switched on compared to that of an *in vivo* situation is not known. Furthermore, it is also not known whether there exists a pool of precursor cells already committed to antibody specificity but not yet antigen sensitive (though perhaps mitogen sensitive).

E. Delayed Assay

When a response is measured in terms of plaque-forming cells (in conventional cultures or microcultures), it is of obvious importance to measure the response on the day the peak is expected to appear. The spot test measures the accummulated product; therefore, the test will be positive even if the clone has disappeared. If, at any time during the culture, antibody was produced, it can be detected. It is a convenient feature of microcultures that the analysis can be postponed for several days beyond the peak, if necessary.

SUGGESTED READING

Lefkovits, I. (1974). Precommitment in the immune system. *Curr. Top. Microbiol. Immunol.* **65**, 21.

Lefkovits, I., Quintáns, J., Munro, A., and Waldmann, H. (1975). T-cell dependent mediator and B-cell clones. *Immunology* **28**, 1149.

Luria, S. E., and Delbrück, M. (1943). Mutation of bacteria from virus sensitivity to virus resistance. *Genetics* **28**, 491.

REFERENCES

Lefkovits, I. (1972). *Eur. J. Immunol.* **2**, 360.

Lefkovits, I., and Kamber, O. (1972). *Eur. J. Immunol.* **2**, 365.

Quintáns, J., and Lefkovits, I. (1973). *Eur. J. Immunol.* **3**, 392.

Quintáns, J., and Lefkovits, I. (1974). *Eur. J. Immunol.* **4**, 617.

Waldmann, H., Lefkovits, I., and Quintáns, J. (1975). *Immunology* **28**, 1135.

28

Establishment and Maintenance of Murine Lymphoid Cell Lines in Culture

Max H. Schreier and Bernd J. Weimann

I. OBJECTIVE

Clones of murine B and T lymphomas provide uniform cell populations, representing distinct stages of lymphoid cell differentiation. Since they are readily propagated *in vivo* or adapted to continous culture *in vitro*, they may be used for the study of any cell-surface receptor, heteroantigen, and alloantigen, thus leading to a better understanding of the structural and functional heterogeneity of the cell populations comprising the immune system. *In vitro* propagation has the advantage that it is free of contamination by host cells or passive absorption of host cell products (e.g.,

IMMUNOLOGICAL METHODS
Copyright © 1979 by Academic Press, Inc.
All rights of reproduction in any form reserved.
ISBN 0-12-442750-2

antibody)—either one a potential source of false interpretations. In addition, cultured cells can be cloned for different features, their growth characteristics and requirements can be defined, and mutants can be selected.

This chapter describes the methods we use to establish *in vitro* cell lines from spontaneously arising AKR thymomas and Abelson murine leukemia virus (A-MuLV)-induced lymphosarcomas. The induction of tumors by A-MuLV *in vivo* will be outlined in detail.

II. PRINCIPLE OF THE METHOD

A. AKR Thymomas

The AKR mouse strain was originally developed as an inbred line with a high incidence of spontaneously arising leukemia. AKR thymomas are caused by the vertical (genetic) transmission of an oncogenic endogenous virus. Thymomas can also be transmitted horizontally, as shown by Gross (1951), by inoculation of cell-free, leukemic extracts of AKR tumors into newborn C3H mice, which have an extremely low incidence of spontaneous leukemia. About 50% of these C3H mice developed leukemia at an age of 8 to 11 months. The incidence of leukemia in different sublines of AKR mice varies considerably (Acton *et al.*, 1973) and can be as high as 90% at an age of 9 months. The tumor cells express the θ-antigen on their surface. Cells of the most frequently used AKR/J subline carry the Thy 1.1 antigen (historical name, θ-AKR), whereas others, for example, AKR-Cum, have the thymus Thy 1.2 antigen (θ-C3H) (Acton *et al.*, 1973).

B. A-MuLV-Induced Lymphosarcomas

After injection of Moloney murine leukemia virus (Mo-MuLV) into a BALB/c mouse, whose thymus was maintained in an atrophic state by corticosteroid injection, Abelson and Rabstein (1970) isolated a new type of virus. Injection of this virus into newborn mice leads to neoplasms in as early as 3 to 4 weeks, affecting bone marrow, meninges, and peripheral lymph nodes. The thymus is not involved. This Abelson virus complex contains two C-type RNA viral genomes, as shown by Scher and Siegler (1975). The Abelson component transforms BALB/c and NIH-3T3 fibroblasts into foci of rounded cells. This transformation can be used as a quantitative assay. The helper activity, Mo-MuLV, in this complex can be quantitated by the XC plaque assay (Rowe *et al.*, 1970).

Neoplastic cells from spleen lymph nodes, or tumors are used for the establishment of cell lines.

III. MATERIALS

A. Salt Solutions and Media

The salt solutions used are as follows:

1. Hank's balanced salt solution (HBSS): 0.14 gm of $CaCl_2$, 0.4 gm of KCl, 0.06 gm of KH_2PO_4, 0.1 gm of $MgCl_2 \cdot 6\ H_2O$, 0.1 gm of $MgSO_4 \cdot 7\ H_2O$, 8.0 gm of NaCl, 0.35 gm of $NaHCO_3$, 0.06 gm of $Na_2HPO_4 \cdot 2\ H_2O$, and 0.01 gm of phenol red per 1 liter of distilled water.

2. Phosphate-buffered saline (PBS): 0.1 gm of $CaCl_2$, 0.2 gm of KH_2PO_4, 0.2 gm of KCl, 0.1 gm of $MgCl_2 \cdot 6\ H_2O$, 8.0 gm of NaCl, and 1.15 gm of $Na_2HPO_4 \cdot 2\ H_2O$ per 1 liter of distilled water.

Dulbecco's modified Eagle's medium (DME) and Eagle's minimum essential medium (MEM) are obtained from Grand Island Biological Company (Gibco) or from Flow Laboratories, Inc. (Irvine, Scotland).

The media are supplemented with 2 mM L-glutamine, 1 mM sodium pyruvate, 10 mM Hepes buffer (pH 7.3), antibiotics, and $5 \times 10^{-5}\ M$ 2-mercaptoethanol. Fetal calf serum and horse serum are heat-inactivated for 30 min at 56°C and used at 10 and 20% final concentrations, respectively.

B. Animals

Aging AKR/J mice as the source of spontaneous tumors and young adult syngeneic mice for *in vivo* serial passages of tumors, as well as BALB/c mice, are commercially available. Newborn mice of many strains, but preferably BALB/c, are used for Abelson tumor induction.

C. Cell Lines

NIH-3T3 cells (clone 1) (Jainchill *et al.*, 1969) are maintained in DME with 10% calf serum. XC cells (Svoboda *et al.*, 1963) (rat tumor cells induced by the Prague strain of Rous sarcoma virus, Pr-RSV) are carried in MEM with 10% fetal calf serum (FCS) as described by Klement *et al.* (1969). SC-1 cells are maintained in MEM with 5% FCS (Hartley and Rowe, 1975).

D. Viruses

Abelson viruses can be obtained either from cell-free extracts of solid tumors or from the medium of A-MuLV-transformed cells in culture. These cells continuously produce and secrete viruses (see Section IV).

IV. PROCEDURE

A. Preparation and Assay of the Virus

1. Virus from Solid Tumors

The preparation of viruses from solid tumors follows the methods of Moloney (1960) and Abelson and Rabstein (1970). About 10 gm of solid tumor in 90 ml of 0.153 M potassium citrate (pH 7.0) and 1.5 mg of hyaluronidase are homogenized with 20 up and down strokes in a Potter–Elveshjem homogenizer. The homogenate is stirred at room temperature for 1 hr and then centrifuged twice at 2500 g for 20 min. The supernatant is centrifuged for 10 min at 10,000 g, the pellet is discarded, and the supernatant is recentrifuged for 1 hr at 100,000 g. The deposited virus is resuspended in 0.05 M sodium citrate, pH 6.8, and centrifuged for 10 min at 10,000 g. Infective virus moves to the middle of the tube.

2. Virus from Cell Culture Medium

A-MuLV-transformed cells in culture continuously produce and secrete virus into the medium from which the virus is pelleted by centrifugation for 1 hr at 100,000 g. Pellets are suspended in a small volume of 0.14 M NaCl, 0.05 M Tris–HCl, pH 7.4, 0.1 mM EDTA and centrifuged in linear 20–60% sucrose gradients for 3 hr at 40,000 rpm in a Beckman Spinco SW 41 rotor. The virus bands at a mean density of 1.16 gm/cm^3. It is convenient first to concentrate viruses from large volumes of cell culture medium in an Amicon filtration device.

3. Direct Transformation of 3T3 Cells by Abelson Murine Leukemia Virus

This method is from Scher and Siegler (1975). BALB/c-3T3 or NIH-3T3 cells are trypsinized 1 day before virus inoculation and 1–2 × 10^5 cells per plastic dish (6 cm) are seeded in fresh medium containing 6–8 μg/ml of Polybrene (Aldrich Chemical Co., Milwaukee, Wisconsin). The medium is removed and cells are inoculated with the virus in 5 ml of fresh medium. Virus stocks are filtered through Millipore filters (0.45-μm pore size) before use. The medium is changed on day 5 and foci are scored on day 8 or 10. Transformed cells appear as foci of rounded cells on the fibroblast layer.

4. XC Plaque Assay

This method is detailed in Rowe *et al.* (1970). BALB/c-3T3, NIH-3T3, or SC-1 cells (Hartley and Rowe, 1975) can be used for the titration of the helper virus in the Abelson virus complex. BALB/c-3T3(A31) and NIH-

3T3 cells are maintained in DME with 10% FCS, and SC-1 cells are maintained in MEM–10% FCS. They are trypsinized and 2×10^5 cells per plastic dish (6 cm) are seeded 1 day before virus inoculation. After 24 hr the medium is removed and 0.5 ml of virus suspension in 5 ml of complete medium is added. The plate is then incubated for 4 days at 37°C. The medium is removed and cells are irradiated with ultraviolet light. The appropriate distance between the ultraviolet lamp and plate as well as the time of irradiation required for cell death should be determined in preliminary.experiments. Irradiated cells are then overlaid with 10^6 XC cells per plate and incubated for 2 days at 37°C in a humidified 5% CO_2 atmosphere. The medium is removed and the plate is washed once with PBS solution. Plaques can be scored under a dissecting microscope or stained for 7 min with 3 parts 1% methylene blue in methanol, 2 parts methanol, and 1 part carboxylfuchsin solution. The plates are rinsed with water and plaques are counted. Intact cells appear dark blue, whereas syncytia will be pinkish.

5. Induction and Development of Abelson Tumors

Mice, 12–24 hr after birth, are injected intraperitoneally with 0.05 ml of virus suspension. After a latent period of 3–4 weeks, tumors are palpable. and appear in the lymph nodes, bone marrow, spleen, and meninges (Fig. 1). Tumors can also be induced in young adult mice by intraperitoneal adminstration of 0.05 ml of the light mineral oil pristane (2,6,10,14-tetramethylpentadecane) followed by virus inoculation (Potter *et al.*, 1973).

B. Establishment and Early Maintenance of Cell Lines

The procedure for establishing cell lines from AKR thymomas and that for Abelson lymphosarcomas are essentially the same. Tumors are removed from the animals under aseptic conditions and placed in plastic tissue culture dishes containing 10 ml of HBSS. Connective tissue is removed and the tumors are minced with forceps and scissors. This method seems preferable to forcing the tumors through a stainless steel sieve since, in our hands, it gives a higher rate of takes *in vitro*. Large cell clumps and remaining pieces of connective tissue (which settle after 2–3 min) are discarded. The cell suspension is centrifuged for 10 min at 170 *g*, washed twice with HBSS, and then seeded in DME medium at cell densities of 2, 5, and 10×10^5 nucleated cells/ml in 25-cm² plastic tissue culture flasks or in petri dishes. Cell viability is measured by the exclusion of 0.05% trypan blue. The cultures are kept at 37°C in a humidified 5% CO_2 atmosphere. Every third day half of the medium is carefully withdrawn with a Pasteur pipette fitted to a suction pump, leaving the cell layer covering the bottom of the culture flask undisturbed.

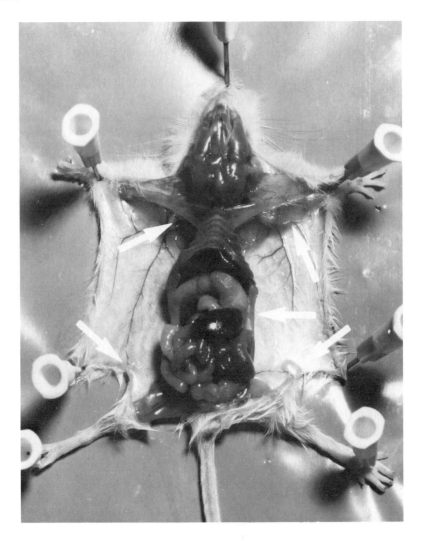

Fig. 1. Tumor formation in the BALB/c mouse after treatment with Abelson murine leukemia virus.

In general, Abelson lymphosarcomas are more readily adapted to *in vitro* growth than are thymomas. After 10–14 days, rapidly dividing cells grow in suspension. They are transferred to new culture flasks at a density of 1×10^5 cells/ml and grow to densities of 4–6×10^6 cells/ml. Higher cell yields are obtainable in roller bottles. Many of our AKR thymoma cells in culture went through a long phase of excessive cell death with only few viable cells remaining after about 10 days. Changing the medium was continued for up to 3 weeks. In most of these cultures clusters of proliferating cells appeared and grew rapidly to saturating densities. In several cases cultures with low viability have been harvested and reinjected subcutaneously into syngeneic recipients. These cells then grew more readily when put into culture once again.

Doubling time and saturation density of cell lines should be determined as soon as possible, by establishing a growth curve. Established lines can be easily lost by overgrowth; in particular, AKR thymomas will die within a few hours after reaching their certain saturation density.

Once a cell line is established, samples should be frozen and stored. About 5×10^6 cells/ml are suspended in medium containing 20% FCS or HS and 10% dimethyl sulfoxide (DMSO) (v/v). Vials are wrapped in foam rubber or paper to ensure slow freezing. After 24 hr at $-70°C$, the vials are transferred into liquid nitrogen. After this procedure the thawed cells showed consistantly high viability. It is advisable to freeze also the original tumor cells to preserve samples with the original characteristics.

V. CRITICAL APPRAISAL

About three-quarters of the AKR thymomas have been successfully adapted to *in vitro* growth on the first attempt; the rest of the thymomas were established after a second passage in the animal. The rate of *in vitro* adaptation of A-MuLV-induced tumors was close to 100%. The high rate of cell death during the first days *in vitro* probably reflects inadequate culture conditions. Growth factors or nutrients, available under *in vivo* conditions, may be limiting or missing.

From numerous comparative studies, that is, initiating cells of the same and different AKR thymomas in media supplemented differently, we conclude that individual AKR thymomas may have different growth requirements. The addition of 2-mercaptoethanol was supportive of the growth of some tumor cells but had no effect on others. A comparison of fetal calf serum, horse serum, and mixtures of both also suggested different requirements for different tumors. Based on the assumption that some thymoma cells might be dependent on thymic hormones, thymic extracts were added during the initiation of some of our thymoma lines. A beneficial effect was obvious in some cases only. This growth-promoting activity, however, was not thymus specific since extracts of other organs, for example, lung, seemed to be even superior (G. Sato and M.H. Schreier, unpublished observations). No correlation was found between the number of *in vivo* passages and the readiness of the tumor cells to adapt to growth *in vitro*. This conclusion is based on our observations made during the establishment of cell lines from AKR tumors, which were maintained in serial *in vivo* passages over several years in our institute (Krammer *et al.*, 1976).

Some features of the thymoma cell lines are remarkably stable. The θ-antigen is expressed over hundreds of *in vitro* passages. The cell line F (Krammer *et al.*, 1976), which was established *in vitro* after 22 *in vivo* passages, expressed the Fc receptor on 40–60% of the cells. Out of fifty clones established from this line four were nearly 100% Fc receptor positive, and one subline (clone 29) was negative (L. Forni, unpublished work). These clones maintained their characteristics over nearly 100 *in vitro* transfers. The surface marker is lost in the progeny cells from overgrown cultures.

Abelson lymphosarcomas are generally easy to adapt to growth *in vitro*. The technique given selects for nonadherent cells. In some cases, however, we obtained a high proportion of adherent cells. Surface markers, such as immunoglobulins, Fc receptors, and θ-antigens, were absent, contrary to other reports (Premkumar *et al.*, 1975). The *in vitro* transformation of mouse spleen, fetal liver, and bone marrow cells has been reported (Rosenberg and Baltimore, 1976).

SUGGESTED READING

Pollack, R., ed. (1973). "Readings in Mammalian Cell Culture." Cold Spring Harbor Lab., Cold Spring Harbor, New York.

Tooze, J., ed. (1973). "The Molecular Biology of Tumor Viruses." Cold Spring Harbor Lab., Cold Spring Harbor, New York.

REFERENCES

Abelson, H. T., and Rabstein, L. S. (1970). *Cancer Res.* **30**, 2213.

Acton, R. T., Blankenhorn, E. P., Douglas, T. C., Owen, R. D., Hilgers, J., Hoffman, H. A., and Boyse, E. A. (1973). *Nature New Biol.* **245**, 8.

Gross, L. (1951). *Proc. Soc. Exp. Biol. Med.* **76**, 27.

Hartley, J. W., and Rowe, W. P. (1975). *Virology* **65**, 128.

Jainchill, J. L., Aaronson, S. A., and Todaro, G. J. (1969). *J. Virol.* **4**, 549.

Klement, V., Rowe, W. P., Hartley, J. W., and Pugh, W. E. (1969). *Proc. Natl. Acad. Sci. U.S.A.* **63**, 753.

Krammer, P. H., Citronbaum, R., Read, S. E., Forni, L., and Lang, R. (1976). *Cell. Immunol.* **21**, 97.

Moloney, J. B. (1960). *J. Natl. Cancer Inst.* **24**, 933.

Potter, M., Sklar, M. D., and Rowe, W. P. (1973). *Science* **182**, 592.

Premkumar, E., Potter, M., Singer, P. A., and Sklar, M. D. (1975). *Cell* **6**, 149.

Rosenberg, N., and Baltimore, D. (1976). *J. Exp. Med.* **143**, 1453.

Rowe, W. P., Pugh, W. E., and Hartley, J. W. (1970). *Virology* **42**, 1136.

Scher, C. D., and Siegler, R. (1975). *Nature (London)* **253**, 729.

Svoboda, J., Chyle, P. P., Simkovis, D., and Hilgert, I. (1963). *Folia Biol. (Prague)* **9**, 77.

29

Clonal Growth of Cells in Semisolid or Viscous Medium

Norman N. Iscove and Max H. Schreier

I. INTRODUCTION

Cell culture in semisolid or viscous medium is widely used for selecting clones, enumerating specific progenitor cells, and studying the control of cellular proliferation and differentiation. Three methods are available: plasma clot (McLeod *et al.*, 1974), agar, and methyl cellulose. This chapter will outline the experimental procedures involved in the use of agar and methyl cellulose.

The properties of agar and methyl cellulose are quite different. Although agar is water soluble at high temperatures, intermolecular hydrogen bonds form as it cools, resulting in gel formation (semisolid state). Methyl cellulose, on the other hand, remains water soluble both at incubator

IMMUNOLOGICAL METHODS
Copyright © 1979 by Academic Press, Inc.

temperatues and in the cold. It immobilizes cells not by gel formation but simply by the high viscosity it imparts to the medium.

The chief advantage of agar over methyl cellulose is its ease of handling. Agar can be pipetted, and can be mixed with other constituents directly in the culture plates. Methyl cellulose solutions, on the other hand, require handling with syringes because of the high viscosity of methyl cellulose and must be mixed with other constituents before plating. However, methyl cellulose offers some advantages over agar. It is chemically better defined and more inert than the crude agar preparations usually used for tissue culture. It contains no contaminating mitogenic activity. Because it is water soluble at room and incubator temperatures, it is relatively easy to recover cells from it for direct study, replating, cytogenetics [see Aye *et al.* (1973) for a method for cytogenetics on single colonies], etc. Finally, scoring of small colonies in methyl cellulose is greatly facilitated by their location in only a single plane at the plastic surface of the culture plate; this occurs because cells are free to sediment slowly through the medium.

II. MATERIALS

A. Double-Strength Medium

Double-strength medium is prepared by dissolving, in only 500 ml of distilled water, the quantities of powdered medium, bicarbonate, and other additives normally required for 1 liter of medium.

B. Preparation of Agar

For cloning purposes a final agar concentration of 0.3% is usually suitable. (0.3% agar is sometimes referred to as "soft" agar. "Harder" preparations, about 0.5%, are used for the preparation of bottom, or feeder, layers, where rigid immobilization of cells is important. However, cell growth is strongly inhibited at these higher agar concentrations.) Agar (Difco Bacto agar), 1.0 gm, is boiled in 100 ml of distilled water in a sterile Erlenmeyer flask. This stock is then maintained at 43°C in a water bath, at which temperature the solution will remain fluid. (The solution will gel at room temperature. It can be stored in this state and later restored to the fluid state by placing the container in a boiling water bath.)

C. Preparation of Methyl Cellulose

One liter of a 2% methyl cellulose solution (2.5× final concentration) is prepared as follows. A sterile 2-liter Erlenmeyer flask is weighed. Distilled water, 450 ml, is then added and brought just to boiling over a Bunsen burner flame. Methyl cellulose powder (Dow Methocel A 4 M, premium grade), 20 gm, is added. The flask is covered loosely with aluminium foil, and the powder is thoroughly suspended by vigorous swirling of the flask until no lumps remain. The flask is heated again just to the boiling point and then immediately removed from the flame. (Methyl cellulose is partially hydrolyzed at high temperatures, resulting in decreased viscosity. Autoclaving or prolonged boiling is therefore to be avoided. The momentary boiling described here has always proved to be sufficient for sterility in our hands.) The suspension is then cooled to 40°–50°C under running water. Double-strength culture medium (at room temperature), 500 ml, is then added, along with any other desired additives, and the contents of the flask are thoroughly mixed by swirling. Finally, distilled water is added to bring the weight of the contents up to 1006 gm (the added water replaces the water lost during heating). After swirling thoroughly again, the flask is immersed in ice for 1–2 hr, during which most, but not all, of the methyl cellulose will hydrate. The solution, now quite viscous, is distributed in 70- to 80-ml aliqots by careful pouring into sterile 100-ml bottles. The bottles are stored at −20°C and will keep indefinitely. For use, bottles should be thawed at 4°C for 2 days, during which time some residual unhydrated methyl cellulose will enter solution to yield the maximum viscosity. However, solution is never complete and some transparent cellulose flakes and fibers will always remain. They do not affect the cultures. The perfectionist can remove them by centrifugation under sterile conditions at 15,000 g for 2–3 hr. The working solution can be stored at 4°C for at least 4–6 weeks.

III. PROCEDURE

This section describes the preparation of 35-mm culture plates, each containing 1 ml of medium and cells, in either agar or methyl cellulose. The particulars of the composition, for example, serum concentration, are arbitrarily chosen.

A. Preparation of Agar Cultures

Complete agar medium, 100 ml, is prepared by combining 30 ml of a 1% agar solution (kept at 43°C) with 70 ml of the mixture shown in the tabulation below (prewarmed to 37°C):

Double-strength medium (including supplemental glutamine, antibiotics, etc., as desired)	30.0 ml
Serum	10.0 ml
Further constituents as required for individual applications	————
Single-strength medium to a total volume of	70.0 ml

The agar medium mixture is maintained at 37°C in a water bath. The cell suspension, in less than 5% of the total volume, is added to the complete agar medium immediately before plating and uniformly dispersed. If several stimulator sources or concentrations are to be tested, they can be placed in the culture dishes before the cell-containing agar mixture is added. The medium must be dispensed quickly to avoid gelling within the pipette. The plates are gently swirled to mix and evenly distribute the materials before gelling has occurred. After allowing 3–4 min for gelling at room temperature, the plates are placed in the incubator. It is important to maintain the humidity of the incubator at near 100% to avoid dehydration of the cultures. Over periods of culture beyond 7 days, it is possible to "feed" agar cultures by adding a 1- to 2-ml overlay of fluid medium.

B. Preparation of Methyl Cellulose Cultures

To a 15-ml Falcon plastic test tube, the following components are added in the sequence indicated: serum, 0.25 ml; stimulator (e.g., LPS, 0.5 mg/ml), 0.25 ml; culture medium, 0.65 ml; 2% methyl cellulose, 1.0 ml. Mix these components gently by hand. Cells in culture medium, 0.1 ml, are then added; mix gently for a few seconds on a Vortex mixer. The volume of culture medium added is chosen to give the mixture a final volume of 2.5 ml, sufficient for two plates.

The methyl cellulose stock is too viscous for pipetting. It is best handled with a disposable plastic syringe fitted with a 15- or 16-gauge needle. The correct amount is deposited *near the bottom* of the plastic tube. The final mixture is also dispensed with a syringe. Since it is less viscous than the methyl cellulose stock, it can be dispensed through a smaller (18-gauge) needle into the culture plates. One milliliter of mixture should be placed in the *center* of the plate. It is then distributed uniformly over the entire surface by tilting the plate in a circular motion to allow the mixture to flow to the edges.

The final concentration of methyl cellulose is about 0.8%. Best growth occurs when the medium is sufficiently fluid to allow the cells to sediment to the bottom of the plate within 24 hr, but sufficiently viscous to prevent visible flowing when the plates are viewed on an inverted microscope. The exact proportion of methyl cellulose stock to achieve this is determined by titrating each individual batch.

IV. APPLICATIONS

A. Cloning of Established Cell Lines

Semisolid or viscous medium can be used for the isolation of clones of anchorage-independent cells. After growth of colonies to a desired size they can be picked from the agar or methyl cellulose with a finely drawn pipette under a dissecting or inverted microscope and transferred to liquid cultures.

It is possible to identify clones of secreting cells among a population of nonsecreting clones by application of an overlay of agar that contains antibody directed against the secretion product (Coffino and Scharff, 1971). Secreting clones are identified by an immune precipitate. Similarly, clones of cells that secrete antibodies can be identified using an overlay of agar that contains suitably coupled red blood cells and complement (Köhler and Milstein, 1975).

To minimize the risk of obtaining overlapping clones, the duration of culture should be kept to a convenient minimum, and the number of cells plated per culture should be as low as possible. The seeding density chosen for a given type of cell will depend on the cloning efficiency of the cells in the given set of culture conditions. Cloning efficiency may be improved by such methods as adding heavily γ- or X-irradiated cells or liquid medium in which the cells have grown ("conditioned medium") or using an agar underlayer containing "feeder" cells.

Some lines may fail to grow in agar. Crude agar contains sulfated polysaccharides and other potentially toxic impurities. DEAE-dextran can be added to complex with the polyanions (Montagnier, 1971). The use of highly purified agarose preparations or methyl cellulose bypasses such problems. A thiol such as β-mercaptoethanol or α-thioglycerol at 5×10^{-5} M can be routinely included, since a number of lymphoid lines are thiol dependent (Broome and Jeng, 1972), and we are unaware of any cells that might be inhibited by thiol at this concentration.

B. B- and T-Cell Cloning

B- and T-cell colonies can be grown in agar or methyl cellulose. B-cell colony growth in methyl cellulose is greatly enhanced by the inclusion of 1%

bovine serum albumin in the culture medium. The albumin should be deionized (Worton *et al.*, 1969) before use. Detailed descriptions can be found in the following references: Metcalf *et al.* (1975a,b, 1976), Metcalf (1976), Johnson *et al.* (1976), and Watanabe *et al.* (1977).

Growth of these cells is dependent on thiols, such as β-mercaptoethanol or α-thioglycerol, and on appropriate mitogens, for example, LPS or PHA, respectively. Crude agar contains a B-cell mitogen (Kincade *et al.*, 1976), but its concentration is not under the control of the experimenter. Adequate stimulation can be ensured by adding optimal quantities of known mitogens to purified agar (agarose) or methyl cellulose.

If the method is to be used to enumerate mitogen-sensitive B and T cells and their precursors, it is important to ensure that there is a linear relationship between the colony number and the numbers of cells plated down to very low seeding densities. For growth of B-cell colonies, this condition appears to be achievable when cultures contain both LPS and agar mitogen, but not with either alone (Kincade *et al.*, 1976; Metcalf, 1976). Under the best available culture conditions, that is, using both LPS and agar mitogen, more than one in eight splenic B cells may be capable of forming colonies or small clusters (Kurland *et al.*, 1977). However, in liquid cultures in which B cells are grown at limiting dilutions, one in three B cells can generate clones in response to LPS alone (Andersson *et al.*, 1977). The colony methods may therefore underestimate the frequency of mitogen-responsive B cells in their present state of development. A linear method for T-cell precursors has not yet been described.

SUGGESTED READING

Ham, R. G. (1972). Cloning of mammalian cells. *Methods Cell Physiol.* **5**, 37–74.
Macpherson, I. (1973). Soft agar technique. *In* "Tissue Culture: Methods and Applications" (P. F. Kruse, Jr. and M. K. Patterson, Jr., eds.), pp 276–280. Academic Press, New York.
Metcalf, D., and Moore, M. A. S. (1971). "Haemopoietic Cells." North-Holland Publ., Amsterdam.

REFERENCES

Andersson, J., Coutinho, A., Lernhardt, W., and Melchers, F. (1977). *Cell* **10**, 27.
Aye, M. T., Till, J. E., and McCulloch, E. A. (1973). *Exp. Hematol. (Copenhagen)* **1**, 115.
Broome, J. D., and Jeng, M. W. (1972). *J. Exp. Med.* **138**, 574.
Coffino, P., and Scharff, M. D. (1971). *Proc. Natl. Acad. Sci. U.S.A.* **68**, 219.
Johnson, G. R., Metcalf, D., and Wilson, H. W. (1976). *Immunology* **30**, 907.
Kincade, P. W., Ralph, P., and Moore, M. A. S. (1976). *J. Exp. Med.* **143**, 1265.

Köhler, G., and Milstein, C. (1975). *Nature (London)* **256**, 495.

Kurland, J. I., Kincade, P. W., and Moore, M. A. S. (1977). *J. Exp. Med.* **146**, 1420.

McLeod, D. L., Shreeve, M. M., and Axelrad, A. A. (1974). *Blood* **44**, 517.

Metcalf, D. (1976). *J. Immunol.* **116**, 635.

Metcalf, D., Nossal, G. J. V., Warner, N. L., Miller, J. F. A. P., Mandel, T. E., Layton, J. E., and Gutman, G. A. (1975a). *J. Exp. Med.* **142**, 1534.

Metcalf, D., Wilson, J. W., Shortman, K., Miller, J. F. A. P., and Stocker, J. (1976). *J. Cell Physiol.* **88**, 107.

Montagnier, L. (1971). *Growth Control Cell Cult., Ciba Found. Symp., 1970* pp. 33–44. *Physiol.* **88**, 107.

Montagnier, L. *Growth Control Cell Cult., Ciba Found. Symp., 1970* pp. 33–44.

Watanabe, T., Fathman, C., and Coutinho, A. (1977). *Immunol. Rev.* **35**, 3.

Worton, R. G., McCulloch, E. A., and Till, J. E. (1969). *J. Cell Physiol.* **74**, 171.

30

Preparation of Sendai Virus for Cell Fusion

Reet Tees

I. GROWTH OF VIRUS

Fertile White Leghorn eggs are set in a hatching incubator (38.5°C, 80–90% relative humidity, rotation every 3–4 hr) for 11 days.

The eggs are candled and a spot near the main umbilical artery free of vessels is marked for inoculation. The shell over this spot is removed with a dental drill, exposing about 2–3 mm ϕ of the shell membrane (breaking of the shell membrane, visible as bleeding, leads to contamination; such eggs should not be used). The eggs are placed on a tray and an area of about 2 cm ϕ centering on the drilled spot is sterilized by painting with hot paraffin wax (melting point, 58°–65°C; kept at approximately 120°C, i.e., just below fuming temperature).

The inoculum of 0.05 ml of saline, containing 10^2–10^3 ID_{50} of Sendai virus, is placed on the waxed surface and the shell membrane is pierced with a flame-sterilized needle. The negative pressure in the allantoic cavity automatically sucks in the inoculum, after which the hole is sealed by swabbing with the hot paraffin wax.

IMMUNOLOGICAL METHODS
ISBN 0-12-442750-2

The eggs are placed in trays (air space = blunt end up!) and kept in an ordinary incubator for 3 days (68–72 hr) at 35°C. They are then chilled (4°C overnight, or at least 3 hr) to stop the circulation and thus bleeding during harvest.

Before harvesting, the shell over the air space is cracked and removed. By piercing the exposed basal membrane with a pair of sterile forceps and using the forceps to keep the embryo to one side, the allantoic fluid is removed with a sterile Pasteur pipette (short tip, preferably wide mouth). The average yield is about 10 ml, with great individual variation. Care should be taken not to damage the amnion, albumen, or yolk sac. Such damage may contaminate the harvested allantoic fluid.

II. TITRATION OF VIRUS

The virus content of allantoic fluids is individually tested in a hemagglutinin test before pooling and inactivation.

The standard test is performed either in 12-mm ϕ round-bottom test tubes or, better, in the WHO hemagglutinin trays (8 rows of 10 spherical cups). The first tube receives 0.50 ml of physiological saline and the other nine tubes receive 0.25 ml. The starting dilution is made up by adding 0.05 ml of allantoic fluid to the first tube (a 1:11 dilution, or 1.04 in log units). By carrying 0.25 ml from cup to cup, a series of twofold dilutions is made up, covering the range of 1:11 to 1:5632 (1.04 to 3.75 in log units). Then 0.025 ml of a 5% fowl red cell suspension in saline is added to each cup, and the trays are shaken and placed in a refrigerator. They are reshaken after 20 min and read after another 40 min at 4°C.

The absence of agglutination (−) is marked by a dense red button in the middle of the cup, whereas complete agglutination (++) is marked by a thin pink film covering the whole bottom of the cup. The conventional end point (+) is a ring whose diameter is one-third the diameter of the cup. By interpolating to this end point, a single test can be read to ±0.033 log (±8%) accuracy; by taking the last tube with complete agglutination as the end point, the precision drops to ±0.27 log unit (±86%).

If the titrations are performed in microtrays (dilution volume, 0.025 ml; starting dilution, 1:2), the red cell concentration is reduced to 1% and the incubation time to 2 × 20 min at 4°C. This test has an accuracy of not better than ±0.20 log unit (±58%).

Calculation of Titers

A hemagglutinating unit (HAU) is the amount of virus that will give the conventional (+) end point against 1.0 ml of 1% fowl red cells, and which contains about 4×10^7 (7.6 in log units) physical virus particles (Fazekas de St.Groth and Cairns, 1952).

Thus, for instance, if a titration starting with the dilution of 1:11 gives (+) end point in the sixth tube, we have 11×32 agglutinating doses in our test system. Since we performed the test in 0.25 ml, we have to multiply this figure by 4, and since we used a 0.5% rather than 1% final red cell concentration, we have to divide by 2, arriving at a titer of 704 HAU/ml, or 2.847 log units. This result can be obtained more simply by adding the log of the starting dilution and the log of the end point (i.e., $0.3 \times$ tube number): $1.04 + 1.8 = 2.84$. (The difference in the third decimal place arises from rounding off the logarithms of both the starting dilution, 1.0414 ... to 1.04, and the multiplier 0.30103 ... to 0.3 = log 2.) This latter method is equally suited to fractional titers. Thus, with a starting point of 1:500 and a pattern of (++) in the second tube and (−) in the third tube, that is, an end point of 2.5 tubes, we have $2.7 + (0.3 \times 2.5) = 3.45$ as log titer, or 2818 HAU/ml.

The average yield of Sendai virus is about 1800 HAU/ml or 3.25 ± 0.20 log units.

III. CONCENTRATION OF VIRUS

Positive allantoic fluids (usually about 300 ml, or the yield of 30–40 eggs) are pooled aseptically and clarified of urates and cell debris by centrifuging for 20 min at 4000 g. The clear supernatant is then transferred to an ultracentrifuge (Beckman Spinco Ti 60 head will take 300 ml in one load) and spun for 30 min at an average g of 60,000 (30,000 rpm for the Ti 60 head).

The pelleted virus is taken up in a minimal volume of Earle's BSS + 1% bovine serum albumin, as recommended by Klebe et al. (1970) to avoid loss during the inactivation step. After dispersion by vigorous pipetting, the virus suspension is once again clarified (20 min at 4000 g) and titrated (starting dilution, 1:500).

IV. INACTIVATION OF VIRUS

This method is from Neff and Enders (1968). β-Propiolactone (Fluka) is diluted to 10% (w/v) in triple-glass-distilled water and then further diluted with 4 parts of saline–bicarbonate (1.68 gm $NaHCO_3$ + 0.02 ml of 1% phenol red + 100 ml of 0.9% NaCl in triple-distilled water). The final stock contains 2% β-propiolactone.

The virus suspension is diluted to 10,000 HAU/ml, made up to 0.05% β-propiolactone (39 parts virus + 1 part β-propiolactone stock), and kept for 10 min at 4°C with continuous shaking, then incubated for 2 hr at 37°C and finally stirred gently at 4°C overnight, to ensure complete hydrolysis of the excess propiolactone.

The inactivated virus is diluted to 4000 HAU/ml with Earle's BSS (2 parts virus + 3 parts BSS), ampuled in 1.1-ml lots, snap-frozen in a mixture of solid CO_2 and ethanol, and stored at -70°C.

For the fusion of 10^7 myeloma cells and 10^8 spleen cells, 1000–2000 HAU/ml are used, that is, about 360 virus particles per cell.

V. ASSAY OF INFECTIVITY

The inactivated virus is diluted in tenfold steps (10^{-1} to 10^{-6}) in Earle's BSS and 0.05 ml of each dilution is inoculated allantoically into a group of three eggs (see Section I). After incubation at 35°C for 68–72 hr, about 0.05 ml of allantoic fluid is removed through the hole of inoculation with a Pasteur pipette and added to 0.25 ml of saline in a titration tray. Then 0.025 ml of 5% fowl red cells is dropped onto each cup, and the tray is shaken and incubated at 4°C for 40 min.

Inactivated virus will give ($-$) patterns even at the lowest dilution (10^{-1}). Active virus of the same concentration will give complete agglutination up to dilutions of 10^{-8}.

REFERENCES

Fazekas de St.Groth, S., and Cairns, H. J. F. (1952). *J. Immunol.* **69**, 173.
Klebe, R. J., Chen, T. R., and Ruddle, F. H. (1970). *J. Cell Biol.* **45**, 74.
Neff, J. H., and Enders, J. F. (1968). *Proc. Soc. Exp. Biol. Med.* **127**, 260.

Fusion of Lymphocytes

Georges Köhler

I. OBJECTIVE

The method provides a tool to generate hybrid lines secreting monoclonal antibodies of different classes and of different predefined antigenic specificities.

II. PRINCIPLE OF THE METHOD

Spleen cells of mice, previously immunized with antigen, are fused to a myeloma line, which grows in tissue culture. The fusion is performed in the presence of Sendai virus (for the preparation of Sendai virus, see Chapter 30).

The myeloma line, which is defective in the enzyme hypoxanthine–guanine phosphoribosyltranferase (HGPRT), cannot survive in tissue culture medium supplemented with hypoxanthine, aminopterin, and thymidine (HAT). Aminopterin blocks the main pathway of DNA synthesis. The rescue pathway that uses, in this case, exogeneous hypoxanthine, depends on the presence of the enzyme HGPRT. Spleen cells die in tissue culture medium. Only hybrids between the myeloma and spleen cells survive in HAT medium since the myeloma provides the ability to

IMMUNOLOGICAL METHODS

grow in tissue culture and the spleen cells contribute the functional HGPRT enzyme necessary to overcome the aminopterin block.

The HGPRT-defective myeloma cells were selected for resistance to the purine killer analogue 8-azaguanine in a single-step selection. Cloning 10^6 myeloma cells (X63) in soft agar in the presence of 20 μg/ml of 8-azaguanine resulted in about 20 resistant clones, which were sensitive to HAT medium. No revertant has been observed for X63-Ag8.

Similar selection procedures can be used to isolate variant myeloma cells defective for the enzyme thymidine kinase (TK), which uses exogenous thymidine and therefore overcomes the central aminopterin block. Such variants are selected for by their resistance to 30 μg/ml of the pyrmidine killer analogue 5'-bromodeoxyuridine (Brd U).

III. MATERIAL

Earle's balanced salt solution (EBSS) (Gibco–Biocult, Paisley, Scotland PA3 4EP)

Dulbecco's modified minimal essential medium ($1\times$) (Flow Laboratories, Irvine, Scotland) supplemented with penicillin–streptomycin (100 U/liter), L-glutamine (4 mM), sodium pyruvate (1 mM), and 20% heat-inactivated horse serum (Gibco) (DMEM)

Sendai virus, 1000 hemagglutinating units (HAU)

10^7 myeloma cells (X63-Ag8); this is a tissue culture line derived from the BALB/c myeloma MOPC-21 and is resistant to 20 μg/ml of 8-azaguanine, dies in HAT medium, and secretes an IgG$_1$ (κ) immunoglobulin

10^8 spleen cells

Aminopterin ($100\times$): To 1.74 mg add 25 ml of distilled water and 1.2 ml of 2 N NaOH; add distilled water to 100 ml and then neutralize slowly with 0.2 ml of 2 N HCl

Hypoxanthine ($100\times$), 136.1 mg/100 ml; heat at 45°C for 1 hr to dissolve

Thymidine ($100\times$), 38.7 mg/100 ml

Costar trays (Costar, Data Packaging Corp., Cambridge, Massachusetts)

Incubator (wet, CO_2, 37°C)

IV. PROCEDURE

The steps involved in the procedure to generate hybrid lines are given in the flow chart (Scheme 1).

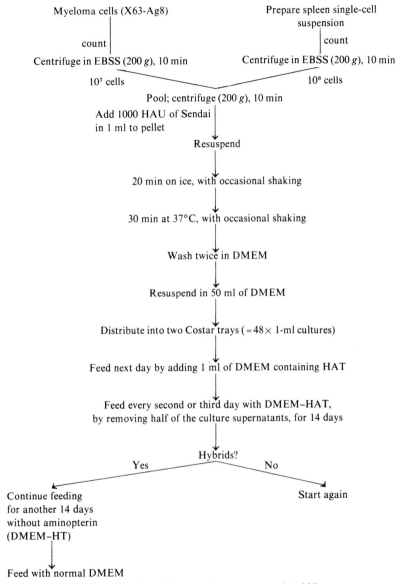

Scheme 1. Flow chart of the procedure to generate hybrid lines.

Controls

Treat both parental lines the same way separately, to rule out growth of either spleen cells or revertants of the HGPRT$^-$ myeloma line.

TABLE I

Analysis of a Typical Fusion Experiment

	Number of cultures	SRBC specificity
Independent cultures	72	
Surviving hybrids	21	
Secretion of X63-Ag8 myeloma (γ_1, κ)	20[a]	
Secretion of new μ and light chains	11	1
Secretion of new γ and light chains	2	1 (γ_{2b})
Secretion of only new light chains	2	
No new Ig chain secreted	6	

[a] One hybrid secreted a new IgM molecule but had lost the ability to express the myeloma IgG$_1$.

A typical positive experiment is summarized in Table I. C57BL/10 mice were immunized intraperitoneally with 20 μl of packed trinitrophenylated SRBC in 0.2 ml of phosphate-buffered saline. Three days after a second injection, given a month later, the spleen cells were removed and the cells from three spleens were pooled. Immediately after fusion we found 10^4 direct, and 10^4 indirect, plaque-forming cells against SRBC in a total of 10^8 spleen cells. Using TNP–SRBC did not increase these numbers, indicating that no TNP-specific response was obtained. Out of 72 1-ml cultures, 21 showed growth of hybrid cells. At this low ratio of positive versus negative cultures, probably not more than 21 independent hybrids were formed.

Radioactively labeled supernatants of all hybrids were analyzed by SDS– and IEF–polyacrylamide gel electrophoreses. Twenty hybrids still secreted the myeloma IgG, eleven secreted an additional IgM, two an additional IgG molecule, two only additional light chains, and six no additional Ig chain. One IgM and one IgG$_{2b}$ showed specific lyses of SRBC. No anti-TNP reactivity was revealed.

V. CRITICAL APPRAISAL

Positive experiments result in 20–80 hybrids, with about 50% secreting new immunoglobulins of the IgM and IgG classes and 10% being specific for the antigen injected into the donor mice. Therefore, about 50% of the (myeloma × spleen cell) hybrids are the result of the fusion of the myeloma with B cells of the spleen.

It is interesting to note that the fusion of myeloma to thymoma cells resulted in the extinction of the thymoma-specific cell-surface antigen θ but in continued secretion of the myeloma IgG (Köhler *et al.*, 1977). No θ-

positive hybrids have been obtained in the myeloma × spleen cell fusions. However, θ was expressed in fusions of the thymoma × spleen cells, indicating successful hybridization to splenic T cells (Hämmerling *et al.*, 1977). No Ig secretion was observed in about 50 thymoma × spleen cell hybrids studied. These observations point to the fact that, in order to rescue the functions of normal cells by fusion, ontogenetically related tumor lines must be used; for example, a thymoma cannot rescue Ig production of normal B cells and a myeloma cannot rescue θ expression of normal T cells.

The following antigens were successfully used in myeloma × spleen cell fusions: SRBC, TNP–lipopolysaccharide, TNP–fowl γ-globulin (Köhler and Milstein, 1976), histocompatibility antigen of the rat fusing the myeloma cell to rat splenocytes (Galfre *et al.*, 1977), and a variety of other antigens including soluble protein and sugar determinants (Hämmerling *et al.*, 1977).

Successful fusions were obtained in syngeneic, allogeneic, and xenogeneic combinations. The advantage of using syngeneic or allogeneic fusions lies in the possibility of growing the hybrid cells as tumors in the appropriate mice and thereby obtaining sera of high titer. The fusion does not invariably work. Often a repetition of the fusion process without obvious changes results in successful hybridization. The use of polyethylene glycol instead of Sendai virus results in similar hybrid frequencies. The procedure described by Galfre *et al.* (1977) is recommended.

REFERENCES

Galfre, G., Howe, S. C., Milstein, C., Butcher, G. W., and Howard, J. C. (1977). *Nature (London)* **266**, 550.

Hämmerling, G. J., Reth, M., Lemke, H., Hewitt, J., Melchers, I., and Rajewsky, K. (1977). *Protides Bio. Fluids, Proc. Colloq.* **25**, 551.

Köhler, G., and Milstein, C. (1976). *Eur. J. Immunol.* **6**, 511.

Köler, G., Pearson, T., and Milstein, C. (1977). *Somatic Cell Genetics* **3**, 303.

32

Soft Agar Cloning of Lymphoid Tumor Lines: Detection of Hybrid Clones with Anti-SRBC Activity

Georges Köhler

I. OBJECTIVE AND PRINCIPLE OF THE METHOD

Heterogeneous mixtures of hybrid or lymphoid tumor lines are separated by localized growth of single cells in soft agar (for the preparation of hybrid lines, see Chapter 31). Clones secreting sheep red blood cell-specific antibodies are revealed by an overlay technique.

II. MATERIAL

Petri dishes, ϕ 9 cm (Falcon, Becton–Dickinson–France, 38100 Grenoble, France)

1% Agar (Difco Laboratories, Detroit, Michigan) in triple-distilled water, autoclaved

Dulbecco's modified Eagle medium (DMEM) (10×) (Gibco Bio-cult, Paisley, Scotland PA3 4EP) made up to 2× DMEM as follows: triple-distilled water, 30 ml; DMEM (10×), 20 ml; penicillin–streptomycin, 5000 U/ml, 4 ml; L-glutamine (200 mM), 4 ml; sodium pyruvate (100 mM), 2 ml; sodium bicarbonate (7.5%), 10 ml; sodium hydroxide

IMMUNOLOGICAL METHODS

(0.1 *M*), 0.6 ml; horse serum, 40 ml; the horse serum is heat-inactivated and screened for mycoplasma

Costar trays (Costar, Data Packaging Corp., Cambridge, Massachusetts)

PBS: 10 m*M* phosphate buffer (pH 7.2), 0.9% sodium chloride

Indubiose A37 (L'Industrie Biologique Française, Gennevilliers, France), 0.6% in PBS, sterile

1× DMEM supplemented with 10% horse serum (made up as for Dulbecco's modified Eagle's medium but adding 20 ml of horse serum and 140 ml of triple-distilled water)

Sheep red blood cells (SRBC) washed three times with saline and made up to 25% in saline

Guinea pig complement (GPC'): Fresh guinea pig serum is absorbed at 4°C with 10% packed SRBC, sterilized by filtration, and kept in 2-ml aliquots frozen at −20°C

Rabbit anti-mouse immunoglobulin, made by injecting a rabbit intraperitoneally with 0.5 mg of purified MOPC-21 (IgG$_1$, κ) emulsified in Freund's complete adjuvant; when a good plaque-developing titer is observed (usually after the third injection given at 3-week intervals), the rabbit serum is absorbed with 10% packed SRBC, filter-sterilized, and kept frozen in 2-ml aliquots at −20°C

III. PROCEDURE

The steps involved in the procedure for soft agar cloning of lymphoid tumor lines are given in the flow chart (Scheme 1).

Figure 1 shows an example of the isolation of hybrid cells secreting an IgM molecule with anti-SRC specificity. The specific cells represent about 3% of the total hybrid population. Figure 1a shows the direct plaques (dark spots) formed by single cells plating 6000 hybrid cells. Figure 1b shows clones (white dots) grown in soft agar for 10 days derived from a cell inoculum of 2000 viable cells. The cloning efficiency was about 50% and 33 clones gave rise to direct lysis (seen as dark halos) in the SRBC overlay lawn. One positive clone was picked, grown in liquid medium, and recloned. In Fig. 1c it can be seen that virtually every clone shows lysis. A higher magnification of such a clone is seen in Fig. 1d.

IV. CRITICAL APPRAISAL

With this method α-SRBC-secreting clones have been isolated from a mixture of hybrids, where only 1 in 500 was specific (Köhler and Milstein,

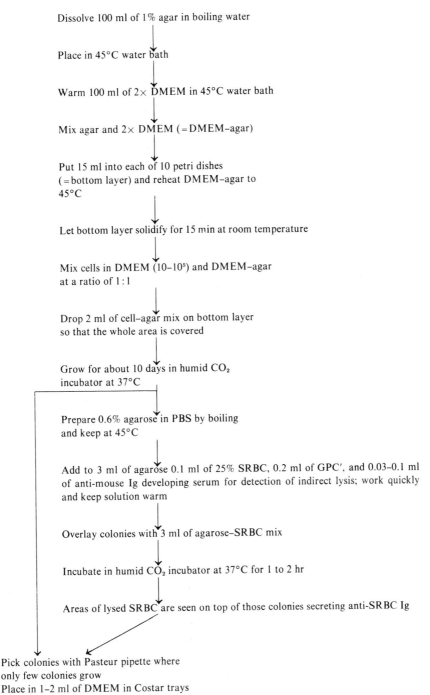

Dissolve 100 ml of 1% agar in boiling water

Place in 45°C water bath

Warm 100 ml of 2× DMEM in 45°C water bath

Mix agar and 2× DMEM (=DMEM–agar)

Put 15 ml into each of 10 petri dishes
(=bottom layer) and reheat DMEM–agar to
45°C

Let bottom layer solidify for 15 min at room temperature

Mix cells in DMEM ($10-10^5$) and DMEM–agar
at a ratio of 1:1

Drop 2 ml of cell–agar mix on bottom layer
so that the whole area is covered

Grow for about 10 days in humid CO_2
incubator at 37°C

Prepare 0.6% agarose in PBS by boiling
and keep at 45°C

Add to 3 ml of agarose 0.1 ml of 25% SRBC, 0.2 ml of GPC', and 0.03–0.1 ml
of anti-mouse Ig developing serum for detection of indirect lysis; work quickly
and keep solution warm

Overlay colonies with 3 ml of agarose–SRBC mix

Incubate in humid CO_2 incubator at 37°C for 1 to 2 hr

Areas of lysed SRBC are seen on top of those colonies secreting anti-SRBC Ig

Pick colonies with Pasteur pipette where
only few colonies grow
Place in 1–2 ml of DMEM in Costar trays

Scheme 1. Flow chart of the procedure for soft agar cloning of lymphoid tumor lines.

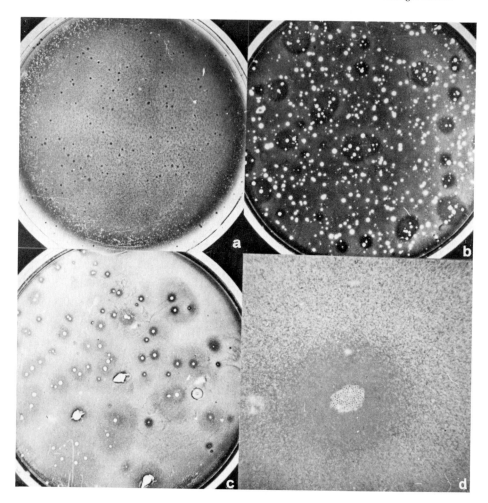

Fig. 1. Selection of hybrid clones secreting an anti-SRBC IgM. For details, see the text. (From Köhler and Milstein, 1975, *Nature (London)* **256**, 495.)

1975). This method has also been used to isolate clones that have lost the unspecific myeloma Ig chains but kept the specific heavy and light chains derived from the spleen lymphocyte (Köhler and Milstein, 1976).

The limitation of the method in isolating specific cells lies in the impossibility of growing more than about 10^4 clones per plate, which allows isolations only for fractions of specific cells not smaller than 1 in 10^4.

If clones that had lost their capacity to lyse SRBC were to be isolated, not more than 100–200 positive clones should be present in one plate since total lysis of the SRBC overlay would mask the negative clones.

This method has been applied successfully using hapten-modified SRBC. It did not work for a reverse-type plaque system, in which an anti-Ig is coupled to the SRBC to allow the detection of unspecific immunoglobulins secreted by the clones. This was found to be due to the presence of the horse serum. The cloning efficiency greatly varies for different hybrid or myeloma cell lines (between 50 and 0.01%), but usually improves after several recloning steps.

REFERENCES

Köhler, G., and Milstein, C. (1975). *Nature (London)* **256**, 495.
Köhler, G., and Milstein, C. (1976). *Eur. J. Immunol.* **6**, 511.

33

Isotope Laboratory

Helmut M. Pohlit, Jürg Widmer, and Ruedi Frech

I. INTRODUCTION

This chapter deals with specific and general aspects of the organization and functioning of a radioisotope laboratory adapted for experiments performed in the field of immunology.

IMMUNOLOGICAL METHODS

II. MATERIALS

A. General Supply and Usage of Radiochemicals

All order for isotopes are placed with the isotope personnel and the incoming material passes through the isotope office, where it is registered (as is required) and stored appropriately (such as cold room or freezer). The personnel requisitioning these materials are immediately informed of the arrival and the place of storage. Thus, the isotope personnel (two trained and two untrained personnel) are aware of the various amounts of isotopes received. In addition, they have an idea where the isotopes are routed and are often, particularly in nonroutine cases (where there might be a higher than normal hazard), informed of the specific usage.

The stocks are kept under appropriate conditions (refrigerator or freezer) within the isotope laboratory area. Part of the stock is accessible to everyone at any time, but a second buffer stock remains accessible only to isotope personnel.

B. Liquid Scintillation Cocktails

All liquid scintillation counting can be done in two types of cocktails. They are prepared by the isotope personnel in 50-liter glass containers that have been painted dark on the outside with a thin vertical strip left unpainted for level observation. The containers are kept in a fume hood, the outlet of which is connected to an adjustable dispenser (Disun, 0–20 ml, manufactured by Struers Scientific Instruments, Copenhagen, Denmark). For mixing during preparation, pneumatic stirrers are used (type M 43100-2200, Pressluft-Goetz, Mannheim, West Germany).

1. Toluene-PPO-POPOP Cocktail

One liter of this cocktail contains 5.0 gm of PPO (No. 2946, E. Merck, D-1600 Darmstadt, Germany), 0.2 gm of POPOP (Merck No. 7249), and toluene (Merck No. 8325 ad), added to a total volume of 1 liter.

2. Toluene-Triton-PPO-POPOP Cocktail

One liter of this cocktail contains 2.7 gm of PPO (Merck No. 2946), 0.1 gm of POPOP (Merck No. 7249), 460 ml of Triton N-101 (Rohm and Haas, Philadelphia, Pennsylvania), and toluene (Merck No. 8325 ad), added to a total volume of 1 liter.

This cocktail allows the addition of up to 5 ml of distilled water or aqueous sample per 10 ml of scintillator volume. However, if the aqueous sample volume is between 200 and 600 μl, the mixture becomes opaque. This can be avoided by adding more distilled water (so that the total volume of aqueous sample is greater than 600 μl). However, with increasing amounts of water present in the vial, the counting efficiency decreases considerably.

C. Standardization of the Liquid Scintillation Counter

The central supply of scintillation cocktails has several advantages (besides saving time and money). The standardization of liquid scintillation counters, which depends on the composition of the scintillation liquid, is necessary for only two different cocktails. Standardization curves are available for every counter, channel, and isotope. The availability and periodic control of standardization for all counters, using the same standards and methods, make it easier for users to switch counters if necessary, thus affording more effective usage of counter time.

D. Special Counting Devices

At various times special counting setups are arranged for special problems. Since these occasions are expected to arise with little overlap, a single but highly flexible counting configuration is appropriate. Thus, a modular counting electronic device consisting of a timer, scaler, discriminator, amplifier, analog-to-digital converter, rate meter, high voltage power supply, diverse photomultiplier tubes, and various NaI crystals has proved to be very useful. This equipment has been used for whole-body (low background) counting of mice, thin-layer chromatography scanning for ^{3}H, ^{14}C, and other isotopes, and determining the incorporation of radioiodine in the thyroid glands of laboratory personnel.

E. Counting Tubes and Vials

Some plastic scintillation vials have been found to vary so much in size (or to change size under the influence of the organic liquids they contain) that they often become jammed in the elevator shaft of the scintillation counter. Some plastic tubes are not stably positioned in the sample holding device so that they may also become stuck in the elevator shaft of gamma counters. Thus, a range of vials (shown in the tabulation below) was tested and is now held for common use in the isotope laboratory.

Vial type	Supplier
Plastic scintillation vials, 20 ml, No. 6008117	Packard Instrument International S.A. (Zürich, Switzerland)
Glass scintillation vials, 20 ml, No. 6000134	Packard Instrument International S.A.
γ-counting tubes, 10 ml, No. TFR-95	Milian Instrument S.A. (Geneva, Switzerland)

III. SPECIAL PROCEDURES

A. Removal of Unbound Radioiodine via Dialysis after Protein Labeling

Many workers in the field prefer to remove unbound radioiodine after the labeling procedure by passing the labeling mixture through a short ion exchange column. This has the advantage that the unwanted radioiodine is concentrated in a small volume (the ion exchange bed), presenting no problems in waste handling. However, this method has given variable results for (radiolabeled) protein and sample volume recovery. The alternative method of choice is dialysis. However, due to the very high speed of diffusion of iodide across the dialysis membrane, the handling of the charged dialysis bag leads to severe contamination of gloves and hands, since these gloves, whether of plastic or rubber, are equally pervious to such small molecules. The setup, shown in Fig. 1, makes it unnecessary to handle the dialysis bag after charging. The sample volume does not usually change. The unbound iodine remains in solution as iodide since excess sodium metabisulfite from the iodination reaction is present. A disadvantage is that the free iodine appears in rather large volume (0.5 to 1 liter). This may be avoided by using a dialysis bag one-half or one-third smaller (a volume of about 20 to 50 ml assures free iodine dilution to less that 5% after the first round of dialysis to equilibrium). The other advantage is that many samples may thus be processed quickly and identically, which may be important for certain kinetic investigations. The difficulties in handling many hot samples often sufficiently inhibit extensive investigations.

1. Procedure

The dialysis tubing (Fig. 1, A) (Union Carbide, size 8 × 100 ft, i.e., 7 mm in diameter) is softened in dialysis buffer, knotted at the appropriate length, and pushed over the end of a Pasteur pipette (Fig. 1, B) (Wilhelm Ulbrich, Bahnhofstrasse 5, D-65 Mainz, West Germany) that has been cut and fire-

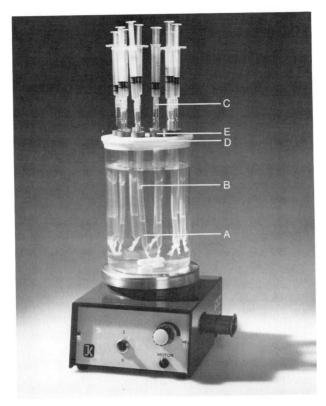

Fig. 1   Multisample dialysis setup (see the text for details).

polished at its tapered part. The Pasteur glass pipette body is fixed in a hole in the plate (Fig. 1, D) by the plug (Fig. 1, E). The plate may be an appropriately perforated lid of a 0.5- or 1-liter bottle, if only one sample is to be dialyzed. Figure 1 shows a specially made, reusable Teflon plate (fitting a one-way plastic container) that holds ten or more samples. The plug may be a cap, usually supplied with plastic tubes of various sizes, into which a hole is drilled that will ensure a snug fit for the glass tube. Dialysis buffer may be added to the container and the dialysis head inserted. The ring gasket (C), made of silicon (Tygon) tubing of the appropriate size to allow a tight fit of the plastic syringe to be inserted, is shown in place. The radioactive sample is then filled through the top with a long-capillary Pasteur pipette. If the dialysis bag has been inserted into the dialysis buffer, it is usually not possible to fill it without simultaneously allowing the liquid to rise into the glass tube by hydrostatic pressure. This is not harmful but may be avoided by adding the dialysis buffer at the end of the procedure. In either case, the bag may be inflated with slight positive pressure after filling it with a 2- to 5-ml disposable syringe. This pressure holds well over 24 hr if everything is done properly.

2. Removal of the Sample

Obviously, there are many ways of removing the sample. However, the simplest seems to be to fix the plate (D) and the dialysis head in a stand, hold the tubing with a tweezer, and cut off the dialysis tubing sufficiently close to the sample liquid level so that the sample may be withdrawn with a short Pasteur pipette. The whole dialysis head is discarded unless one is sure it or parts of it can be reused.

B. Indirect Iodination of Proteins, Nucleic Acids, Etc., with Tagit (Bolton–Hunter Reagent)

To avoid possibly harmful effects on the substances to be radioiodinated by the chemicals involved in the iodination reaction, an indirect radioiodine labeling method has been divised by Bolton and Hunter (1973; see also Rudinger and Ruegg, 1973). The rather stable activated ester 3-(p-hydroxyphenyl)propionic acid is iodinated, and the resulting molecule, in a separate step, is coupled to free amino groups of the substances to be labeled. We have used this method to attach iodine to proteins. The following procedure has afforded us a high degree of reproducibility.

1. Procedure

The iodination reaction is carried out in a glass tube that preferentially may be fitted to a lyophilizer or used as a low-speed centrifuge tube. All operations must be carried out in a fume hood until the completion of the first lyophilization cycle.

Twenty microliters of a Tagit solution [20 mg in 50 μl of dimethylformamide (DMF)] is added to 20 μl of phosphate buffer (PB, 0.05 M pH 7.2) containing the radioiodine[1] (in the glass tube). Quickly 10 μl of 5 mg/ml of chloramine-T in PB is added and, after 10–15 sec, 10 μl of 1 N HCl is added. The liquid is then frozen instantly by immersing the tube in a liquid nitrogen or dry ice–acetone bath (or the equivalent). The tube is connected to a lyophilizer and, after 3 or 4 hr (after completion of lyophilization), the contents are immersed in about 200 μl of benzene, and

---

[1] Radioiodine may be obtained from three different suppliers: Amersham/Searle (Amersham, England), Würenlingen (Switzerland), and New England Nuclear (Boston, Massachusetts). Contrary to assertions in the literature (e.g., Hunter, 1971), we have never had any indication that the failure of any protein iodinations was due to the materials.

the remaining solid is removed by low-speed centrifugation. The supernatant containing the iodinated Tagit is placed in a second glass tube and lyophilized again. The contents of the tube are then dissolved in an appropriate volume of DMF (1 ml). The labeled Tagit may be kept at 4°C or lower for several months without appreciable loss of coupling efficiency.

2. Comments

a. DMF. The use of DMF during iodination avoids an inhomogeneous reaction medium, since Tagit is only slightly soluble in water.

b. Reaction Time. The reaction time of 10 sec is not critical because this activated ester is relatively stable to hydrolysis. On the other hand, 10 sec is sufficient, and nothing is gained by lengthening the reaction time.

c. Lyophilization. Lyophilization (see Section III,C) removes DMF and water in 2–3 hr, but it also removes unbound, molecular iodine. Since oxidation of iodide to I_2 proceeds faster at lower pH, and because at lower pH the activated ester is more stable, acidification of the reaction mixture before lyophilization is advantageous.

d. Benzene Passage. Passage through benzene reduces drastically the amount of chloramine-T (and the inorganic salts) otherwise carried along.

e. DMF as Final Solvent. Dissolving the iodinated Tagit in DMF has the following advantages. DMF is less volatile than benzene, is compatible with some common plastics (such as polypropylene and polystyrene, but not Lucite and others), has a high solubility for Tagit, and, most important, is infinitely miscible with water. The latter fact makes a quick dispersion possible and thus affords a high reaction efficiency with protein, nucleic acids, etc. On the other hand, DMF (together with unbound Tagit) may be easily dialyzed. DMF at concentrations not exceeding 10% in aqueous buffers does not seem to have any deleterious effects on biological materials (see Chapter 11). However, there may be conditions under which water-immiscible benzene would be a more suitable intermediate solvent.

f. Noncovalent Binding. We, as well as others (Cuatrecasas and Hollenberg, 1976), have made several observations that led us to conclude that Tagit in its free acid form binds to some proteins, such as the serum albumins, probably noncovalently. Thus, despite an addition of ethylene diamine (in amounts sufficient to inactivate the activated ester by 98% or more) to a Tagit–[125]I-labeled DMF aliquot prior to performing the protein coupling reaction, the apparent uptake of ^{125}I may be as high as 30% or more. Indeed, using the free acid of Tagit, radiolabeled identically to Tagit (except that the benzene passage has been omitted since the acid is only slightly soluble in benzene), yields uptakes of about 30%. The observation that the homologous *p*-hydroxyphenylacetic acid shows a reduced degree of nonconvalent binding appears to be compatible with its lower degree of hydrophobicity.

g. Test for Coupling. To ensure that the labeled Tagit is bound covalently, a sample of the material to be Tagit-labeled should also be incubated with an ethylene diamine (or other readily available primary amine)-pretreated sample of Tagit–^{125}I and then dialyzed.

As a test protein, 0.05% gelatin has been used (Cuatrecasas and Hollenberg, 1976). We have used 500 μl of 10% polylysine (MW greater than 20,000) plus 50 μl of 1 M NaHCO$_3$ in distilled water, to which 10 μl of the Tagit–^{125}I-labeled sample is added. This mixture is dialyzed (after 20 min) for 24 hr against PBS. The content of iodine before and after dialysis yields the coupling efficiency.

Polylysine has an advantage over tyrosine- and histidine-containing proteins in that it cannot be accidently iodinated via transiodination or residual chloramine-T.

h. High Specific Activity Tagit. Obviously only a small number of Tagit molecules become iodinated, even when the iodination efficiency is 100%. One millicurie of ^{125}I corresponds to about 6×10^{-9} mole of I, and 3 mg of Tagit corresponds to about 6×10^{-5} mole. Thus, only 1 in 10,000 molecules of Tagit carries ^{125}I. It is clearly unnecessary to use an excess of Tagit, and for some applications one might be particularly interested in as high a specific activity as possible. We have therefore tested both iodination and coupling efficiencies under conditions of lower Tagit concentration during iodination. By lowering the Tagit concentration as much as 1000-fold, the percentage of iodine uptake on Tagit fell from 80 to about 40% and the chemical coupling efficiency (to polylysine—Section III,B,2,g) decreased from 50 to 25%. Thus, the specific activity of Tagit–^{125}I may be increased effectively by a factor of 500 (to a labeling ratio of 1 in 20 molecules of Tagit, at a final Tagit–DMF concentration of 50 μM) while the chemical coupling efficiency is still acceptable.

C. Lyophilization of Radioiodine or Other Volatile Isotope-Containing Material

When materials containing such volatile radiochemicals as molecular iodine are lyophilized, gross contamination of some of the apparatus cannot be avoided. It is important, therefore, to confine the contamination either to inexpensive, replaceable parts or to parts that may be decontaminated easily. The intake (manifold) must be placed inside a hood to avoid breathing the possible iodine volatilizations. Tubing connecting the sample container with the vacuum pump should therefore be kept as short as possible. The sample tube must be connected directly to a hose (i.e., it must not be placed inside a larger vessel, which would lead to heavy contamination of the outside surface of the sample tube). In our procedure, at worst, only the upper rim of the flask is contaminated. The piece of connecting rubber tubing should be renewed each time.

A liquid nitrogen trap does collect some iodine, but a much more effective way of reducing the amount of radioiodine entering the pump is to use a filter between the sample and the cold trap. The filter is an ordinary gas mask carbon filter (R51, American Optical Corp., Southbridge, Maine) mounted as shown in Fig. 2. This filter is extremely effective in keeping trap and pump oil contamination at almost negligible levels. After volatilizing 1 mCi of ^{125}I in a tube at the lyophilizer and operating the pumps for about 10 hr, the first filter contained all the activity and a second equal filter in line with the first contained only 1/80,000th of the input activity. After operating the lyophilizer for a period of over 1 year and admitting between 10 and 20 mCi of ^{125}I, the pump oil containing only 0.05 μCi of ^{125}I per liter. The pump speed is not affected by the filter. Despite the good performance of the filter,

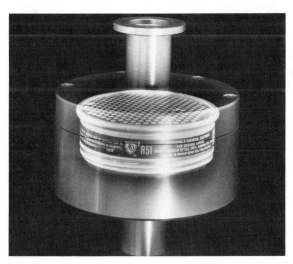

Fig. 2 Photograph of the vacuum line carbon filter: The R51 (see text) gas mask filter is held inside the brass housing by O-rings appropriately placed so that all air must pass through the filter. Air flow is from top to bottom. The flanges at both ends are "normed" flanges (Pneurop 20 KF, 20-mm i.d., Leybold–Heraeus GmbH, D-5000, Köln).

the outlet of the vacuum pump must be connected to the exhaust system of the building.

IV. RADIATION AND CONTAMINATION SURVEILLANCE

A. Ingestion and Contamination

Danger to health of personnel arises from exposure to and incorporation of radiation from radioactive material (see Suggested Reading on this problem). It is our experience that the incidence of incorporation (however infrequent) is not related to the amount of isotope used in the experiment; instead, it is almost always traceable to an unforeseen or unforeseeable cause. Radioiodine has never been detected in individuals after experiments involving large amounts of isotopes; if it is found at all, it is found in individuals connected only peripherally with such operations. We have reason to believe that this is caused, for example, by slow evaporation of iodine from waste (not necessarily very hot) or from samples. Reducing the residence time of waste in the lab, regardless of whether considered hot or "cold," and actively ventilating the mobile hot waste containers by connecting them to the general laboratory exhaust system by a flexible tube have proved (according to monitoring the radioiodine content of the laboratory air) to be sufficiently effective in reducing the overall content. A high local concentration, which is potentially dangerous, could possibly go unnoticed.

Other suspected avenues of ingestion have been via hands and mouth. Protective devices, such as gloves, are often used in a sloppy manner. The reason for this is quite clear: Plastic gloves prevent contamination of the skin; thus, people do not worry about the contamination of their gloves. They seem to work unperturbedly with them, opening doors and handling equipment, etc. As a result one finds activity in certain places that would indicate gross contamination of the researcher's hands. Had gloves *not* been worn, more attention would have been directed to the avoidance of hand contamination. Gloves should therefore be used only in experiments with *definite* risk of contamination and only for those specific steps; gloves then should be changed more frequently between risky steps and/or monitored. The same applies to breathing masks and shields, which must be (or are unconciously) handled and fingered during hot operations. They sometimes become mediators for ingestion. In general, protective equipment tends to increase the risk of accident by reducing agility and dexterity.

B. Portable Monitors

The liberal use, supply, and strict maintenance of simple, battery-powered hand monitors, particularly in normal (D-level) laboratories, are of utmost importance. Information about the detection sensitivity in terms of tolerable contamination levels for the different isotopes should be supplied with these monitors to the users of this equipment.

Many different makes of monitors are equivalent. We have found that the followings models fill our needs well.

For γ-ray emitters
   Mini Monitor, type 5-40 (with a NaI scintillation probe, type 5-42)
For β-ray emitters
   Mini Monitor, type 5-10E (Mini Instruments, Ltd., London, England), with a Geiger–Muller tube (Mullard Limited, Mullard House, Torrington Place, London, England)

C. Personal Monitors

1. Film Badge

Even though required by law only for regular users of laboratories with radiation danger levels above the (ordinary) D-level, every employee of the Basel Institute may and is encouraged to wear such a badge. Badges are renewed on a monthly bases.

2. Thermoluminescence Detectors (TLD)

The thermoluminescence dosimeter has recently been introduced in Switzerland. It is undoubtedly an improved personal monitor. Accumulated dose evaluation is done by a central federal agency every 3 months.

3. Other Personal Monitors

For short-term usage (vistors), or under circumstances where the exposure dose is expected to be unusually high and rates of exposure should be known immediately, a few electrometer-type monitors are available (BF-Verbriebs GmbH f. Messtechnik, D-75 Karlsruhe; type LB 1300 or LB 1400, 0–200 mR).

D. Urine Sampling

All urine analyses are performed by a federal agency. Very little evidence has been accumulated thus far. However, it becomes apparent that urine

TABLE I

Thyroid Test Setup

	^{125}I	^{131}I
Counting efficiency[a] (cpm)	$2.4 \times 10^5 (2.4 \times 10^4)^b$	$8.3 \times 10^3 (8.3 \times 10^2)$
Background (cpm)	120	170
Sensitivity with respect to PEP tolerance level[c]	$2000 \ (200)^b$	50 (5)
Tolerance incorporation for PEP (and non-PEP) (μCi)	$1.1 \ (0.11)^b$	0.15 (0.15)

[a] Corresponding to an incorporation of isotope equal to the tolerance level, as in the last row. For example, 2.4×10^5 cpm (first row) would be registered at this particular setup if 1.1 μCi (last row) of I-125 had been incorporated.

[b] Values in parentheses are those for non-PEP (professionally exposed persons).

[c] The units are the respective tolerance incorporation levels. Thus, "2000" means that our setup will register a signal equal to background (second row) if the incorporation is 1/2000th of the tolerance amount.

sampling serves as a sensitive indicator for negligent operations or behavior by scientists and technicians at a sufficiently early stage—in a way similar to the film or TLD badges, except that in the urine samples the otherwise undetectable low-energy electron emitters (such as ^3H) are also detected.

E. Thyroid Test

To check on radioiodine incorporation, direct monitoring of the thyroid gland is much more pertinent and sensitive than urine analysis. We use a NaI-scintillation crystal (1 × 1.75-in. diameter, 0.001-in. aluminum window; Harshaw Chemie B. V., De Meern, Holland) on an EMI 9656 detector (EMI, Hayes, Middlesex, England). Measurements on phantoms[2] show that the level of detection sensitivity is as indicated in Table I.

F. Surveillance of Laboratories and Laboratory Air

1. Wipe Tests

Wipe tests are found to be quite effective for general surveillance because their sensitivity is far superior to that of portable monitors. The frequency of testing (approximately once every 1 to 3 months for a D-level laboratory)

[2] "Phantom" is the technical term in radiology for models of parts of the human body, which have all the properties of the body as far as radiation absorption, etc., is concerned. With these one can determine exact radiation intensities under simulated conditions.

depends again on past history of contamination of the lab and the amount and types of isotopes used there.

Tests with intentional spills have shown that the efficacy of pickup in a wipe test of a given amount of radioisotope ranges between 10 and 70%, depending on the material and condition of the contaminated surface, as well as on the chemical nature of the spilled material.

Instead of the usual alcohol–water mixture, an aqueous solution of a detergent is often used to do smear tests in hot labs. This has the advantage of decreasing the volatility and thus the higher solubility for inorganic or insoluble contaminants.

2. Air Monitoring

To detect vaporized radioiodine in the hot lab atmosphere, air samples are taken continuously at various points (see Table II) and sucked through a charcoal filter (Schleicher and Schuell AG, Feldbach, CH-8000 Zürich, Switzerland). The pump speed is 3 liters/min (Aerosol collector, type 720, Pedrolit GMBH, CH-8000 Zürich, Switzerland). The filters are removed once per week and counted in a γ-scintillation counter. The collection efficiency of such a filter was estimated to be 25% by observing that a second, serial filter in the line contained about 50% of the activity of the first. For special purposes a high-speed pump (Pedrolit, type 710, 800 liters/min) is used. However, the filter is now a gas mask filter cartridge. Its

TABLE II

^{125}I **Aerosol Monitoring**

	^{125}I [a]	
Location	Net cpm/30 m^3	μCi/m^3
B-level laboratory	5,300 (110,000)[b]	1×10^{-4} (2×10^{-3})
Isotope office	1,600	3×10^{-5}
Library of the Basel Institute	100	2×10^{-6}
Exhaust air downstream from hood filters of the B-level laboratory	1,600 (11,000)	3×10^{-5} (2×10^{-4})
Three miles away from the Basel Institute	60	1×10^{-6}
Counter background	100	
Permissible concentration for PEP[c]	530,000	1×10^{-2}
Permissible concentration for non-PEP	18,000	3.3×10^{-4}

[a] Count rate in the ^{125}I window (with a counting efficiency of 80%) of carbon filters from air samplers. Period of measurement, 1 week; sampled air volume, 30 m^3.

[b] Figures in parentheses refer to peak values of the past 2 years. Other figures refer to the mean counts per minute during the past 2 years minus the counter background.

[c] PEP, professionally exposed persons.

collection efficiency is about 99%. The smaller carbon filter papers are not suitable for such high flow rates. On the other hand, the gas mask cartridges are too impractical for routine monitoring.

Considering the results of air monitoring in Table II, it may be concluded that (1) air monitoring in the B-level laboratories is important and (2) despite institutionalized precautions and all technical arrangements to prevent leakage in high-activity areas, some (although much less than maximally admissable) ^{125}I still enters the B-level laboratory and seemingly also the atmospheres of other laboratories; we believe this is due to sources that are, according to the usual rational approach, "nonsources" (e.g., gloves, low-active waste, and tubes).

3. Hoods

Originally the fume hoods of the isotope laboratory did not have built-in filters. Emanation of radioiodine vapors in the hoods resulted in an ever-increasing deposition of radioiodine in air ducts. When the ventilation system was modified, more powerful fans were installed, which allowed the insertion of carbon filters between the hoods and air ducts (type CP-CG 1/25, CEAG–Dominit, Dortmund, West Germany) and a prefilter, Astrocel (type A 11-J6-R2, CEAG–Dominit; installation by Sulzer AG, CH-8400 Winterthur, Switzerland). These filters have been in place, with the exhaust system running 24 hr a day, for 1 year. Table II shows that even in the exhaust air downstream from the filters the permissable limit has never been reached.

G. Decontamination

1. Glassware

Heavily contaminated utensils are most efficiently decontaminated with chromic and sulfuric acids. Laboratory glassware can be effectively decontaminated to low background in this way. Fumes from the acid bath must be ventilated.

Less severe or easily soluble contamination may be efficiently removed by special decontaminating agents such as Deconex 11NS (Borer Chemie, CH8000 Zürich).

2. Floors

Particularly in the hot laboratories the use of too strong detergents should be avoided because they tend to make the floor cover more porous so that subsequent contamination by spillage becomes more difficult to remove. Liquid soap seems to be both efficient and sufficiently gentle.

3. Lab Benches

For general cleaning, any mild household detergent suffices. However, to remove actual, heavy contamination, a foam-producing spray (3M Office Cleaner, 3M Co., Switzerland AG, Ch-8000 Zürich) very effectively keeps the cleaning medium concentrated on the contaminated area.

ACKNOWLEDGMENTS

We are grateful to Mr. Holloway of the MRC laboratory at Mill Hill, London, who advised us at the very beginning of operations. We also wish to acknowledge the contributions of the early staff members of the isotope laboratory, Pierre Lix and the late Reto Jaeggi.

SUGGESTED READING

Faires, R. A., and Parks, B. H. (1958). "Radioisotope Laboratory Techniques." George Newnes Limited, London.
Steere, N., ed. (1971). "Handbook of Laboratory Safety." Chem. Rubber Publ. Co., Cleveland, Ohio.
U.S. Department of Health, Education and Welfare. (1970). "Radiological Health Handbook," rev. ed. Public Health Serv., Rockville, Maryland. USDHEW.
Wilson, B. J., ed. (1966). "The Radiochemical Manual," 2nd ed. The Radiochemical Centre, Amersham, England.

REFERENCES

Bolton, A. E., and Hunter, W. M. (1973). *Biochem. J.* **133**, 529.
Cuatrecasas, P., and Hollenberg, M. (1976). *Adv. Protein Chem.* **30**, 295.
Hunter, W. M. (1971). *In* "Radioimmunoassay Methods" (K. E. Kirkham and W. M. Hunter, eds.), pp. 16 and 61ff. Churchill, London.
Rudinger, J., and Ruegg, U. (1973). *Biochem. J.* **133**, 538.

34

Analysis of Immunological Data

Alberto Piazza

IMMUNOLOGICAL METHODS
Copyright © 1979 by Academic Press, Inc.
All rights of reproduction in any form reserved.
ISBN 0-12-442750-2

I. INTRODUCTION

Several excellent books dealing specifically with the applications of statistics to biological problems have appeared in recent years (see, e.g., Armitage, 1971; Bliss, 1970; Colton, 1974; Mather, 1972; Sokal and Rohlf, 1973), but there are some peculiar facets of the analysis of data in immunology that may be usefully brought together between two covers. Mathematics, statistics, and genetics are the ingredients of what follows, but they will be kept at an elementary level, the philosophy being that of *how to cook*, not of *how to prove it*. Given the nature of this chapter, the references are not extensive and are meant to encourage further reading rather than presenting an unwieldy bibliography.

The various statistical techniques will be demonstrated on worked examples, drawn from the literature or from everyday work of an immunological laboratory.

II. WORKED EXAMPLES

A. A Serological Survey

Hsia *et al.* (1977) published an interesting study concerning viral antibody responses in families. Antibodies to adenovirus, cytomegalovirus, herpes simplex virus, influenza type A virus, and others were measured from 584 humans belonging to 21 Indiana Amish families. The problem was to assess the relevance of sex and age on antibody responses and to test for familial associations.

1. Non-normal and Normal Distributions

Antibody titers usually show an extremely asymmetric distribution. The left part of Table I records the frequency distribution of the cyto-

TABLE I

**Frequency Distribution of CMV Antibody Titers and
Transformations**[a]

Original data		Transformations		
Frequency (n_i)	Titer^{-1} (x_i)	Harmonic $(100/x_i)$	Square root $(\sqrt{x_i})$	Logarithmic $(\log_2 x_i)$
23	2	50	1.41	1
53	4	25	2	2
90	8	12.5	2.83	3
110	16	6.25	4	4
60	32	3.125	5.66	5
34	64	1.563	8	6
10	128	0.781	11.31	7

[a] Data are from Hsia *et al.* (1977).

megalovirus (CMV) antibody titers taken from Hsia *et al.* (1977). Nearly
65% (380 individuals) of the entire population has measurable CMV serum
antibody. Figure 1 displays the corresponding bar diagram. It can be seen
that the distribution is asymmetric about the *mode* (the titer value of
maximum frequency). An asymmetric distribution is called *skew*. When the

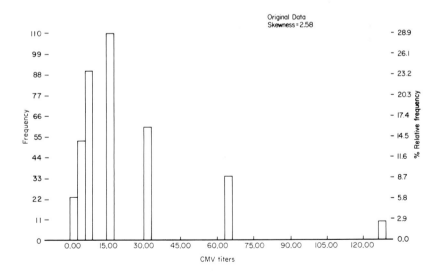

Figure 1

upper tail is longer than the lower, as in Fig. 1, we say that the skewness is positive.

Imagine that the titers were determined much more accurately. There would then be many more bars in Fig. 1. In the limit the bars would be so narrow that the tips of the bars would define a continuous curve. Such a curve is called a *continuous frequency distribution*.

A continuous distribution that has only one mode (unimodal) and is symmetric (in such a case the mode and the mean are the same) is the *normal distribution*. This distribution exhibits a shape rather like a bell, with a pronounced peak in the middle and a gradual falling off of the frequency in the two tails. The normal distribution was originally derived as a theory of errors in physical measurements: If an event is influenced by a large number of small random perturbances, most of the effects will tend to cancel out and the observations will cluster about the mean; outlying observations, in either direction, become less likely the farther away they are from the mean value. The importance of the normal distribution lies not so much in any claim to represent a wide range of observed frequency distributions, but in the central place it occupies in tests of hypotheses. In fact, even though there is no formal proof that natural events are normally distributed, it can be proved that their means *are*. The probability of a normally distributed variable x to fall between x and $x + dx$ is

$$f(x)dx = \frac{1}{\sigma(2\pi)^{1/2}} \exp[-(x - \mu)^2/2\sigma^2]dx \tag{1}$$

$f(x)$ is called the *probability density* of a continuous distribution; μ and σ^2 are two parameters. A plot of $f(x)$ versus x gives the bell-shaped curve, with μ defining its position along the x-axis and σ its width. Tables of the normal distribution $f(x)$ defined by Eq. (1) and its integral are to be found in each of the statistical tests listed in the books by Armitage (1971), Bliss (1970), Cotton (1974), Mather (1972), and Sokal and Rohlf (1973).

2. Measures of Location and Dispersion

Experimental data, that is, a limited number of observations as those collected in Table I, will not fall exactly on the theoretical curve: One of the problems of statistical inference is to know whether this lack of fitting is due to simple sampling errors or to a true non-normality of the population of measures from which we are sampling. In any case, it is important to give in a single figure some indication of the general "trend" of a series of measurements. Such a figure is called a measure of *location*, and the most familiar among the measures of location is the *arithmetic mean*. If there are N observations of the variable x, they will be denoted by x_i ($i = 1, 2, \cdots,$

N). The arithmetic mean of x_i is defined by m_x:

$$m_x = \frac{\sum_{i=1}^{N} x_i}{N}$$

More generally, if each x_i is observed n_i times, we have

$$m_x = \frac{\sum_{i=1}^{N} n_i x_i}{\sum_{i=1}^{N} n_i} = \sum_{i=1}^{N} f_i x_i \qquad (2)$$

where $f_i = n_i / \Sigma n_i$.

The mean of the reciprocal antibody titers in Table I is

$$m_x = \frac{23 \cdot 2 + 53 \cdot 4 + \cdots + 128 \cdot 10}{23 + 53 + \cdots + 10} = \frac{8114}{380} = 21.35$$

The mean of the reciprocal $\log_2$ antibody titers $y_i = \log x_i$ is

$$m_y = \frac{\sum_{i=1}^{N} (\log x_i) n_i}{\sum_{i=1}^{N} n_i} = \frac{1413}{380} = 3.72$$

The arithmetic mean m_y can be transformed back to the original scale of titers by taking

$$m_x^* = \text{antilog}_2 \, m_y$$

m_x^* is called the *geometric mean* of x.

When the mean value of a series of measurements has been obtained, it is usually a matter of considerable interest to express the degree of variation or scatter around this mean. We therefore require what is variously termed a measure of *variation*, *scatter*, *spread*, or *dispersion*. The most common measure of dispersion is the mean value of the squared deviations from the mean:

$$s^2 = \frac{\sum_{i=1}^{N} (x_i - m_x)^2}{N}$$

which is called *variance*. More generally, if each x_i is observed f_i times, we have

$$s^2 = \frac{\sum\limits_{i=1}^{N} n_i(x_i - m_x)^2}{\sum\limits_{i=1}^{N} n_i} = \sum\limits_{i=1}^{N} f_i(x_i - m_x)^2 \qquad (3)$$

where

$$f_i = \frac{n_i}{\sum\limits_{i=1}^{N} n_i}$$

The total number of observations [the denominator of Eq. (3)] is usually subtracted by 1, when the mean (one parameter) has already been calculated from the sample.

The variance is measured in the square of the units in which x is measured. It is convenient, therefore, to have a measure of variation expressed in the original units of x, and this can be done easily by taking the square root of the variance, s. This quantity is known as the *standard deviation*. Equations (2) and (3) are easily generalized to the case of continuous distributions by substituting summation with integration over all the space of the (continuous) variable x:

$$m(x) = \int_{-\infty}^{\infty} xf(x)dx \qquad (2')$$

$$s^2(x) = \int_{-\infty}^{\infty} [x - m(x)]^2 f(x)dx \qquad (3')$$

In the case of the normal distribution, by integration of Eqs. (2') and (3') with $f(x)$ given by Eq. (1), it can be found that (i) the mean of the normal distribution is given by the parameter μ and (ii) the variance of the normal distribution is given by the parameter σ^2.

3. Normalizing Transformations and Tests of Inference

The distribution of Fig. 1, positively skewed, is obviously far from being normal. As many statistical tests are based on the assumption of normality, it is often convenient to look for ways to transform skewed data to approximate normal distribution. Three of the most used normalizing transformations are given on the right side of Table I and their effect is shown in the bar diagrams of Figs. 2–4.

The success of normalization is assessed by the statistic

$$\text{skewness} = \frac{\Sigma(x_i - m)^3}{s^3}$$

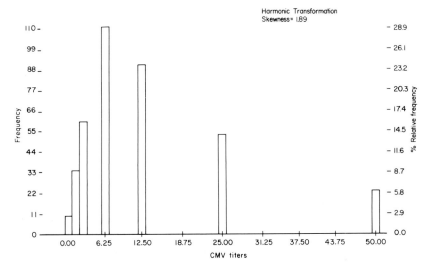

Figure 2

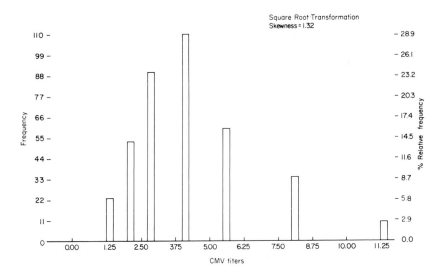

Figure 3

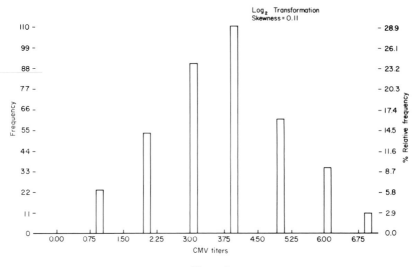

Figure 4

which in the absence of skewness equals zero, whereas positive or negative values indicate positive or negative skewness, respectively.

It is evident that, while both the harmonic and square root transformations reduce skewness, the transformation appropriate to this set of data is the logarithmic.

If the distribution of the reciprocal $\log_2$ values of antibody titers is found to fit a normal curve, the transformed data can be used for statistical inference. The simplest question we may like to answer is the following: Given two groups of individuals, for instance, males and females, is there any evidence that the mean antibody response of the females is significantly different from the antibody response of the males? In statistical terms the question must be formulated as follows: Is there a test that gives us the probability error in rejecting the hypothesis that the two samples are drawn from the *same* population, any difference between them being due to random sampling fluctuations?

The Student t test is appropriate for this problem. If m_1 and m_2 are the means of the two samples and n_1, n_2 and s_1^2, s_2^2 their sample sizes and their variances, the quantity

$$t = \frac{m_1 - m_2}{\left\{ \left[\dfrac{(n_1 - 1)s_1^2 + (n_2 - 1)s_2^2}{n_1 + n_2 - 2} \right] \left(\dfrac{n_1 + n_2}{n_1 n_2} \right) \right\}^{1/2}} \tag{4}$$

is a distribution that depends on the associated degrees of freedom $n_1 + n_2 - 2$ and gives the probability shown above. It is tabulated in any textbook on statistics and in statistical tables. Let us suppose that in our example we have for the females (group 1) and the males (group 2) the following data on the antibody response (expressed in $\log_2$ values of titers):

$$m_1 = 3.742 \qquad n_1 = 296 \qquad s_1^2 = 0.04$$
$$m_2 = 3.701 \qquad n_2 = 288 \qquad s_2^2 = 0.04$$

By applying Eq. (4) we have

$$t_{582} = \frac{0.041}{(0.000274)^{1/2}} = 2.48$$

Looking at the table of t, a value of 2.48, corresponding to df = 582 ($\simeq \infty$, the last row of the table), is associated with a probability value of less than 0.001. Hence, we reject the hypothesis of equal means (the two samples are drawn from the same population). In other words, we can conclude that the observed difference in the means is almost certainly due to a real difference in the populations from which the two samples are drawn: The fluctuations due to sampling effects could *not* explain these different responses in the two sexes.

4. Test for Associations

Hsia *et al.* (1977) also describe a simple analysis of variance for investigating the possible association of viral antibody response with haplotypes within a family. Let us assign the parental haplotypes as *ab* (father) and *cd* (mother). In the absence of recombination, each child has one of the four possible combinations of parental haplotypes: *ac*, *ad*, *bc*, or *bd*. Assuming that the haplotype effects on antibody response are additive and that the action of each haplotype is independent of the other three, each person's titer would be the sum of his two haplotype effects.

Let us first consider all individuals in a family with haplotype *a* and let us suppose that the sum of the titers of these individuals is S_a and that the haplotypes *a*, *b*, *c*, and *d* are present in numbers n_a, n_b, n_c, and n_d, respectively. The haplotype effects are assumed to be described by a linear equation:

$$\beta_a n_a + \beta_b n_b + \beta_c n_c + \beta_d n_d = S_a \tag{5}$$

where β_a, β_b, β_c, and β_d are unknowns to be estimated from the data. Writing similar equations for the haplotypes *b*, *c*, and *d* we have a linear system of four equations in four unknowns that can be handled easily.

As an example, consider the following family from the Amish data:

			Sibs					
	Father	Mother	1	2	3	4	5	6
Haplotype	ab	cd	bd	bc	bc	ad	bd	ad
Log_2 (titer^{-1})(to CMV)	0	5	0	2	0	3	0	3

The system of equations of type (5) is the following:

$$3\beta_a + 1\beta_b + 0\beta_c + 2\beta_d = 6$$
$$1\beta_a + 5\beta_b + 2\beta_c + 1\beta_d = 2$$
$$0\beta_a + 2\beta_b + 3\beta_c + 1\beta_d = 7$$
$$2\beta_a + 2\beta_b + 1\beta_c + 5\beta_d = 11$$

For the first equation, $n_a = 3$ because there are three individuals with haplotype a (father, sib 4, and sib 6), $n_b = 1$ because only the father has haplotype ab, $n_c = 0$ because the haplotype ac is not represented in this family, and $n_d = 2$ because sibs 4 and 6 carry the haplotype ad. The sum of the titers of these individuals contributing a is $S_a = 3 + 3 = 6$. The other three equations are derived in the same way considering the contributions of the individuals to the haplotypes respectively: b, c, and d. The algebraic solution to this system of equations is

$$\beta_a = 1.42 \qquad \beta_b = -1.75 \qquad \beta_c = 2.92 \qquad \beta_d = 1.75$$

The problem is how can we test whether the observations fit our model or are due to random, chance phenomena.

The technique is a good introduction to the *analysis of variance*, which will be developed in the worked examples below, and it consists mainly in comparing two variances and testing for their equality.

The sum of squares from the mean of the measured antibody levels for n individuals can be written as

$$\sum_{i=1}^{n} (Y_i - m)^2 = \sum_{i=1}^{n} (Y_i - Y_i^{exp})^2 + \sum_{i=1}^{n} (Y_i^{exp} - m)^2$$

where Y_i is the measured antibody level of the ith individual, m is the mean titer of all n individuals, and Y_i^{exp} is the antibody level of the ith individual expected when the additive contribution of two among the four calculated β_a, β_b, β_c, and β_d haplotype effects are taken into account. The first sum of squares gives the error of the model: If it is zero, expected and observed levels of antibody are coincident, and the model is absolutely correct. Therefore, the second sum of squares represents the part of the variability explained by the model itself: Its magnitude compared to the magnitude of the error is a measure of the goodness of fit of the model. Since the sum of squares is proportional to the variance and the ratio

$$\frac{\text{variance due to the model}}{\text{variance due to the error}}$$

when sampled from a normal population is a known statistical distribution, called F distribution, or variance ratio, it is possible to test whether such a ratio is statistically different from 1, that is, to calculate the probability of being in error when the hypothesis of two variances estimated through samples drawn from the same population is rejected. In the family above the following is true:

$$\text{Variance due to the model} = 23.5$$
$$\text{Variance due to error} = 2.33$$
$$F_{3;4} = 13.5$$

Entering in the F probability table (see Section II,B for the meaning of the indices 3 and 4 attached to F), we find the associated probability P to fall in the range $0.01 \leq P \leq 0.05$. The conclusion is that the data fit with the model, because the hypothesis of two variances estimated by samples taken from the same population is rejected with a very small error, $P \leq 0.05$.

B. Comparison of Cell Yields

Spleen cells of BALB/c or BALB/c *nu/nu* mice were collected by either of two techniques, the erythrocytes were lysed, and the remaining cells were counted. We wish to find out whether there is a difference (i) between the two techniques of collecting cells and (ii) between the two strains of mice.

1. Computation of Statistics

The experimental data are shown in Table II. Table III shows all the calculations required to investigate the problem.

On inspection, the two groups of mice seem to differ greatly, whereas the difference between techniques A and B is small. To assess these differences, we first perform t tests within each strain of mice. For the BALB/c$^+$/$+$ group we have

$$t_{(22)} = \frac{101.92 - 194.42}{[(2351.64 + 2705.37)/12]^{1/2}} = 0.369$$

which corresponds to a probability of $0.7 < P < 0.8$; that is, the same

TABLE II

Splenic Cell Counts[a]

BALB/c +/+ mice[b]		BALB/c *nu/nu* mice[b]	
Technique A	Technique B	Technique A	Technique B
178	204	99	78
212	165	93	88
257	158	104	104
191	200	130	113
177	137	94	84
210	147	112	78
107	208	86	96
180	334	94	106
168	211	118	122
196	218	89	96
286	157	107	98
.262	194	97	97

[a] The cells were collected in Earle's saline, and the erythrocytes were lysed by the $(NH_4)Cl$ technique, washed, and counted in a Coulter counter. The numbers per spleen are given in millions.

[b] Technique A: Spleens were diced to a cube size of approximately 2 mm and passed through a stainless steel mesh. Technique B: The splenic capsule was opened at both ends and the cells were teased out with a sterile spatula.

TABLE III

Calculations from the Data in Table II

	+/+		*nu/nu*	
	A	B	A	B
Sum of x, Σx	2,424	2,333	1,223	1,160
Sum of x^2, Σx^2	515,516	483,333	126,481	114,118
Sum of squares, S_{xx} [a]	25,868.0	29,758.9	1,836.9	1,984.7
Mean, m	202.00	194.42	101.92	96.67
Variance, s^2	2,351.64	2,705.37	166.99	180.42

[a] $S_{xx} = \Sigma(x_i - m)^2$.

result could have been obtained in three out of four cases by chance. For the nude mice we have

$$t_{(22)} = \frac{101.92 - 96.67}{[(166.99 + 180.42)/12]^{1/2}} = 0.976 \qquad 0.3 < P < 0.4$$

2. Pooling of Data

Since the differences between the two techniques are not significant ($P >$ 0.05), the observations may be pooled. Thus, for the BALB/c^+/+ mice, $m = (2424 + 2333)/24 = 198.21; s^2 = 2433.56$.

For the nude mice, $m = 99.29; s^2 = 173.35$.

Comparing now the pooled values of the two strains:

$$t_{(46)} = \frac{198.21 + 99.29}{[(2433.56 + 173.35)/24]^{1/2}} = 9.49 \qquad P \ll 0.001$$

Since such an outcome would occur by chance in less than 1 in 1000 cases, the difference between the two strains is highly significant.

The best estimate of the average number of splenic cells obtained from BALB/c mice is 198.21×10^6 and is 99.29×10^6 for nude mice.

3. Analysis of Variance

The t test compares two means at a time: We had to perform two such tests to justify pooling the data and then a third to assess the difference between the two strains of mice. While two means may still be compared conveniently by a t test, the effective tool for multiple comparisons is the *analysis of variance*. The principle here is to obtain the total sum of squares (as if all observations came from the same population) and then take out partial sums of squares for meaningful subsets of observations.

We consider the simplest situation in which there is just one observation at each combination of a technique and a strain, simply the mean of the 12 observations calculated in Table III. The data can be ordered as shown in Table IV.

TABLE IV

Means from the Data in Table II

	Strain		
	+/+	*nu/nu*	Row mean
Technique A	202.00	101.92	151.96
Technique B	194.42	96.67	145.55
Column mean	198.21	99.30	General mean, 148.75

A more general notation for our analysis of variance is

			Column						
		1	$\cdots$ 2	$\cdots$	j	$\cdots$	c	Total	Mean (R_i/c)
	1 $\cdots$	Y_{11}	Y_{12}	$\cdots$	Y_{1j}	$\cdots$	Y_{1c}	R_1	$\bar{Y}_{1.}$
	2	Y_{21}	Y_{22}	$\cdots$	Y_{2j}	$\cdots$	Y_{2c}	R_2	$\bar{Y}_{2.}$
	$\vdots$	$\vdots$	$\vdots$		$\vdots$		$\vdots$	$\vdots$	$\vdots$
Row	j	Y_{i1}	Y_{i2}	$\cdots$	Y_{ij}	$\cdots$	Y_{ic}	R_i	$\bar{Y}_{i.}$
	$\vdots$	$\vdots$	$\vdots$		$\vdots$		$\vdots$	$\vdots$	$\vdots$
	r	Y_{r1}	Y_{r2}	$\cdots$	Y_{rj}	$\cdots$	Y_{rc}	R_r	$\bar{Y}_{r.}$
Total		C_1	C_2	$\cdots$	C_j	$\cdots$	C_c	T	
Mean (C_j/r)		$\bar{Y}_{.1}$	$\bar{Y}_{.2}$	$\cdots$	$\bar{Y}_{.j}$	$\cdots$	$\bar{Y}_{.c}$		$\bar{Y} = T/rc$

The total sum of squares

$$\text{SS}(t) = \sum_{i=1}^{r} \sum_{j=1}^{c} (Y_{ij} - \bar{Y})^2$$

can be partitioned into various parts. For any one of these deviations from the mean, $Y_{ij} - \bar{Y}$, the following holds:

$$Y_{ij} - \bar{Y} = (\bar{Y}_{i.} - \bar{Y}) + (\bar{Y}_{.j} - \bar{Y}) + (Y_{ij} - \bar{Y}_{i.} - \bar{Y}_{.j} + \bar{Y})$$

The three terms on the right-hand side reflect the fact that Y_{ij} differs from $\bar{Y}$, partly due to a different characteristic of the ith row, partly because of a difference characteristic of the jth column, and partly by an amount that is not explicable by either row or column differences. Summing and squaring over all $N = rc$ observations, we find

$$\sum_i \sum_j (Y_{ij} - \bar{Y})^2 = \sum_i (\bar{Y}_{i.} - \bar{Y})^2 + \sum_j (\bar{Y}_{.j} - \bar{Y})^2$$
$$+ \sum_i \sum_j (Y_y - \bar{Y}_{i.} - \bar{Y}_{.j} + \bar{Y}) \tag{7}$$

The three sums of squares (SS) on the right-hand side of Eq. (7) are called the "between rows" (in our example, techniques) SS(r), the "between columns" (in our example, strains) SS(c), and the "residual" SS.

The first two sums of squares (SS) are used to test for evidence of significant differences between the groups defined by their belonging, respectively, to the rows or to the columns. Suppose that the observations in the ith group form a random sample from a population with mean μ_i and variance σ^2. To examine the evidence for differences between the μ_i, we shall test the null hypothesis that the μ_i *do not* vary, being equal to some common unknown value μ. Three ways of estimating σ^2 suggest themselves:

(a)   From the "total" sum of squares we can calculate the variance

$$s^2_{\text{total}} = \frac{SS(t)}{N-1}$$

(b)   From the "between rows" sum of squares we can calculate the variance

$$s^2_{\text{rows}} = \frac{SS(r)}{r-1}$$

(c)   From the "between columns" sum of squares we can calculate the variance

$$s^2_{\text{columns}} = \frac{SS(c)}{c-1}$$

The denominators of these three variances express the *degrees of freedom* of the corresponding sources of variation: They tell how many independent deviation squares are used to estimate the variance. Under the null hypothesis of no differences among groups, the variances s^2_{rows} and s^2_{columns} do *not* differ from the variance due to the uncontrolled source of variation (residual) described by the third sum of squares in the right-hand side of Eq. (7). As mentioned in Section II,A,4, the hypothesis of two variances s^2_1 and s^2_2 being sampled from the *same* normal population is tested by their ratio

$$F = s^2_1/s^2_2 \tag{8}$$

whose probability distribution depends on the degrees of freedom of the two variances. The analysis of variance we are discussing can thus be summarized in the following tabulation:

Source of variation	Degrees of freedom	Sum of squares	Variance	F
Between rows	$r-1$	$SS(r)$	$s^2_{\text{rows}} = \dfrac{SS(r)}{r-1}$	s^2_{rows}/s^2
Between columns	$c-1$	$SS(c)$	$s^2_{\text{columns}} = \dfrac{SS(c)}{c-1}$	s^2_{columns}/s^2
Residual	$(r-1)(c-1)$	SS	$s^2 = \dfrac{SS}{(r-1)(c-1)}$	
Total	$rc-1$	$SS(t)$		

This tabulation can be filled in as follows by using the data of Table II and the calculations of Table III.

Source of variation	Degrees of freedom	Sum of squares	Variance	F
Between techniques	1	41	41	21.5
Between strains	1	9784	9784	4892
Residual	1	2	2	
Total	3	9827		

The degrees of freedom of F are in this case 1;1 $(f_{1;1})$ and the corresponding probability is found in the appropriate tables (e.g., Fisher and Yates, 1963; Documenta Geigy, 1962). As we see, only the F value corresponding to the variation between strains is significant, providing the same answer as obtained earlier by the t test.

In Section II,A,4 the degrees of freedom associated with the model sum of squares are 3 (one less than the predicted number of haplotypes) and the degrees of freedom associated with the error sum of squares are 4, since the total sum of squares has 7 degrees of freedom (one less than the number of observations). This is why the F ratio there is written as $F_{3;4}$.

C. Estimating the Quantity and Quality of Antibodies

The equilibrium test, taken from Fig. 2 of Chapter 1, will serve as an example of *curve fitting* and *regression analysis*. We are not concerned here with the measurements themselves and shall deal only with the transformed values $(x_1, y_1; x_2, y_2)$, which, theoretically, should fall on a straight line. The first problem is how to decide whether or not the theory is contradicted. The second problem, provided the observations passed the fundamental *test of validity*, is to estimate the *parameters of the regression*, namely, the slope and intercept of the best-fitting straight line.

1. Regression Analysis

Unlike the preceding sections, in which single variables (x) were dealt with, here we have pairs of variables (x, y). Apart from the added computational labor caused by the extra dimension, the principles (and even the practice) of analysis are much the same.

Of the two variables, one is usually taken as independent (i.e., free from error) and conventionally plotted on the x-axis. The other is the dependent variable, y, subject to experimental error. The relation of the two variables is, in statistical parlance, the *regression of y on x*. In this section we shall deal with *linear regression*, which has the functional form of $y = a + bx$, where a is the y intercept (the point where the regression line cuts the ordinate; i.e., where $x = 0$) and b is the slope (the first derivative of the function x, or the tangent of the angle enclosed by the regression line and the abscissa).

2. Linear Regression

The first question, whether the variables are correlated, that is, whether the regression is significant, and, if so, whether it is linear, is answered by the same technique as used in Section II,B,3: The total variation is partitioned into components due to regression, linearity, and error. To this end, we need first to find the regression line, that is, its slope b and its intercept a, which fit in the "best way" our data. Theoretical arguments lead to the following rule: The regression line is drawn through the n points on the scatter diagram so as to minimize the sum of squares of the distances $y_i - y_i^*$ of the observed points y_i from the expected points y_i^* on the line. It can be shown by elementary calculus that a and b are given by the formulas

$$a = \frac{\Sigma y_i - b\Sigma x_i}{n} \tag{9}$$

$$b = \frac{S_{xy}}{S_{xx}} \tag{10}$$

where the sum of squares S_{xx} and the sum of products S_{xy} are defined by

$$S_{xx} = \Sigma(x_i - \bar{x})^2 = \Sigma x^2 - (\Sigma x)^2/n$$
$$S_{xy} = \Sigma(x_i - \bar{x})(y_i - \bar{y}) = \Sigma xy - \Sigma x \Sigma y/n$$
$$\bar{x} = \frac{\Sigma x_i}{n} \qquad \bar{y} = \frac{\Sigma y_i}{n}$$

Suppose now that our fitted regression line of y on x has the equation

$$y = a + bx \tag{11}$$

with a and b given by Eqs. (9) and (10). The deviation of y_i from the mean $\bar{y}$ can be divided into two parts:

$$y_i - \bar{y} = y_i - y_i^* + y_i^* - \bar{y} \tag{12}$$

where y_i^* is the value of y calculated from the regression line of Eq. (11) with $x = x_i$. When both sides of Eq. (12) are squared and summed over all the observations, the following relation holds:

$$\Sigma(y_i - \bar{y})^2 = \Sigma(y_i - y_i^*)^2 + \Sigma(y_i^* - \bar{y})^2 \tag{13}$$

The term on the left is the total sum of square S_{yy}. The first term on the right is the sum of squares of deviations of observed y's about the regression line (the error term), and the second is the sum of squares about the mean of the values y_i^* predicted by the regression line (the regression term). From Eqs. (9) to (13), the analysis of variance of linear regression is laid out as shown in the following tabulation.

Source of variation	df	Sum of squares	Variance	F
Regression	1	S_{xy}^2/S_{xx}	S_{xy}^2/S_{xx}	$S_{xy}^2/s^2 S_{xx}$
Error	$n - 2$	$S_{yy} - S_{xy}^2/S_{xx}$	$s^2 = \dfrac{1}{n - 2}(S_{yy} - S_{xy}^2/S_{xx})$	
Total	$n - 1$	S_{yy}		

A significant F value validates the regression.

3. Computational Procedure

The experimental data as well as their squares and products are listed in Table V. It should be noted that only the sums are required for the calculations so that, in practice, only the total values are of further interest.

From the totals we obtain

$$S_{xx} = 119.07 - (35.71)^2/12 = 12.802$$
$$S_{xy} = 73.68 - 35.71 \times 27.9/12 = -9.343$$
$$S_{yy} = 71.74 - (27.9)^2/12 = 6.876$$

and the analysis of variance yields the following data.

Source of variation	df	Sum of squares	Variance	F	P
Regression	1	6.818	6.818	1136.67	≪0.001
Error	10	0.057	0.0057		
Total	11	6.876			

The significance of the regression or, more precisely, of the *correlation* between the variables may be assessed also in another way. Instead of comparing variances, the sum of squares for regression is divided by the total sum of squares. This ratio, conventionally denoted by r^2, shows what fraction of the variability is accounted for by the regression:

$$r^2 = \frac{S_{xy}^2}{S_{xx}S_{yy}} \tag{14}$$

TABLE V

Experimental Data Taken from Chapter 1, Fig. 2, to Test
Their Fitting to a Straight Line

x	y	x^2	xy	y^2
4.47	1.13	19.9809	5.0511	1.2769
4.57	1.19	20.8849	5.4383	1.4161
3.92	1.62	15.3664	6.3504	2.6244
3.94	1.64	15.5236	6.4616	2.6896
3.25	2.22	10.5625	7.2150	4.9284
3.21	2.14	10.3041	6.8694	4.5796
2.57	2.60	6.6049	6.6820	6.7600
2.60	2.74	6.7600	7.1240	7.5076
2.02	3.01	4.0804	6.0802	9.0601
2.01	2.93	4.0401	5.8893	8.5849
1.57	3.29	2.4649	5.1653	10.8241
1.58	3.39	2.9664	5.3562	11.4291
35.71	27.90	119.0691	73.6828	71.7438

Note that this treatment does not distinguish between independent and dependent variables: The value of r^2 is the same whether the regression sum of squares is defined as S_{xy}^2/S_{xx} or as S_{xy}^2/S_{yy}, that is, whether a regression of y on x or x on y is assumed. The test of correlation is appropriate to the present example. The original equilibrium equation is quadratic, with the concentration of epitopes as the independent variable. By using linearizing transforms, the dependent variable (the fraction of epitopes occupied) appears in some form on both sides of the equation and x becomes a compound variable, subject to error.

The significance of the correlation may be found in tables of the *correlation coefficient, r*:

$$r = \frac{S_{xy}}{(S_{xx}S_{yy})^{1/2}} \tag{14'}$$

It varies between -1 and $+1$, the absolute magnitude indicating the closeness of correlation and the sign its direction.

For our data $r^2 = 6.818/6.876 = 0.9916$, and the probability associated with $r = (0.9916)^{1/2} = -0.9958$ for 10 degrees of freedom is $P \ll 0.001$.

4. Linearity

Both the variance ratio for regression and the correlation are highly significant, but that in itself does not answer the question whether the regression is also linear. This can be tested within the same analysis by separating a sum of squares for variation among the six pairs of replicates and subtracting from it the already computed component for linear regression. This provides a *test for linearity* and completes the analysis of variance (Table VI). The deviations from linearity are not significant and thus the validity of the model is not contradicted.

The parameters of the regression are estimated next. The slope is

$$b = -9.32/12.8 = 0.730$$

The y intercept is

$$a = (27.9 + 0.73 \cdot 35.71)/12 = 4.498$$

Thus, the data fit to the linear model given by the equation

$$y = 0.730x + 4.498$$

D. Estimating the Number of Precursor B Cells

1. Probability Models

Köhler (1976) describes a method for detecting anti-β-galactosidase antibodies and evaluating the frequency of B precursor cells specific for the enzyme in BALB/c mice. The number of precursor cells is determined by transferring a limited number of syngeneic spleen cells into lethally or sublethally irradiated host mice and observing the distribution of clonal antibodies in the recipient sera. The distribution of recipient sera with either none, one, two, three, four, or more clonal antibodies in two selected experiments is shown in the following tabulation.

Number of spleen cells transferred	Number of clones/serum				
	0	1	2	3	≥ 4
2×10^6	4	3	4	3	5
1×10^7	7	1	3	1	7

The problem is: How can we calculate the average number of different clones per recipient sera? To do this, we need a model by which we can estimate the *expected* number of sera with 0, 1, 2, 3, or 4 and more antibodies. Such a model is called a *probability model* because it associates to the ith outcome of the experiment, x_i, a function $f(x_i)$ that tells how many times (with what *frequency*) we expect (expected frequency = probability) that outcome to occur. The expected frequency or probability is obviously different from the experimental or observed frequency, but we can postulate that, when the observations are sampled from the correct

TABLE VI

Test for Linearity and Analysis of Regression Applied to the Data of Table V

Source of variation	df	Sum of squares	Variance	F	P
Regression	1	6.818	6.8180	1763.40	≪0.001
Deviations from linearity	4	0.035	0.0087	2.23	~0.2
Between replicates	5	6.853			
Error	6	0.023	0.0039		
Total	11	6.876			

probability model, the observed frequency distribution approaches the probability distribution as the trials we do to produce the outcomes are repeated an infinite number of times. The probability is thus a long-run concept. Probabilities and frequencies $f(x_i)$ are usually normalized to the total number of outcomes, say N (i.e., $i = 1, 2, \ldots, N$), so we have:

$$\sum_{i=1}^{N} f(x_i) = 1$$

$$0 \leq f(x_i) \leq 1$$

When all the $f(x_i)$ are specified by a model, the function f is called a *probability distribution*, while the expression *frequency distribution* is usually reserved to the analogous *observed* distribution. When all outcomes occur with the same probability, we have the simple *uniform* distribution:

$$f(x_i) = 1/N \qquad i = 1, 2, \ldots, N \qquad (16)$$

2. Parameters

A distribution is characterized by its position and its spread. The more common measure of position is the *mean*, defined by

$$m = \sum_{i=1}^{N} x_i f(x_i) \qquad (17)$$

which, in the case of equiprobable outcomes [Eq. (16)], simplifies to

$$m = \frac{\sum_{i=1}^{N} x_i}{N} \qquad (18)$$

The more common measure of spread or dispersion is the variance, defined by

$$s^2 = \sum_{i=1}^{N} f(x_i)(x_i - m)^2 = \sum_{i=1}^{N} x_i^2 f(x_i) - \left[\sum_{i=1}^{N} x_i f(x_i) \right]^2 \qquad (19)$$

In the common case of equiprobable outcomes [Eq. (16)], this expression becomes

$$s^2 = \frac{\sum_{i=1}^{N} (x_i - m)^2}{N} \qquad (20)$$

or, if the mean is estimated from the data:

$$s^2 = \frac{\sum_{i=1}^{N} (x_i - m)^2}{N - 1} \qquad (20')$$

Its square root is called the *standard deviation*.

3. Construction of a Model

The problem in hand demands a reasonable probability model to which we can compare our observed distribution frequency. The model must be *discrete*, since the number of precursor cells can take only integer values 0, 1, 2, . . . , n. To build such a model we start from the simplest case. Instead of considering a suspension of millions of cells, one or two of which are the precursor cells we are looking for, we shall first consider an urn that contains, say, one black ball and nine white balls. The chance of drawing the black ball is $p = 1/10$ and the chance of drawing a white ball is $q = (1 - p) = 9/10$. The chances remain the same if our urn contained a million balls, one-tenth of which were black. However, we cannot expect to draw exactly one black ball in every ten trials; what we can expect is that, in a very large number of trials, on the average, about one-tenth of the balls will be black.

What happens then if we draw, say, four balls at a time? We may draw four black balls, and the probability of doing so is $p \cdot p \cdot p \cdot p = p^4 = 10^{-4}$. Three black balls have the probability of $p^3 q$, multiplied by 4 (since the white ball could occupy any of four places: $pppq$, $ppqp$, $pqpp$, or $qppp$). In general, w out of n balls can be drawn with a probability $f(x) = \binom{n}{x} p^x q^{n-x}$, where the term $\binom{n}{x}$ represents the number or arrangements for x successes and $(n - x)$ failures and it is given by $\binom{n}{x} = \dfrac{n!}{x!\,(n - x)!}$ [the symbol $n!$, called n factorial, stands for the product $n(n - 1)\,(n - 2)\cdots2.1$; $0! = 1$, by definition].

The sum of such probabilities,

$$\binom{n}{0}p^0q^n + \binom{n}{1}p^1q^{n-1} + \binom{n}{2}p^2q^{n-2} + \cdots + \binom{n}{n-1}p^{n-1}q^1 + \binom{n}{n}p^nq^0$$

is the binomial expansion of $(p + q)^n$, and the discrete probability distribution comprising these terms is hence called the *binomial distribution*. It satisfies the criteria of a probability distribution since the $n + 1$ terms add up to unity and each term falls between 0 and 1. From Eqs. (17) and (19), the mean of the binomial distribution is np and its variance is npq.

4. The Poisson Distribution

The binomial distribution could serve directly as our probability model, because it specifies with what frequency we should expect 0, 1, 2, . . . clones in the recipients. However, with the number of cells transferred (2×10^6 or 10^7), the arithmetic work would prove prohibitive. We therefore examine the general term of the binomial distribution, looking for some simplifying approximation valid under the conditions of our tests. We note that, while the number of transferred cells (n) is very large, the fraction of specific precursor cells (p, the probability of success) is very small. Given these conditions, it can be shown that

$$\binom{n}{x}p^xq^{n-x} \xrightarrow[\substack{n\to\infty \\ p\to0}]{} \frac{(np)^x}{x}\,e^{-np} \qquad (e = 2.71828 \ldots)$$

that is, when n tends to infinity and p tends to zero, the binomial distribution tends to its *Poissonian limit*.

The corresponding limit for the variance could be obtained by a similar procedure, but it should be intuitively clear that, when p is very small, $(1 - p) = q$ will approximately equal unity and we may write directly

$$npq \xrightarrow[p\to0]{} np$$

that is, the variance equals the mean.

We are dealing with a *Poisson distribution*. Coming back to our immunological data, we have n units of cells transferred from a Poisson-distributed population with an average number p of different clones per unit. The effective number of clones in a unit of cells, which may be denoted by x, will vary from one sample to another. In fact, it is a random variable, the possible values of which are 0, 1, 2, . . . , etc. What is the probability of a particular value x? We have simply shown that if p is negligible as compared to n, this probability is

$$f(x) = \frac{\mu^x e^{-\mu}}{x!} \qquad (x = 0, 1, 2, \ldots) \tag{21}$$

where $\mu = np$ is the average number of different clones in the recipient sera.

Equation (21) defines the Poisson probability distribution. The variable x takes the values 0, 1, 2, . . . with the corresponding probabilities obtained by putting these values of x in Eq. (21). Thus,

$$f(0) = e^{-\mu} \tag{22}$$

$$f(1) = e^{-\mu}$$

$$f(2) = \frac{\mu^2}{2} e^{-\mu}$$

etc.

Equation (22) rewritten as $\mu = -\log[f(0)]$ gives an estimate of the average number of different clones per recipient sera from the percentage of number of sera with no antibodies. In the first experiment of our example, 4 over 19 sera have no clones, so the average number of different clones is $\mu_1 = -\log(4/19) = 1.56$. In the second experiment, we have $\mu_2 = -\log(7/19) \simeq 1$.

By substituting Eq. (21) in Eqs. (17) and (19) we find that the mean and the variance of a Poisson distribution are both μ.

5. The Poisson Truncated Distribution

An additional common problem is the *ascertainment bias*. As we can see from the data, each mouse is classified as having 0, 1, 2, 3, 4, or more clones. This is due to the fact that, using isoelectric focusing as the test criterion, clones can be told apart only when their number is small, say, less than 4.

In this case we speak of a *truncated* Poisson distribution. We could estimate the mean by $\mu = -\log[f(0)]$, but this clearly would not use all the information contained in the data. We could assume that the mice with k or more clones had exactly k clones and calculate the mean in the usual way (i.e., the total number of clones divided by the total number of mice), but this "fictitious mean" μ^* would obviously be inaccurate. Steinberg (1976) proposed a useful iterative formula:

$$\mu_t = \frac{\mu^*}{1 - [(n_k/n)Q]} \tag{23}$$

where μ^* is the mean assuming that mice with k or greater than k clones have exactly k clones, n is the total number of mice, and n_k is the number of mice with k or greater than k clones.

$$Q = 1 - \frac{k}{\mu_t} + \frac{\mu_t^{k-1}/(k-1)!}{e^{\mu_t} - [1 + \cdots + \mu_t^{k-1}/(k-1)!]} \tag{24}$$

Using μ^* as a first approximation to μ_t, a value of Q is obtained by Eq. (24). This value of Q is used in Eq. (23) to obtain a second approximation to μ_t, the procedure being repeated until successive approximations do not differ significantly. Once the μ_t is estimated from the data, Eq. (21) with $\mu = \mu_t$ is used to obtain the *expected* number of sera with the 0, 1, 2, 3, 4, and more than 4 antibodies. The results of the two experiments above are given in Table VII.

6. Test of a Model

Now the question is how can we test whether the differences between observed and expected frequency values might or might not be due to chance fluctuations. The statistician gives this kind of answer: I can calculate the probability of being in error in refusing a "true" hypothesis. If this probability P is below a conventional level (usually 5%, sometimes 1 or 0.1%), the hypothesis is refused at that probability level; otherwise the hypothesis is not refused. This way of reasoning is called *test of the hypothesis*, and when, as in our example, the hypothesis concerns the fitting of an observed distribution frequency to a theoretical probability model, one

TABLE VII

The Truncated Poisson Distribution to Evaluate the Frequency of B Precursor Cells[a]

Number of spleen cells transferred	μ_t	Observed (O) and expected (E) number of sera with 0, 1, 2, 3, 4, or more antibodies									
		0		1		2		3		4 or more	
		O	E	O	E	O	E	O	E	O	E
2×10^6	2.27	4	2.08	3	4.49	4	5.10	3	3.86	5	3.42
1×10^7	2.22	7	2.06	1	4.48	3	5.08	1	3.77	7	3.51

[a] Data are from Köhler (1976).

speaks of *testing the goodness of fit*. The theoretical distribution used to test the goodness of fit is called the χ^2 *distribution*. It is tabulated in any book of statistical tables (e.g., Fisher and Yates, 1963; Documenta Geigy, 1962); it depends on the so-called *degrees of freedom* (df), which is the number of independent comparisons made to test the goodness of fit. The formula to calculate χ^2 is

$$\chi^2_{df} = \sum_{i=1}^{c} \frac{(n_{obs_i} - n_{exp_i})^2}{n_{exp_i}} \tag{25}$$

where n_{obs_i} and n_{exp_i} are the number of cases observed and expected, respectively (on the basis of the hypothesis), in the class of frequency i. The sum is extended over all the c classes, and df, the number of degrees of freedom, is given by c minus the number of constraints. For the first experiment of our example, where the goodness of fit to a Poisson distribution is to be tested, we have

$$\chi^2_3 = \frac{(4 - 2.08)^2}{2.08} + \frac{(3 - 4.49)^2}{4.49} + \frac{(4 - 5.10)^2}{5.10}$$
$$+ \frac{(3 - 3.86)^2}{3.86} + \frac{(5 - 3.42)^2}{3.42} = 3.36$$

We have five comparisons, but they are not all independent because they depend on (i) the total number of sera and (ii) μ_t estimated by the same sample of date; therefore, only 3 degrees of freedom are left for testing. A χ^2 with 3 df at a probability level of 5% is expected to be 7.81 as it can be read in the third row of any χ^2-distribution table. As 3.36 (observed) is less than 7.81 (expected), we do not reject the hypothesis of a Poisson distribution for the first experiment's data. On the other hand, for the second experiment, we have

$$\chi^2_3 = \frac{(7 - 2.06)^2}{2.06} + \frac{(1 - 4.48)^2}{4.48} + \frac{(3 - 5.08)^2}{5.08}$$
$$+ \frac{(1 - 3.77)^2}{3.77} + \frac{(7 - 3.51)^2}{3.51} = 21.0$$

In this case, 21.0 is greater than 7.81 and we reject the hypothesis of a Poisson distribution, since the observed data do *not* fit with the Poisson model. The reason for such a poor fit and further details are discussed in the original paper by Köhler (1976): It is suggested that T cells are frequently the limiting factor.

Note that the χ^2 test [Eq. (25)] can be applied to any theoretical model able to provide the *expected* outcomes for the experiment. Some care is required in allocating the correct number of degrees of freedom.

E. Competition between Clones with Different Generation Times

1. Exponential Growth

In a population of 10^3 antibody-producing hybrid myeloma cells growing exponentially with a mean generation time of $T = 18$ hr, a nonproducing mutant arises for which the mean generation time is 12 hr. How long will it take for the mutant to overtake the parental clone? What is the total population at that time?

Consider the number of cells in the population, N, as a continuous variable that changes with time. If the change of N, ΔN, is proportional to N as well as to the time elapsed, Δt, we have

$$\Delta N = kN\Delta t \tag{26}$$

where k is a constant. By dividing Eq. (26) by Δt and taking the limit $\Delta t \to 0$, we obtain a *differential equation*,

$$\frac{dN}{dt} = kN \tag{27}$$

whose solution (or integral) is given by

$$N(t) = N_0 e^{kt} \tag{28}$$

where N_0 represents the number of cells in the population at $t = 0$. The constant k, called the *specific growth rate*, is related to the time interval taken by the population to double itself. This time interval is called the *doubling time*, and, if there are no cell deaths, it is the same as the *mean generation time*, which is the mean lifetime of a single cell. Calling this doubling time T, we have

$$2N_0 = N_0 e^{kT} \quad \text{or} \quad k = \frac{\log 2}{T} \tag{29}$$

By substituting Eq. (29) into Eq. (28) we obtain

$$N(t) = N_0 2^{t/T} \tag{30}$$

The number of parental cells may be calculated, for any time t, by substituting their initial number and the mean generation time into Eq. (30), in our case $N_0 = 10^3$ and $T = 18$ hr. Let $t = 0$ represent the instant at which a mutant is born. For the mutant the population number at time t, $N_m(t)$, is given by

$$N_m(t) = 2^{3t/2T} \tag{31}$$

because the initial number of mutants is 1, and the mutant's generation time is $(2/3)T$. The time t at which the two cell populations are equal is determined by the condition $N_m(t) = N(t)$ or, from Eqs. (30) and (31),

$$2^{t/2T} = 10^3 \tag{32}$$

By taking the log of both sides of the last equation, we find

$$t = \frac{3}{\log 2} \, 2T \simeq 20T = 360 \text{ hr} = 15 \text{ days}$$

The total population size at the time when the number of parental and mutant cells is equal will be $2N(t)$, where $N(t)$ is given by Eq. (30) and t satisfies Eq. (32):

$$2N(360) = 2 \times 10^3 \cdot 2^{360/18} \simeq 2 \times 10^9 \text{ cells}$$

F. Comparison of Two Assays for Testing an Antibody Response

1. Contingency Tables

Quintans and Lefkovits (1973) have described how to use a microculture method to estimate the number of precursor cells responsive to sheep red cells *in vitro* from the fraction of nonresponding cultures of spleen cells from normal mice. The method applies the Poisson formula [Eq. (21)] to calculate the mean number of precursors from the observed proportion of negative culture, as shown in Section D. In their paper, however, some experiments are tabulated where the spot assay (Lefkovits, 1972) is compared with the plaque-forming cell (PFC) assay in order to confirm the number of responding cells in the microculture. The number of wells responding in both, in one or the other, or in neither of the two assays is shown in the tabulation below. The data are from two trays of 60 wells each, taken from two different experiments.

		Experiment 1 Spot test					Experiment 2 Spot test		
		+	−	Row totals			+	−	Row totals
PFC	+	3	0	3	PFC	+	30	6	36
test	−	2	55	57	test	−	16	8	24
Column totals		5	55	60			46	14	60

Tabulations such as the two above are called *2 × 2 contingency tables*. In experiment 1, there are 3 wells that respond in both assays, 2 wells that respond in the spot but not in the PFC assay, no well that responds in the

PFC but not in the spot assay, and 55 wells that do not respond in both assays. Generally, we can write the 2×2 table in the following form:

	Factor 1		
	Present	Not present	Row totals
Factor 2 Present	a	b	$R_1 = a + b$
Not present	c	d	$R_2 = c + d$
Column totals	C_1 $= a + c$	C_2 $= b + d$	$N = a + b + c + d$

Two main problems are worth discussing: (i) Is there any association between the two factors? (ii) How can we measure it?

2. χ^2 *Test for Association*

The first problem can be answered by testing the hypothesis of *no* association between factors 1 and 2. In fact, if we assume no association, the *expected* number of individuals α for which both factors are present must satisfy the proportion

$$\frac{\alpha}{C_1} = \frac{R_1}{N}$$

By analogy:

$$\beta = \frac{R_1 C_2}{N} \; ; \qquad \gamma = \frac{R_2 C_1}{N} \; ; \qquad \delta = \frac{R_2 C_2}{N}$$

As the expected numbers α, β, γ, and δ of the 2×2 table can be explicitly calculated from the observed numbers a, b, c, and d, the χ^2 test for the goodness of fit [Eq. (25)] can be used:

$$\chi^2 = \frac{(a - \alpha)^2}{\alpha} + \frac{(b - \beta)^2}{\beta} + \frac{(c - \gamma)^2}{\gamma} + \frac{(d - \delta)^2}{\delta} \tag{33}$$

This χ^2 has only one degree of freedom because we have four comparisons and three independent parameters calculated from the data: one row total, one column total, and the total number of individuals. With some manipulation Eq. (33) gives

$$\chi_1^2 = \frac{(ad - bc)^2 N}{R_1 R_2 C_1 C_2} \tag{34}$$

If the probability associated to the observed χ^2 is less than 5%, the probability of erroneously rejecting the hypothesis of no association is so small that we conclude that the *existence of a significant association* (at a 5% probability level) is not due to chance fluctuations. In our example, we have, for experiment 2,

$$\chi_1^2 = \frac{(30 \cdot 8 - 6 \cdot 16)^2 \, 60}{46 \cdot 14 \cdot 36 \cdot 24} = 2.236$$

For one degree of freedom, this value corresponds to a probability P within the interval 0.1–0.2. Thus, we conclude that the association between the PFC and spot assay for this tray is *not* statistically significant.

3. Correction for Continuity

The following method, the *continuity correction for fourfold tables*, was described by F. Yates (1934) and is often called *Yates' correction*. The χ_1^2 distribution has been used as an approximation to the distribution given by Eq. (33) or (34) on the null hypothesis of no association and subject to fixed marginal totals. But with 2×2 tables, with low frequencies, the possible number of sets of values satisfying a given marginal (generated by increasing or decreasing one of the entries by one unit at a time, until either that entry or some other reaches zero) is small, so that the resultant distribution is discontinuous, whereas the χ^2 distribution, which approximates to it, is continuous. The continuity-corrected version of Eq. (34) proposed by Yates is

$$\chi_1^2 \, (\text{Yates}) = \frac{(|ad - bc| - \frac{1}{2} \, N)^2}{R_1 R_2 C_1 C_2} \tag{35}$$

In our example, we have, for experiment 2,

$$\chi_1^2 \, (\text{Yates}) = \frac{(|30 \cdot 8 - 6 \cdot 16| - \frac{1}{2} \, 60)^2}{46 \cdot 14 \cdot 36 \cdot 24} = 1.401$$

This value corresponds to a probability P within the interval 0.20–0.30. By comparing this result with that obtained above on the same data, one can see that the χ^2 test *without* continuity correction underestimates the probability of association: The null hypothesis could be falsely rejected.

4. The Exact Test for Fourfold Tables

Unfortunately, when a, b, c, or d is very small, say less than 5, the theory that supplies the χ^2 distribution for testing the goodness of fit is too approximate and should not be used for testing a 2×2 contingency table like that of experiment 1. In the mid-1930s Fisher suggested a test for calculating the *exact* probability of error in rejecting the no-association hypothesis in the 2×2 contingency table. This exact probability is given by the formula

$$P = \frac{R_1! \, R_2! \, C_1! \, C_2!}{N! \, a! \, b! \, c! \, d!} \tag{36}$$

and the method is usually referred to as the *exact test for fourfold tables* (see also Fisher, 1950). Applying this test (as we must) to the data for experiment 1, we have

$$P = \frac{5! \cdot 55! \cdot 3! \cdot 57!}{60! \cdot 3! \cdot 2! \cdot 55! \cdot 0!} = \frac{3 \cdot 4 \cdot 5}{58 \cdot 59 \cdot 60} = 0.00029$$

This P value is so low that we conclude that in this tray there is a very significant association between the two assays.

The exact formula, Eq. (36), defines the probability of a table with given frequencies a, b, c, and d. To assess its significance and to test the null hypothesis of no association, we must measure the extent to which this probability falls into the tail of the distribution *by summing* the probability of that table to the probabilities of the more extreme configurations with the same marginals.

Taking again our example of experiment 2, we must sum up the probabilities corresponding to the following seven fourfold tables with the same marginals:

30	6		31	5		32	4		33	3		34	2		35	1		36	0
16	8		15	9		14	10		13	11		12	12		11	13		10	14

By applying Eq. (36) to these tables and by summing up the corresponding probabilities, we obtain $P = 0.212$, which is an *exact* result. Consider how Yates' correction calculated above leads in this case to an acceptable approximation to this exact probability. For a quick calculation of Eq. (36) the Documenta Geigy (1962, pp. 109–123) tables can be used.

5. Correlation

The second problem with which we must deal concerns how to measure the extent of the association. Note that the extent of association is not the same as the significance of the association. It is quite possible to have data with either a high association that is not statistically significant ($P > 0.05$) or a low association that is statistically significant ($P < 0.05$). For the $2 \times$ 2 contingency tables, a convenient measure of association is given by the *correlation coefficient*:

$$r = \frac{(ad - bc)}{(R_1 R_2 C_1 C_2)^{1/2}} \tag{37}$$

(Note that $\chi^2 = Nr^2$; that is, the correlation coefficient depends only on relative frequencies, and this is essentially the difference between the extent and significance of an association.) When $b = c = 0$ (the two factors are either both present or both absent) we have the maximum *positive* association and $r = 1$. When $a = d = 0$ (i.e., when the two factors are mutually exclusive) we have the maximum negative association (anticorrelation) and $r = -1$. For any other combination, r lies within these two limits: Its absolute value is a measure of the extent of the association; its sign identifies concurrence (positive) or discordance (negative) of the two factors. A zero value of r means no correlation: In such a case, $\chi^2 = 0$, too.

For experiment 1 we calculate $R = 0.76$: The lack of complete association ($R = 1$) is due to the two wells that respond in the spot test and not in the PFC assay. For experiment 2, we have $r = 0.06$: The two assays are not associated.

G. Typing MLC Determinants

1. Nonparametric Estimates

When lymphocytes from two genetically different individuals are brought together in a mixed lymphocyte culture (MLC) test, proliferation is usually observed. The responding cells are a subclass of T lymphocytes, whereas the activating determinants are governed by genes of the major histocompatibility region. Conventional MLC tests consist of one unidirectional set of responses (given by the so-called "responder" cells) activated by a particular set of "stimulator" cells. The actual response in a given responder–stimulator combination is influenced by several factors, the most important of which is the differential capacity of the cells to stimulate or to respond, this capacity varying greatly from experiment to experiment. Therefore, the method of evaluation must be "robust" enough to normalize the responses of all the experiments (Thorsby and Piazza, 1975, and references therein). The following example was chosen to illustrate such a technique.

Let us consider 24 responses given by 8 sets of responder cells and 3 sets of stimulator cells. The experimental data shown in the following tabulation are given in counts per minute:

Stimulator cells	Responder cells								Median
	1	2	3	4	5	6	7	8	
1	22	100	150	1,000	200	2,000	2,100	50	175
2	3,000	3,000	3,000	3,000	10,000	3,000	3,000	100,000	3,000
3	200	250	1,000	1,000	14,000	81,000	5,000	500	1,000

To extract robust estimates from data like these, statistics that do not depend on outlier values of the data are usually used. The most common among them is the *median*, used instead of the usual *mean*. More generally, the common practice is the use of *nonparametric* instead of *parametric* estimators. If the observations are arranged in increasing (or decreasing) order, the median (or 50th percentile) is the middle observation. If the number of observations, n, is odd there will be a unique median. If n is even, the median is defined as the mean of the two middle observations. For instance, the median of the observations 1, 2, 3, and 10,000 is 2.5; the mean 2500.75 is strongly affected by the extreme value 10,000.

2. Normalization of Data

These variabilities among stimulator and responder cells are "normalized" in two stages. First, the observed counts of any stimulating cell are expressed as a fraction of the corresponding median; that is, each entry in a row is divided by the row median:

Stimulator cells	Responder cells							
	1	2	3	4	5	6	7	8
1	0.13	0.57	0.86	5.71	1.14	11.43	12.00	0.29
2	1.00	1.00	1.00	1.00	3.33	1.00	1.00	33.33
3	0.20	0.25	1.00	1.00	14.00	81.00	5.00	0.50
Median	0.20	0.57	1.00	1.00	3.33	11.43	5.00	0.50

In the second stage the normalization is applied in the other dimension; that is, each entry in a column is divided by the column median:

Stimulator cells	Responder cells							
	1	2	3	4	5	6	7	8
1	0.65	1.00	0.86	5.71	0.34	1.00	2.40	0.58
2	5.00	1.75	1.00	1.00	1.00	0.09	0.20	66.66
3	1.00	0.43	1.00	1.00	4.20	7.09	1.00	1.00

Such a "double normalization" procedure (responderwise and stimulatorwise) was found useful in scoring the reactions for cell typing. The median has no monopoly in this procedure; in fact, an even better scale for scoring was obtained when data were normalized to the 75th percentile. (The *Qth percentile* is the upper value of the lowest *Q*% of observations; for example, the median is the 50th percentile.)

H. Haplotype Frequencies and Linkage Disequilibria

1. Estimation of Haplotype Frequencies from Population Data

Let N individuals be typed for two markers A and B controlled by two genes each with two alleles A, a and B, b, where lowercase denotes the recessive or "silent" (negative) allele. The following 2×2 table gives the *phenotypic* distribution.

		Marker A reaction		
		Positive	Negative	Marginals
Marker B	Positive	f_{AB}	f_{aB}	f_B
reaction	Negative	f_{Ab}	f_{ab}	$1 - f_B$
	Marginals	f_A	$1 - f_A$	1

where f_{AB} is the fraction of individuals positive with A and B, etc. The marginal totals f_A and f_B are the *phenotypic frequencies* of the two markers. A common problem is to estimate from these population data the frequencies of the four haplotypes (or gametes). The following 2×2 table represents the gametic or haplotypic distribution.

		Gamete A		
		Present	Absent	
Gamete B	Present	p_{AB}	p_{aB}	p_B
	Absent	p_{Ab}	p_{ab}	$1 - p_B$
		p_A	$1 - p_A$	1

where p_{AB} is the fraction of gametes with the haplotype AB, etc., and p_A and p_B are the allele frequencies of the two markers. Since the allele A is dominant to a, and B is dominant to b, we can write on the hypothesis of the Hardy–Weinberg equilibrium:

$$p_{ab}^2 = f_{ab}$$

$$(1 - p_A)^2 = (p_{aB} + p_{ab})^2 = 1 - f_A = f_{aB} + f_{ab}$$

$$(1 - p_B)^2 = (p_{Ab} + p_{ab})^2 = 1 - f_B = f_{Ab} + f_{ab}$$

$$p_{AB} = 1 - p_{aB} - p_{Ab} - p_{ab}$$

which, after some manipulation, gives

$$
\begin{aligned}
p_{AB} &= 1 - p_{Ab} - p_{aB} - p_{ab} \\
p_{Ab} &= (f_{Ab} + f_{ab})^{1/2} - (f_{ab})^{1/2} \\
p_{aB} &= (f_{aB} + f_{ab})^{1/2} - (f_{ab})^{1/2} \\
p_{ab} &= (f_{ab})^{1/2}
\end{aligned}
\tag{38}
$$

These equations express the *haplotype frequencies*, p_{AB}, p_{Ab}, p_{aB}, and p_{ab}, which are usually not observable directly, as a function of the observable *phenotypic frequencies*, f_{Ab}, f_{aB}, and f_{ab}.

2. Linkage Disequilibrium

It is interesting to compare the frequency of the haplotype AB with that expected by random association of the two alleles. The random expectation is obviously $p_A p_B$, so the quantity

$$\Delta = p_{AB} - p_A p_B \tag{39}$$

is usually calculated to assess the deviation from a random association of alleles and is called the *linkage disequilibrium* parameter. From the identity

$$\Delta = p_{AB} - p_A p_B = p_{AB} p_{ab} - p_{Ab} p_{aB} \tag{40}$$

and the expressions of Eq. (38), we can write

$$\Delta = (f_{ab})^{1/2} - [(f_{Ab} + f_{ab})(f_{aB} + f_{ab})]^{1/2} \tag{41}$$

which estimates the gametic association from the usually measured phenotypic frequencies. It varies between -0.25 and $+0.25$. From Eq. (40) a positive Δ value indicates a preponderance of gametes AB and ab, whereas a negative Δ points to an excess of Ab and aB gametes. The significance of an estimated Δ (i.e., whether it is significantly different from zero) may be assessed by the usual 2×2 χ^2 test based on the observed phenotypes.

The *correlation* ρ between the markers A and B is given by

$$\rho = \frac{f_{AB}f_{ab} - f_{Ab}f_{aB}}{[(f_{AB} + f_{aB})(f_{AB} + f_{Ab})(f_{Ab} + f_{ab})(f_{aB} + f_{ab})]^{\frac{1}{2}}}$$

$$= \frac{\Delta[\Delta + 2(1 - p_A)(1 - p_B)]}{\{(1 - p_A)^2(1 - p_B)^2[1 - (1 - p_A)^2][1 - (1 - p_B)^2]\}^{\frac{1}{2}}}$$

From the form of ρ, it is easily seen that the 2×2 χ^2 is given by

$$\chi^2 = N\rho^2$$

3. Treatment of Field Data

The example below is taken from Piazza *et al.* (1973), who collected data on the human histocompatibility HLA polymorphism on the island of Sardinia, a very isolated geographic region of the Mediterranean. The HLA complex, such as H-2 in the mouse, is controlled by many linked genes, each of them with several alleles. We shall consider here only two loci of the complex, *HLA-A* and *HLA-B*, and test the distribution of the two alleles *Aw30* (locus *A*) and *B18* (locus *B*). The 403 individuals tested gave the following observed *phenotypic* distribution:

	Aw30+	*Aw30-*	
B18+	131 $f_{AB} = 131/403 = 0.326$	76 $f_{aB} = 0.188$	207 $f_B = 0.514$
B18-	8 $f_{Ab} = 0.019$	188 $f_{ab} = 0.467$	196 $1 - f_B = 0.486$
	139 $f_A = 0.345$	264 $1 - f_A = 0.655$	403

The allele frequencies of *Aw30* and *B18* are

$$p_A = 0.191$$

$$p_B = 0.303$$

The frequency of the haplotype (*Aw30*, *B18*) is given by Eq. (38):

$$p_{AB} = 0.177$$

The linkage disequilibrium parameter is given by Eq. (41):

$$\Delta = \sqrt{0.467} - \sqrt{(0.655)(0.486)} = 0.119$$

The corresponding χ^2 is

$$\chi_1^2 = \frac{(131 \cdot 188 - 76 \cdot 8)^2 \, 403}{207 \cdot 196 \cdot 139 \cdot 264} = 15.62$$

establishing the significance of the antigenic association, since such a high value would be obtained in less than 1 in 1000 cases by chance. The correlation of the phenotypes is, in this example:

$$\rho = \left(\frac{\chi^2}{N}\right)^{\frac{1}{2}} = \left(\frac{15.62}{403}\right)^{\frac{1}{2}} = 0.62$$

It is interesting to notice that the haplotype ($Aw30$, $B18$) is maintained at this very high linkage disequilibrium by the Sardinians only; all the Caucasian populations living around are lacking it. They usually carry another chromosomal combination ($A1$, $B8$), which also shows a very high linkage disequilibrium parameter, usually 0.08. Linkage disequilibria between genes at different linked loci are a characteristic feature of the histocompatibility complex in mammals (HLA in humans, H-2 in mice, etc.). Such disequilibria have no simple explanation: Linkage, natural selection, migration, and genetic drift are the forces that can keep a linkage disequilibrium stable in time, but the relative weight of each of these pressures is difficult to assess. It is suggested that the interaction between genes tightly linked for functional reasons, with natural selection that favors such genetic linkages, is the major factor responsible for selecting and perpetuating such disequilibria.

For more information on the subject, the interested reader may consult Chapter 5 of the book by Cavalli-Sforza and Bodmer (1971).

ACKNOWLEDGMENTS

Professor Fazekas de St.Groth kindly read and copiously commented on an earlier version of this chapter. Most of his valuable suggestions have been incorporated into the text. While I am deeply indepted to him for his generous contributions, I acknowledge that any errors or omissions are mine alone. The CNR, Centro di Studio per l'Immunogenetica e l'Istocompatibilità, Torino, Italy, is also acknowledged for its support.

REFERENCES

Armitage, P. (1971). "Statistical Methods in Medical Research." Wiley, New York.
Bliss, C. I. (1970). "Statistics in Biology." McGraw-Hill, New York.

Cavalli-Sforza, L. L., and Bodmer, W. F. (1971). "The Genetics of Human Populations." Freeman, San Francisco.

Colton, R. (1974). "Statistics in Medicine." Little, Brown, Boston.

Documenta Geigy—Scientific Tables, 6th ed. (1962). Geigy Pharmaceutical Co. Ltd., Manchester.

Fisher, R. A. (1950). "Statistical Methods for Research Workers." Oliver and Boyd, Edinburg.

Fisher, R. A., and Yates, F. (1963). "Statistical Tables for Biological, Agricultural and Medical Research." Oliver and Boyd, Edinburg.

Hsia, S., Howell, D. N., Amos, B., and Woodbury, M. A. (1977). *J. Immunol.* **118**, 1659.

Köhler, G. (1976). *Eur. J. Immunol.* **6**, 340.

Lefkovits, I. (1972). *Eur. J. Immunol.* **2**, 360.

Mather, K. (1972). "Statistical Analysis in Biology." Smith, Gloucester, Massachusetts.

Piazza, A., Belvedere, M. C., Bernocco, D., Conighi, C., Contu, L., Curtoni, E. S., Mattiuz, P. L., Mayr, W., Richiardi, P., Scudeller, G., and Ceppellini, R. (1973). *In* "Histocompatibility Testing 1972" (J. Dausset and J. Colombani, eds.), p. 73. Munksgaard, Copenhagen.

Quintans, J., and Lefkovits, I. (1973). *Eur. J. Immunol.* **3**, 392.

Sokal, R. R., and Rohlf, F. J. (1973). "Introduction to Biostatistics." Freeman, San Francisco.

Steinberg, C. (1976). *Eur. J. Immunol.* **6**, 346.

Thorsby, E., and Piazza, A. (1975). *In* "Histocompatibility Testing 1975" (F. Kissmeyer-Nielsen, eds.), p. 414. Munksgaard, Copenhagen.

Yates, F. (1934). Contingency tables involving small numbers and the χ^2 test. *J. R. Stat. Assoc.* **29**, 51.

Subject Index

A

A-variant streptococcal vaccine, 129
Abelson
  lymphosarcoma, 375
  murine leukemia virus, 372, 374
  tumors, induction and development of, 375
  viruses, 373
Acidic separation gels, 101
Acidic spacer gels, 101
Acrylamide monomer, polymerization of, 82
Acrylic acid, 141
Actin, 177
Adenovirus, 420
Adherent cells, 332
  removal of, 220
Adipic acid, 143
Adsorbent, preparation of, 270
Affinity chromatography, 44
  columns, 140
  on Sepharose immunoadsorbents, isolation
    of antibody, 51
  on Sepharose 4B, 55
Agar
  anticomplementary property of, 283
  bottom layer, 280
  cultures, preparation of, 381
  preparation of, 380
  top layer, 280, 361
Agarose, 281, 383
  block electrophoresis, 48
    pattern, 50
  preparation of, 49
Air monitoring, 415
AKR thymoma, 372
AKR tumor, 372
Alkaline separation gels, 101
Alkaline spacer gels, 101
Allantoic cavity, 387
Allantoic fluid, 388
Alloantigen-binding cells, assay for, 300
Alloantigen-binding T cells, assay for, 291
Alloantisera, preparation of, 295

Allogeneic
  cells, irradiation of, 362
  complementation, 362
  cultures, 294
  lymphoctyes, 227
Alloreactive lymphoctyes, 235
Allotype assay, 338
Amberlite, 110
Amino acid chain
  (Phe,G)-A--L, 319
  (T,G)-A--L, 319
  (T,G)-Pro--L, 319
p-Aminocaproic acid, 184
6-Aminocaproic acid, 132
Aminopterin, 391
Ampholine, 109, 112, 132
  electrofocusing kit, 125
Ampholytes, 108
  separation of, 128
Analysis of variance, 431
Analytical isoelectric focusing, 107
Anti-allotype
  antibodies, isolation of, 55
  antisera
    assay of, 197
    production of, 197
  sera, 341
  serum, quantification of, 201
Anti-DNP-forming clones, 351
Anti-H-2 antiserum, 213, 266, 295
  production of, 208
Anti-hapten antibodies, 154
  isolation of, 57
Anti-HLA antibodies, 222
Anti-Ia antisera, 166
Anti-idiotypic antibodies, isolation of, 55
Anti-idiotypic antisera, 119
Anti-immunoglobulin serum, 267
Anti-lymphocyte serum (ALS), 253
Anti-*Proteus* antisera, preparation of, 199
Anti-SIII pneumococcal antiserum, 54
Anti-SJL alloantibody, 307
Anti-SRBC